Sergio Canavero (Ed.)
Textbook of Cortical Brain Stimulation

Sergio Canavero (Ed.)

Textbook of Cortical Brain Stimulation

Managing Editor: Magdalena Wierzchowiecka

Language Editor: Brent Roberts

DE GRUYTER
OPEN

Published by De Gruyter Open Ltd, Warsaw/Berlin
Part of Walter de Gruyter GmbH, Berlin/Munich/Boston

ISBN: 978-3-11-041261-1
e-ISBN: 978-3-11-041262-8

Bibliographic information published by the Deutsche Nationalbibliothek
The Deutsche Nationalbibliothek lists this publication in the Deutsche Nationalbibliografie; detailed bibliographic data are available in the Internet at http://dnb.dnb.de.

Editor: Sergio Canavero
Managing Editor: Magdalena Wierzchowiecka
Language Editor: Brent Roberts

www.degruyteropen.com

Cover illustration: © Sergio Canavero

To my children, Serena and Marco

"I would like to see the day when somebody would be appointed surgeon somewhere who has no hands for the operative part is the least part of the work"

Harvey Cushing

Contents

List of Contributing Authors

Anne Beuter

University of Bordeaux

Chapter 17

Jeffrey E. Arle

Department of Neurosurgery, Beth Israel Deaconess Medical Center, Harvard University, Boston, MA

Chapter 3, Chapter 6, Chapter 7

Sharona Ben-Haim

Department of Neurosurgery, Ichan School of Medicine of Mount Sinai, New York, NY,USA

Chapter 14

Olivier Bodart

Coma Science Group, Cyclotron Research Center and Neurology Department, University of Liège and University Hospital of Liège, Liège, Belgium

Chapter 13

Domenico Bosco

Department of Neurology, General Hospital San Giovanni di Dio, Crotone, Italy

Chapter 10

Jeffrey A. Brown

Division of Neurosurgery, Mercy Medical Center, Rockville Centre, New York, USA

Intorduction

Sergio Canavero

Turin Advanced Neuromodulation Group, Turin, Italy

Intorduction, Chapter 1, 8, 10, 12, 13, 16, 18

Miryam Carecchio

Department of Neurology, Amedeo Avogadro University, Novara, Italy

Chapter 11

Roberto Cordella

Unit of Functional Neurosurgery, Fondazione IRCCS Istituto Neurologico "Carlo Besta", MIlan, Italy

Chapter 11

Sergio Dantas

Pain Clinic of the University Hospital of the Federal University of Rio Grande do Norte, Natal-RN, Brazil

Chapter 9

Dirk De Ridder

Department of Surgical Sciences, Section of Neurosurgery, Dunedin School of Medicine, University of Otago, New Zealand

Chapter 15

Marisa De Rose

Department of Neurosurgery, University Hospital of Germaneto, "Magna Graecia" University, Catanzaro, Italy

Chapter 10

Walter Fagundes-Pereyra

Department of Neurosurgery of University Hospital of the Federal University of Espirito Santo, Vitoria-ES, Brazil

Chapter 8, 9

Angelo Franzini

Unit of Functional Neurosurgery, Fondazione IRCCS Istituto Neurologico "Carlo Besta", MIlan, Italy

Chapter 11

Giusy Guzzi

Department of Neurosurgery, University Hospital of Germaneto, "Magna Graecia" University, Catanzaro, Italy

Chapter 10

Sung Chan Jun
School of Information and Communication, Gwanju Institute of Science and Technology (GIST)
Chapter 19

Donghyeon Kim
School of Information and Communication, Gwanju Institute of Science and Technology (GIST)
Chapter 19

Hyoung-Ihl Kim
School of Mechatronics, Gwanju Institute of Science and Technology (GIST) and Department of Neurosurgery, Presbyterian Medical Center, Jeonju, Republic of Korea
Chapter 12, 19

Brian Harris Kopell
Departments of Neurosurgery, Neurology, Psychiatry and Neuroscience,Ichan School of Medicine of Mount Sinai, New York, NY,USA
Chapter 14

Berthold Langguth
Interdisciplinary Tinnitus Clinic, Department of Psychiatry and Psychotherapy, University of Regensburg, Regensburg, Germany
Chapter 15

Steven Laureys
Coma Science Group, Cyclotron Research Center and Neurology Department, University of Liège and University Hospital of Liège, Liège, Belgium
Chapter 13

Angelo Lavano
Department of Neurosurgery, University Hospital of Germaneto, "Magna Graecia" University, Catanzaro, Italy
Chapter 10

Jean Pascal Lefaucheur
Service de Physiologie, Groupe Henri Mondor, Créteil, and Faculté de Médecine, Université Paris Est Créteil, Créteil, France
Chapter 2, Chapter 5

Sara Marceglia
Centro Clinico per le Neuronanotecnologie e la Neurostimolazione, Fondazione IRCCS Ospedale Maggiore, Università di Milano, Milan, Italy
Chapter 20

Giuseppe Messina
Unit of Functional Neurosurgery, Fondazione IRCCS Istituto Neurologico "Carlo Besta", MIlan, Italy
Chapter 11

Jean Paul Nguyen
Service de Neurochirurgie, Centre Hospitalier Universitaire, Nantes, France
Chapter 2, Chapter 5

Alberto Priori
Centro Clinico per le Neuronanotecnologie e la Neurostimolazione, Fondazione IRCCS Ospedale Maggiore, Università di Milano, Milan, Italy
Chapter 20

Dirk Rasche
Department of Neurosurgery, University of Lübeck, University Hospital of Schleswig-Holstein, Campus Lübeck, Lübeck, Germany
Chapter 4

Michele Rizzi
Unit of Functional Neurosurgery, Fondazione IRCCS Istituto Neurologico "Carlo Besta", MIlan, Italy
Chapter 11

Elena Rossi

Centro Clinico per le Neuronanotecnologie e la Neurostimolazione, Fondazione IRCCS Ospedale Maggiore, Università di Milano, Milan, Italy

Chapter 20

Hyeon Seo

School of Information and Communication, Gwanju Institute of Science and Technology (GIST)

Chapter 19

Jay L. Shils

Department of Neurosurgery, The Lahey Hospital and Health System, Tufts University, Boston, MA, USA

Chapter 3, Chapter 6

Jae-Jin Song

Department of Otorhinolaryngology Head-and-Neck Surgery, Seoul National University Bundang Hospital, Korea

Chapter 15

Aurore Thibaut

Coma Science Group, Cyclotron Research Center and Neurology Department, University of Liège and University Hospital of Liège, Liège, Belgium

Chapter 13

Volker M. Tronnier

Department of Neurosurgery, University of Lübeck, University Hospital of Schleswig-Holstein, Campus Lübeck, Lübeck, Germany

Chapter 4

Sven Vanneste

Laboratory for Auditory & Integrative Neuroscience, School of Behavioral and Brain Sciences, University of Texas at dallas, USA

Chapter 15

Giorgio Volpentesta

Department of Neurosurgery, University Hospital of Germaneto, "Magna Graecia" University, Catanzaro, Italy

Chapter 10

Jeffrey A. Brown, Sergio Canavero

Introduction

Nanos, gigantium humeris insidentes

Implantable cortical stimulation (ICS) was officially introduced to medical practice in a 1991 publication by Prof. Tsubokawa's group in Japan. Since then, hundreds of cases have been published (although the exact number cannot be extrapolated due to duplicate publications), spanning the whole field of functional neurosurgery: pain, movement disorders, psychiatry, epilepsy and neurorehabilitation, with an apparent acceleration over the past few years. The primary reason for investigating ICS, given the general success of deep brain stimulation (DBS), is three-fold: first, both patients and physicians are more comfortable considering surgery if the risk of a potentially lethal intracerebral hemorrhage and infection is eliminated: the bleeding risk for DBS is <2% (range: 0.2% - 9.5%) vs virtually 0% for extradural ICS. Second, the benefit in some conditions is significant and superior to DBS (e.g. central pain). Third, ICS appears to be more cost-effective than DBS surgery. Double blind evaluations of ICS effectiveness are possible because the stimulation is subthreshold for either sensory or motor discrimination: such studies consistently show efficacy only when the device is on. Yet, despite an extensive literature, ICS remains an unapproved modality worldwide. It is true that many questions regarding ICS remain unanswered, but the same conclusion applies to other forms of neurostimulation.

What has become clear in recent years, though, is that ICS is superior in clinical efficacy to non-implantable cortical stimulation, e.g. trancranial magnetic stimulation (TMS) and transcranial direct current stimulation (tDCS). And yet, it was non-invasive methods of cranial electrotherapy that opened the way to modern neurosurgical ICS (for a historical account, see Mottelay 1922, Finger 1994; see also Canavero 2009). Here, we summarize the key steps. One caveat is in order. Is the concept of "non-invasive" really a misnomer? Is not anything that involves modulation of brain function inherently invasive?

History

The word "electricity" was introduced by William Gilbert (1546-1603), President of the Royal College of Physicians, from the Greek word for amber, which he used to produce frictional electricity. In the middle of the XVII century, special machines for creating electricity appeared and paralysis was one of the first therapeutic applications, if not the first. As major advances were made in the development of machines that could produce electrical charges, scientists became increasingly willing to try out their new devices in therapeutic settings. The invention and dissemination of the Leyden Jar in 1745 made these efforts easier. The inventor was Pieter van Musschenbroek (1692-1761) of the University of Leiden. This jar allowed electricity to be built up and conserved until released, a marked advance over machines that simply produced sparks by friction. Non-physician John Wesley (1703-1791), the founder of the Methodist Church, grew so enthusiastic over the new technology that he wrote "*there is no remedy in nature for nervous disorders of every kind, comparable to the proper and consistent use of the electrical machine*" and suggested that 50-100 shocks should be used for most conditions. For paralysis, he recommended that "*the palsey be electrified, daily, for three months, from the places wherein the nerves sprang*". Other two non-physicians, colonial American scientist and founding father, Benjamin Franklin (1706-1790) and French revolutionary Jean-Paul Marat (1743-1793) were among the many who grew enamored with electrotherapy (although Franklin expressed later doubts about electricity as a treatment for paralysis, while suggesting applying shocks to the head for depression). A Dutch physician, Jan Ingen-Housz, discoverer of photosynthesis, corresponded with Franklin regarding his electrical mishap:

"*The flash...entered my forehead...I was struck down, I lost all my senses, memory, understanding and even sound judgment....*" but, later "*I felt the most lively joye in finding as I thought at the time my judgment infinitely more acute... a liveliness in my whole frame, which I never had observed before.*" Small wonder that static machines soon found their way into many major hospitals, e.g. in England (1767-1777). British physician John Birch, who founded a department of electricity at St. Thomas's Hospital, treated a "*melancholic porter*" and a "*suicidal singer*" in 1787. He reported that the singer then returned to practice "*boldly, without any serious inconvenience to the brain.*"

These reasoned approaches towards the treatment of depression and motor deficits thus originated more than two and one-half centuries ago.

Modern electrophysiology was born on September 20 1786 when Luigi Galvani (1737-1798), a professor of anatomy at the University of Bologna, in Italy, hung some fresh frog legs on brass hooks from the iron railings of his garden, and unexpectedly discovered the powers of "bimetallic electricity". He looked upon the nerve as a conductor of electricity, much like a wire from a generator and actually substituted electricity for so-called "animal spirits". Intense scientific debate then ensued between Galvani and Alessandro Volta who argued that the electrical currents in tissue derived from external metals, until Alexander Von Humboldt (1769-1859) finally settled the matter in favor of Galvani. However, in 1800, Volta invented the wet cell battery ("*la pila*"), consisting of the dissimilar metals zinc and silver, which allowed whole streams of current to be produced – a marked improvement over previous electrotechnology.

Galvani's nephew, Giovanni Aldini (1762-1834), who also lived in Bologna, showed that electrical stimulation of the exposed brain could produce movements in decapitated criminals and demonstrated these rather "theatrical" feats both in Paris and London. Here, the media coverage of the time would be such as to later inspire –along with similar experiments by others- Mary Wollstonecraft Shelley (1792-1851)'s Frankstein novel. However, exploiting Volta's battery, Aldini introduced what we would now designate as tDCS to the field of psychiatry by treating the first depressive (melancholic) subject with a modern stimulation set-up (Fig.1).

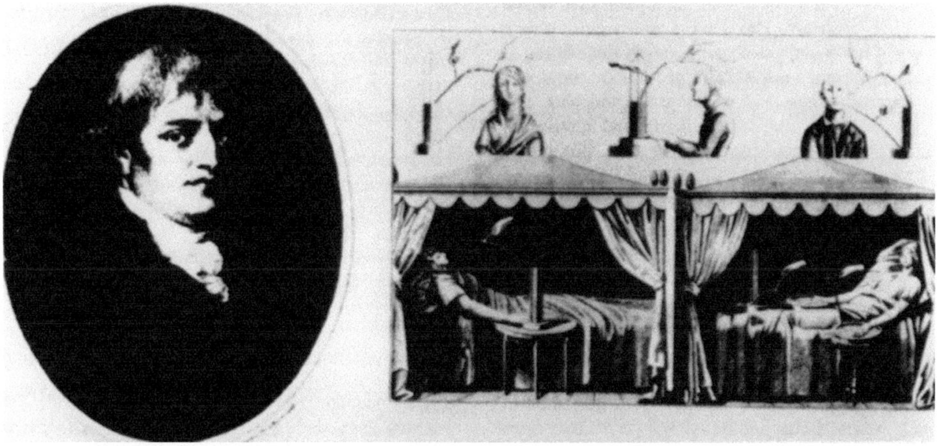

Fig. 1: Giovanni Aldini's experiments with the forerunner of transcranial direct current stimulation for the treatment of "melancholia".

The XIX century witnessed an explosion of applications of galvanism to nervous system conditions, including paralysis, aphasia, pain, epilepsy, visual and auditory loss and insanity. Critics emerged, though, including Sigmund Freud (1856-1939).

In 1938, Ugo Cerletti and Lucino Bini developed electroconvulsive therapy. The focus of electroconvulsive therapy, however, was not on delivery of an electric stimulus per se, but on the induction of a cerebral convulsion. Certainly Cerletti's description of his first patient was sufficiently theatrical to command attention:

> *"All had their hearts in the mouths...during the tonic phase with apnea, ashy paleness, and cadaverous facial cyanosis...which...now seemed painfully never ending-until at the first deep, stertorous inhalation, and first chronic shutters, the blood ran more freely in the bystanders veins as well: and, lastly, to the immense relief of all concerned, was witnessed a characteristic, gradual awakening by step. The patient sat up of his own accord, looked about him calmly with a vague smile...*
> *I asked him "what has been happening to you?" He answered, with no more gibberish: " I don't know, perhaps I have been asleep.'"*

In the 1950's, deep brain stimulation (DBS) started its initially slow, yet later "brushfire" ascent into the Olympus of clinical neurology and psychiatry: DBS gained Food and Drug Administration (FDA) approval as a treatment for essential tremor in 1997, for Parkinson's disease in 2002 and dystonia in 2003, and chronic, severe obsessive-compulsive disorder (OCD) in 2009. The huge success of DBS has eclipsed the related field of cortical stimulation which (re)started its slow ascent in 1985 with the introduction by Anthony Barker of TMS. Used initially as a diagnostic tool to measure conduction time, in the 1990's its use extended to therapeutic trials for neuropathic pain, Parkinson's disease, depression and then nearly the whole field of clinical neurology and psychiatry: in 2008 it was FDA-approved for the treatment of depression. At the end of the 1990's, tDCS was reintroduced, after a short revival in the 1960-1970's, especially in the former Soviet Union (Kropotov 2009). Yet, benefits from non-invasive cortical stimulation are transitory and sometimes even questionable (see full discussion in Canavero 2009).

ICS too had an early start. Alberts had already quenched Parkinsonian tremor using Delgado cortical stimulation paddles in the early 1970's and, in 1979, Woolsey et al wrote: "*Subthreshold electrical stimulation through implanted electrodes might be used to control marked tremor and strong rigidity in Parkinsonian patients*". The first clinical application of ICS was to be central pain, though, 10 years later, at the hands of Tsubokawa's group, in Japan. They also noted improved movements in post-stroke patients. In 1998, Canavero implanted the first Parkinsonian according to Woolsey's suggestion and in 2002, both the authors introduced ICS for stroke rehabilitation. In 2004 De Ridder treated tinnitus and around 2010 Kopell and others relieved depression. In 2008 Canavero announced initial results for the vegetative state. Finally on November 14, 2013, the FDA approved the closed-loop NeuroPace RNS® System for the adjunctive treatment of adults with uncontrolled partial seizures.

Issues

If we look at the results of ICS for some applications, we are stricken by the apparent dichotomy between more or less positive studies (the majority) and a handful of completely negative ones (e.g. pain and Parkinson). The fact is that, unlike DBS, ICS directly targets the cortex, a vast expanse of organic matter with myriad cyto- and neuro-chemical differences between individuals. The simple perception of polarity-specific neuronal modulation so rife in the ICS field is an oversimplification of complex effects, which are currently far less predictable than currently assumed (Krause and Kadosh 2014). ICS –as well as TMS/tDCS- effects are moderated by the pre-existing baseline excitation/inhibition (glutamate/GABA) balance (EIB), so called *state-dependency*. This is affected by factors such as individual differences in cortical morphology (gyri and sulci), pre-existing different interhemispheric connectivity patterns, age-related changes in EIB across the lifespan (decline of GABA levels, but also NMDA receptors, in the aged), circadian influences that are as yet to be clarified (e.g. time of day: morning vs night stimulations, sleep deprivation), interactions with other neurotransmitters, medications, fatigue, attention, even smoking and hormonal fluctuations (in women). The actual state of brain functioning at the subject level and previous experiences can influence –and even flip- polarity-dependent effects: "more stimulation" may not lead to "more benefit", but rather the opposite. Networking in the brain is such that stimulating one area may negatively interfere with another; even worse, while artificially enhancing plasticity one may actually "overshoot" the threshold of homeostatic plasticity and damage the patient more or less irreversibly (e.g. Canavero et al 1999). Thus, if baseline excitation is already high, ICS may add little or even be detrimental. It is suggested that for each patient his or her GABA and glutamate levels be assessed with MR spectroscopy (MRS) (Krause and Kadosh 2014). This adds in terms of cost, but may better guide programming.

Future

Where lies the future of ICS? Suppose that non-implantable transcranial (TMS, tDCS, tACS...) therapy requires physician-supervised re-treatments once monthly for a chronic condition. How long before its cost effectiveness comes into question? Three months? One year? Ten years? What if a procedure with low morbidity that requires a few hospital days can provide years of benefit before any further procedures are needed, especially since the advent of rechargeable devices? Is the cost-benefit ratio within reason when compared to repeated "non-invasive" procedures over the same period? Or is it better to be "tied" to the chair for repeated transcranial treatment? Studies have shown ICS to be safe. Surgical implantation frees the patient from the physician and frequent office visits, once he or she has been adequately trained in use of the device. Arguably, freeing the patient from the physician and giving over control of their health is a reasonable goal of modern health care and a psychological goal for health recovery. Moreover, Zaghi et al (2009) showed that tDCS (followed by rTMS) is the most cost-effective approach for pain therapy at 1 year, but ICS leads at 5 years! In our view, ICS, without ongoing side effects, enjoys the upper hand. It relieves the patient of the burden imposed by the need to call oneself ill.

That said, we dare venture into uncharted territory. Given initial promising results from non-invasive CS (Oliveira et al 2013, Floel 2014), can we expect ICS, a technique already demonstrated to be safe, to be deployed for permanent cognitive and memory enhancement – in the young as well as in the elderly? Can ICS, again a safe technique, be brought to bear on controlling deviant minds, such as psychopaths – a sort of Delgadian mind control (Canavero 2014)? Can the accidental generation of additional subjective limbs (Canavero et al 1999) or out-of-the-body experiences (DeRidder et al 2007) in the course of ICS (or even vivid memories as found by Penfield) portend a time when ICS will be harnessed to create new synesthetic "virtual realities"?

We must wait for the next generation of scientist/physicians to answer these questions. The field remains nascent even after so long a birthing.

Acknowledgement: the editor wishes to thank Dr. Magdalena Wierzchowiecka at DeGruyter Open for her much appreciated help.

References

Alberts WW. A simple view of Parkinsonian tremor. Electrical stimulation of cortex adjacent to the Rolandic fissure in awake man. Brain Res 1972; 44: 357-369

Barker AT, Jalinous R, Freeston IL. Non-invasive magnetic stimulation of human motor cortex. Lancet 1985;1:1106-1107.

Canavero S, Bonicalzi V, Castellano G, et al. Painful supernumerary phantom arm following motor cortex stimulation for central poststroke pain. Case report. J Neurosurg 1999;91:121-3.

Canavero S (ed) Textbook of therapeutic cortical stimulation. New York: Nova Science, 2009

Canavero S. Criminal minds: neuromodulating the psychopathic brain. Front Hum Neurosci 2014: 8: art.124

Cerletti U. Old and new information about electroshock. Am J Psych 1950;107:87-94.

DeRidder D, Van Laere K, Dupont P, et al. Visualizing out-of-body experience in the brain. NEJM 2007; 357: 1829-1833

Finger S. Origins of neuroscience: A history of explorations into brain function. New York: Oxford University Press, 1994

Floel A. tDCS-enhanced motor and cognitive function in neurological diseases. Neuroimage 2014;85:934-947

Krause B, Kadosh RC. Not all brains are created equal: the relevance of indivisual differences in responsiveness to transcranial electrical stimulation. Front Systems Neurosci 2014; 8: art.25

Kropotov JD. Quantitative EEG, event-related potentials and neurotherapy. San Diego: Academic Press, 2009

Mottelay PF. Bibliographical history of electricity and magnetism. London: C. Griffin, 1922

Oliveira JF, Zanao TA, Valiengo L, et al. Acute working memory improvement after tDCS in antide-pressant-free patients with major depressive disorder. Neuroscience letters. 2013;537:60-64.

Tsubokawa T, Katayama Y, Yamamoto T, et al. Treatment of thalamic pain by chronic motor cortex stimulation. Pacing and clinical electrophysiology : PACE1991;14:131-134.

Woolsey CN, Erickson TC, Gilson WE. Localization in somatic sensory and motor areas of human cerebral cortex as determined by direct recording of evoked potentials and electrical stimulation.J Neurosurg 1979;51:476-506.

Zaghi S, Heine N, Fregni F. Brain stimulation for the treatment of pain: A review of costs, clinical effects, and mechanisms of treatment for three different central neuromodulatory approaches. J Pain Manag. 2009;2:339-352.

PART I: **Techniques**

Sergio Canavero

1 Anatomical Localization

Early studies suggested that the precision of electrode placement for chronic stimulation significantly influences the therapeutic efficacy of motor cortex (primary motor cortex, M1, Brodmann's area 4, BA 4) stimulation (MCS) for pain relief, i.e. relief is generally obtained in the territory corresponding to the cortical region that is stimulated (somatotopically) as per Penfield's motor homunculus. Several problems arise that make this assumption moot, if not untenable.

Contrary to standard teaching, the cortical representation of the lower limb musculature, classically located on the mesial wall of the hemisphere (motor area folding into the longitudinal fissure), actually extends to the lateral surface of the hemisphere (and can thus be targeted extradurally). Experience with other indications, namely Parkinson's disease, shows that targeting part of the surface of M1 on one side only is enough to improve symptoms body-wide (chapter 10) and cases of bilateral pain relief exist from unilateral M1 stimulation (chapters 8-9). Besides, a large portion of BA4 occupies the posterior wall of the precentral gyrus in the depth of the anterior bank of the central sulcus, with only a relatively small dorsomedial portion found on the exposed surface of the precentral gyrus. Therefore, the epidural approach should be inadequate for the stimulation of motor cortical targets, which is not the case.

Methods of localizing cortical landmarks – e.g. the central sulcus (CS), a.k.a. Rolando's Fissure, which separates the motor strip (precentral gyrus) anteriorly from the primary sensory cortex posteriorly, and the lateral (Sylvian) sulcus (LS)-based on the relationship of cortical fissures and convolutions as they project to the cranial bony structures have been developed and utilized since the XIX century (Box 1.1). These basic craniocerebral localization techniques play an important role in therapeutic electrical cortical stimulation. In this chapter, I present the more well-known and widely utilized techniques for the localization of the CS and the LS, as well as the more recent techniques of identifying the precentral knob, or the hand representation, in M1 for the purpose of therapeutic ICS.

Pterion: region of approximation of the frontal, parietal, temporal and sphenoid (greater wing) bones; it lies approximately 2 finger-breadths above the zygomatic arch, and a thumb's breadth behind the frontal process of the zygomatic bone.
Asterion: junction of the lambdoid, occipitomastoid and parietomastoid sutures. It overlies the junction of transverse and sigmoid sinus.
Lambda: junction of the lambdoid and sagittal sutures.
Stephanion: junction of the coronal suture and the superior temporal line.
Glabella: the most forward projecting point of the forehead at the level of the supraorbital ridge in the Midline.
Opisthion: the posterior margin of the foramen magnum in the midline.

Box 1.1: Craniometric Points

1.1 Craniometric Methods

These are reviewed in depth by Park et al (2009). These are the methods of Broca-Championnière (1896), Reid (1884), Poirier (1891) and Taylor-Haughton (1900) (Fig.1.1-1.4). In 1980, the Taylor-Haughton line was re-evaluated using CT imaging for localization of the CS and LS (Taylor et al 1980). The study concluded that the Taylor-Haughton line provides a good approximation of the CS and "*the motor and sensory cortex can be accurately located for planning surgical procedures for anatomic studies*". In 1995, Albert L. Rhoton, Jr. published his procedure for localizing CS and LS based on a large number of cadaver studies (Rhoton 2002, Reis et al 2008) (Fig.1.5).

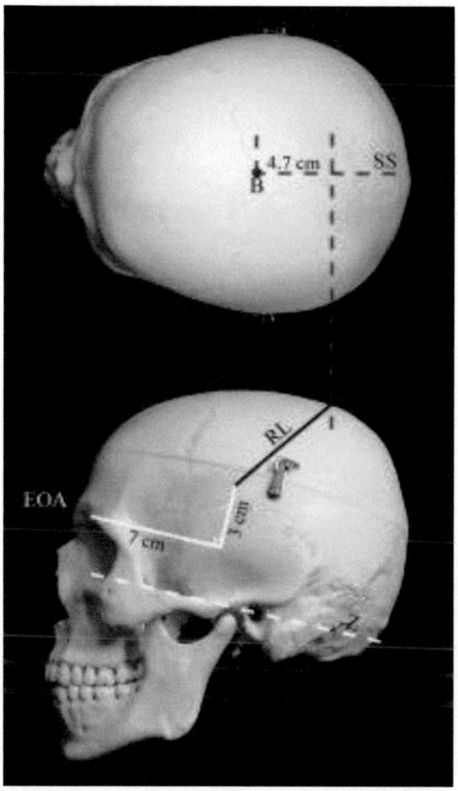

Fig. 1.1: Top and lateral views of the skull illustrating Broca-Championnière method of central sulcus or Rolandic fissure localization. B: bregma (black dot), EOA: external orbital apophysis, IE: inferior end (inferior Rolandic point), RL: Rolandic line (solid black line), SP: superior point (superior Rolandic point), SS: sagittal suture, Z: Zygomatic arch line (white dashed line). Here, "*l'extrémité inférieure*" or the inferior Rolandic point is localized by determining a 7-cm line which starts at the external orbital apophysis of the frontal bone, parallel to the zygomatic arch, and "*le point supérieur*" or the superior Rolandic point (SRP) is located on average 4.7 cm behind the bregma. The central sulcus is located on the line connecting the two points.

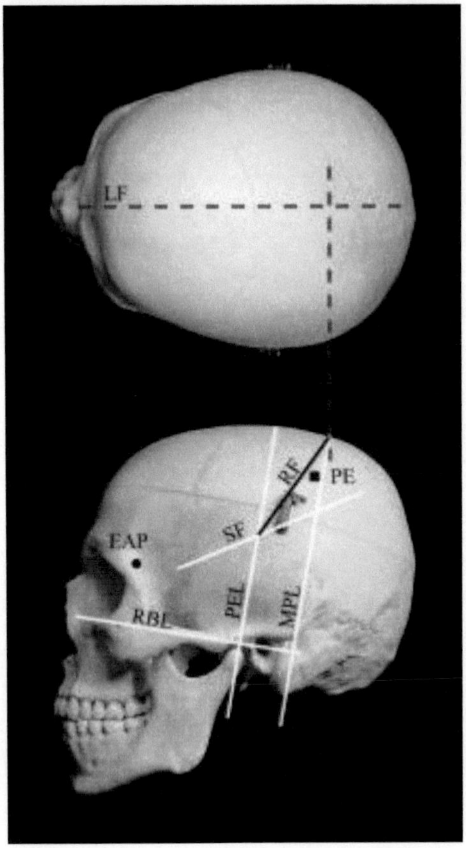

Fig. 1.2: Top and lateral views of the skull illustrating Reid's method of central sulcus or Rolandic fissure localization. EAP: external angular process of the frontal bone (black dot), LF: longitudinal fissure, MPL: mastoid process line, PE: parietal eminence (black square), PEL: pre-external auditory meatus line, RBL: Reid's base line, RF: Rolandic fissure (solid black line), SF: Sylvian fissure. The base line, known as Reid's base line, is defined as that which "*runs through the lowest part of the infraorbital margin and the middle of the external auditory meatus*". The Sylvian fissure is localized by drawing a line "*from a point one inch and a quarter behind the external angular process of the frontal bone to a point three-quarters of an inch below the most prominent part of the parietal eminence*". The Rolandic fissure is localized by drawing a pair of perpendicular lines to Reid's base line. The first line is drawn "*from the depression in front of the external and auditory meatus*" and the second line is drawn "*from the posterior border of the mastoid process at its root*". This creates a "*four-sided fig.*", bounded above and below by the lines for the longitudinal fissure and horizontal limb of the fissure of Sylvius respectively, and in front and behind by the two perpendicular lines. The diagonal line of this four-sided fig. represents the fissure of Rolando.

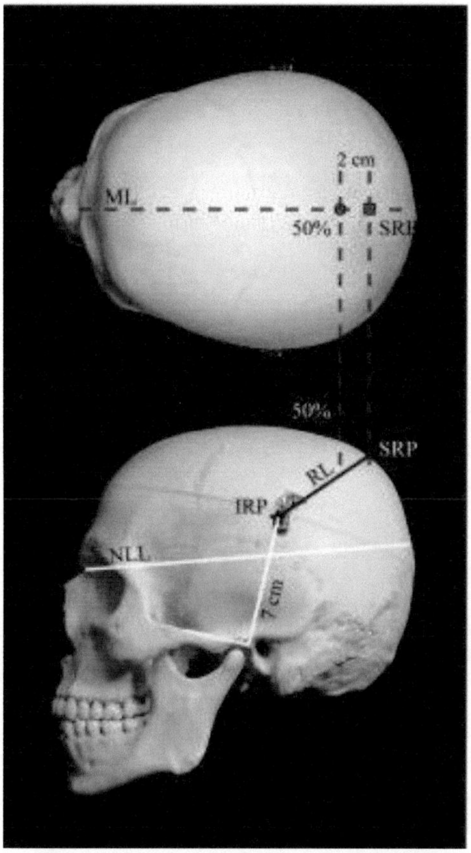

Fig. 1.3: Top and lateral views of the skull illustrating Poirier's method of central sulcus or Rolandic fissure localization. IRP: inferior Rolandic point (black star), ML: midline, RL: Rolandic line (solid black line), SRP: superior Rolandic point (black open square), 50%: halfway point between nasion and inion. The superior Rolandic point is 2 cm behind the midpoint between the nasion and inion on the midline. The inferior Rolandic point is 7 cm above the zygomatic arch immediately anterior to the tragus, perpendicular to the zygomatic arch. The LS lies on the nasion-lambda line which starts at the temporal canthus to a point 1 cm anterior to the lambda on the midline.

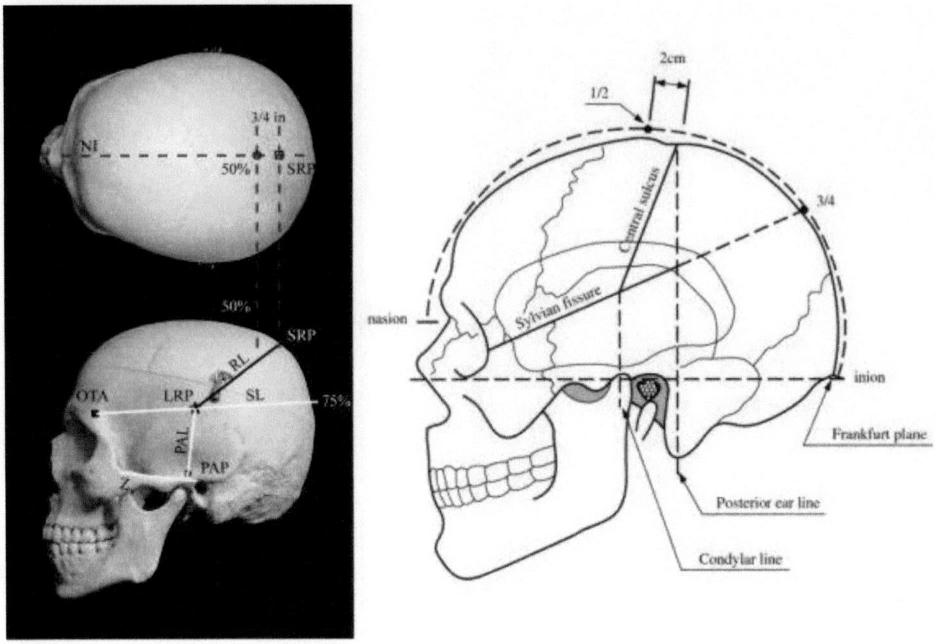

Fig. 1.4: Top and lateral views of the skull illustrating Taylor-Haughton method of central sulcus or Rolandic fissure localization. Central sulcus (RL) is the line connecting the SRP and IRP. IRP: inferior Rolandic point (black star), NI: Nasion-inion line, OTA: orbito-temporal angle (solid black square), PAL: pre-auricular line, PAP: pre-auricular point (solid black dot), RL: Rolandic line (black line), SL: Sylvian line, SRP: superior Rolandic point (open black square), Z: zygomatic arch (upper margin) line, 50%: halfway point on the naso-inion line (open black dot), 75%: three-quarters point on the nasion-inion line. *"In the adult take a point (superior Rolandic) three-quarters of an inch behind the centre of the naso-inion line. This will usually be found to correspond to 53 to 55 per cent of the naso-inion distance, measuring from before backwards. The lower Rolandic point is found by erecting a perpendicular to the upper margin of the zygoma, starting from the pre-auricular point to meet the Sylvian line. Should, however, the upper margin of the zygoma be difficult to determine, the perpendicular (pre-auricular line) may be erected on a line connecting the center of the infra-orbital margin with the center of the external auditory meatus or auricular point. The Rolandic line may now be drawn by connecting these two points".*

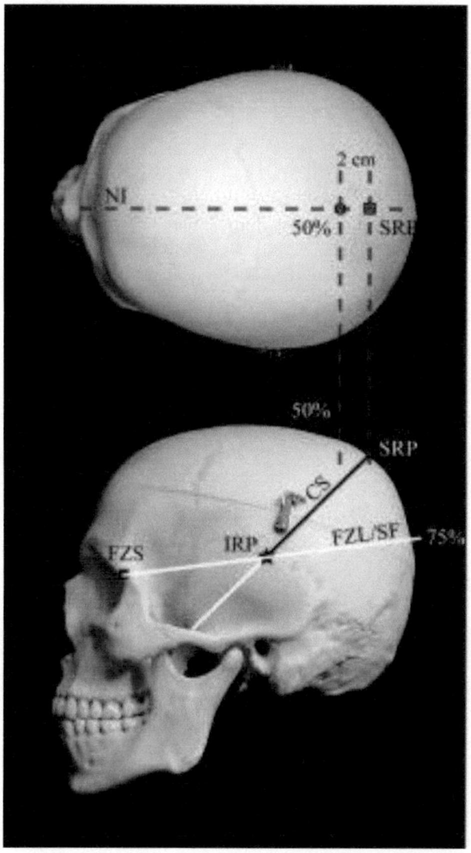

Fig. 1.5: Top and lateral views of the skull illustrating the method of CS and LS localization as described by Dr. Albert L. Rhoton, Jr. CS: central sulcus (solid black line), FZL/SF: frontozygomatic line / Sylvian fissure, IRP: inferior Rolandic point (black star), NI: Nasion-inion line, SRP: superior Rolandic point (open black square), 50%: halfway point on the nasion-inion line, 75%: three-quarters point on the nasion-inion line. The LS is located on the frontozygomatic line which connects the frontozygomatic suture to the 75% point of the naso-inion line. The SRP is located 2 cm behind the 50% point of the naso-inion line. Another line is drawn from the midportion of the zygomatic arch to the SRP where IRP is the point of intersection with the LS or frontozygomatic line.

1.2 Image-Guided Methods

Kido et al (1980), using CT axial views of cadaveric brain specimens with specially marked superior frontal, precentral and central sulci, as well as that of live patients (86 hemispheres, 50 patients), concluded that the approximate location of CS - even when it cannot be visualized on the scan- is a point 4.6 cm behind the coronal suture and 2.1 cm from the midline, and then drawing a line through this point at an angle of 67.9° from the midline (Fig.1.6). However, they did not extend their localization to a specific landmark, such as the precentral knob (see ahead). Using CT and MRI axial views, Iwasaki et al (1991) described a method of identifying the precentral and postcentral gyri on the basis of the medullary branches of the cerebral white matter. The superior frontal gyrus, which runs parallel to the sagittal plane, will form an angle with the precentral gyrus; the CS will be localized posterior to it. Using magnetic resonance (MR) sagittal images, Naidich et al (1995) described the cingulate sulcus as a landmark for recognition of the CS. The cingulate sulcus can be followed in a midline sagittal image posteriorly, where its ascending segment is known as the marginal ramus or sulcus. The notch formed immediately anterior to it (at the vertex) is formed by the central sulcus. The MR lateral sagittal image is also used to localize the CS. The anterior horizontal and anterior ascending rami of the inferior frontal gyrus are identified. They have a Y-shaped appearance. The major descending sulcus immediately posterior to the "Y" is the precentral sulcus, followed posteriorly by the CS. The precentral sulcus is formed by two discontinuous grooves called the inferior precentral sulcus (Ebeling et al 1989) and the superior precentral sulcus. The CS courses approximately parallel to the zigzag precentral sulcus and almost never intersects the Sylvian fissure. Rather, the bottom end is closed by the fusion of the precentral and postcentral gyri. The CS runs uninterrupted in 92% of the cases, while the precentral sulcus is regularly interrupted in 100% of the cases (Yasargil 1994).

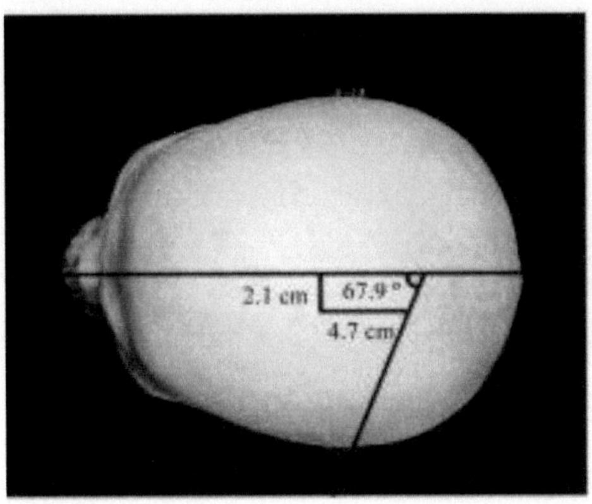

Fig. 1.6: Top view of the skull illustrating the position of the central sulcus based on the measurements of Figure 8 in Kido et al (1980). The lines and measurements are superimposed onto the skull to estimate the location of the central sulcus.

Yousry et al (1997) proposed a new landmark corresponding to the neural elements involved in motor hand function. Using functional MRI, the segment of the precentral gyrus that most often contained motor hand function was a knob-like, broad based, posterolaterally directed structure. It usually (90% of cases) has an inverted omega

(Ω) shape and sometimes a horizontal epsilon (ε) shape in the axial plane with a mean diameter of 1.4 cm. On average it is located about 23 mm from the midline, just posterior to the junction of the superior frontal sulcus with the precentral gyrus and 19 mm from the lateral surface. In the sagittal plane, this knob has the form of a posteriorly directed hook (92% of the cases), with a mean depth and height of 17 and 19 mm, respectively. It is located in the sagittal plane on the same section on which the insula can be identified, perpendicular to its posterior end. On the cortical surface of cadaver specimens, this precentral knob corresponded precisely to the characteristic 'middle knee' of the CS that has been described by various anatomists in the XIX century. This "precentral" knob is a reliable landmark for identifying the precentral gyrus directly, in particular the neural elements involved in motor hand function (Boling et al 1999). It faces and forms the 'middle knee' of the CS, is located just at the cross point between the precentral sulcus and the CS, and is therefore also visible on the cortical surface. Based on measurements from the MRI, this hand area can thus be localized to an area 30 mm lateral to the midline and posteriorly following the superior frontal sulcus until it intersects with the precentral sulcus. Above this knob, the cortical portion subserving the chest and inferior limb can be found, with extension to the medial edge of the hemisphere or even in the interhemispheric part of the strip.

Classically, the CS has been described as having three curves in the axial plane: the superior and inferior genua, which are convex anteriorly, and the middle genu, which is convex posteriorly. A 43-patient study confirmed this arrangement (Campero et al 2011). On anatomic specimens, this Ω (Omega) is 11.2 +/-3.35 mm in height, on average, and 18.7 +/-2.49 mm in width, at the base. The average distance from the medial limit of the Ω to the medial edge of the hemisphere is 24.5 +/-5.35 mm. Most importantly, the anatomical identification of the CS on a normal brain approaches 100%. Caulo et al (2007) obtained structural brain MR images from 257 right-handed healthy men and women and identified new variants of the hand M1 besides the omega and epsilon shapes described above. In particular they observed a medially asymmetric ε (epsilon), a laterally asymmetric ε and a null variant in respectively 2.9%, 7% and 1.8% of the study subjects (Fig.1.7). Also, the ε variant was twice as frequent in men, and an interhemispheric concordance for morphologic variants was observed only for women.

On a CT, the precentral knob on MI is consistently located 45.1 ± 5.2 mm posterior with respect to the coronal suture line and 33.9 ± 3.4 mm lateral to the midline on the right hemisphere, and 44.6 ± 5.7 mm posterior and 33.2 ± 2.5 mm lateral on the left hemisphere (Park et al 2007). This can also be transposed onto the skull to provide the approximate location of the precentral knob on M1 with respect to the external skull markings (Fig.1.8). The approximate location of the precentral knob based on CT is in agreement with the previously described methods and appears capable of replacing MR scanning when this is not available or contraindicated (e.g. in the presence of an implanted cardiac or neural pacemaker, metal debris or metal fragments in the body).

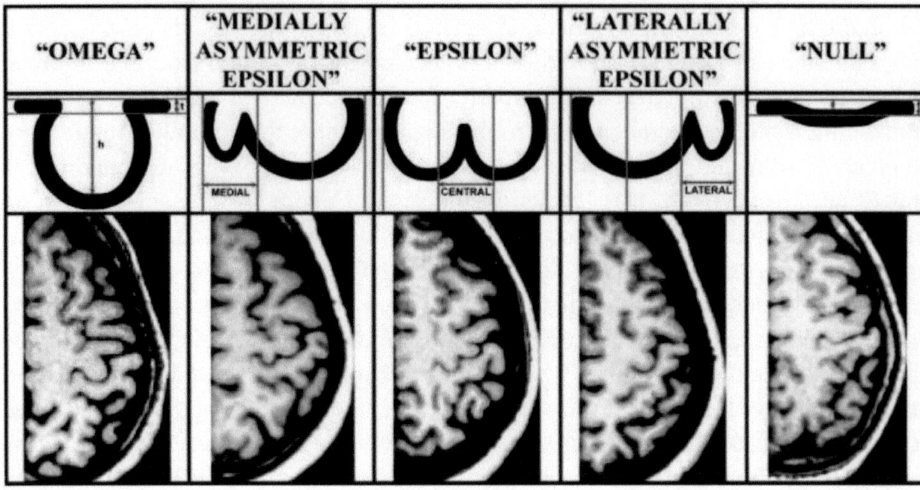

Fig. 1.7: Schematic representation of the criteria used for morphologic classification and corresponding MR image of a typical example. The position of the third fissure, which segments the knob, modifying its appearance from an omega to an epsilon in the lateral, central, or medial part of the hand knob indicates a medially asymmetric epsilon, epsilon, and laterally asymmetric epsilon, respectively. To distinguish an omega from a null, the height of the knob must be greater than the thickness of the precentral gyrus measured at the base of the knob. If the height is smaller than the thickness, the HMC is classified as null. Multiplanar reformatted MR imaging axial sections were obtained from left hemispheres 50 ± 2 mm above the Talairach ACPC plane. The red area in the MR images highlights the morphologic variant (from Caulo et al 2007).

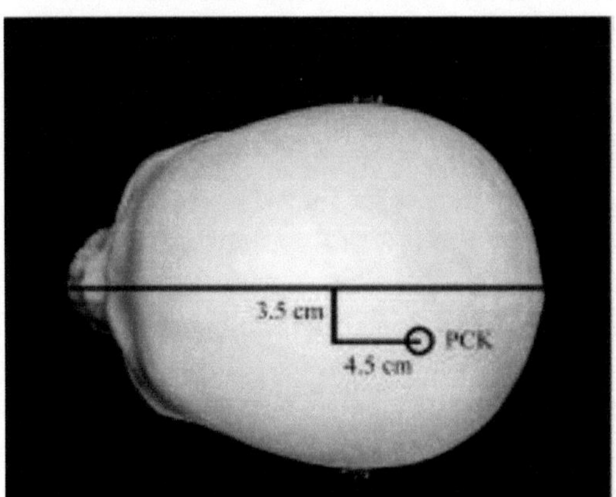

Fig. 1.8: Top view of the skull illustrating the position of the precentral knob of the primary motor cortex with respect to skull landmarks, based on the measurements from CT of the brain (Park et al 2007). PCK: precentral knob.

Anatomical localization of MI can also be accomplished using image-guided neuronavigation systems, based on standard MRI, functional MRI(fMRI), positron emission tomography (PET) or magnetoencephalography (MEG) (Sobel et al 1993, Mogilner and Rezai 2001) (Fig.1.9). 3D image-guided navigation systems help to determine the exact location of anatomical reference points, CS, LS, interhemispheric sulcus, superior and inferior frontal sulci, which can be clearly visualized on the reconstructed images. The superior frontal sulcus separates the superior frontal gyrus from the middle frontal gyrus, coursing anterior to posterior and perpendicular to the precentral sulcus. The next sulcus posteriorly may be identified as the CS. Referring to the cortical representation of body parts (cortical homunculus), the face area lies below the inferior frontal sulcus, the neck at the level of the inferior frontal sulcus, the arm and hand between the inferior and superior frontal sulci and the upper chest at the level of the superior frontal sulcus (Velasco et al 2002).

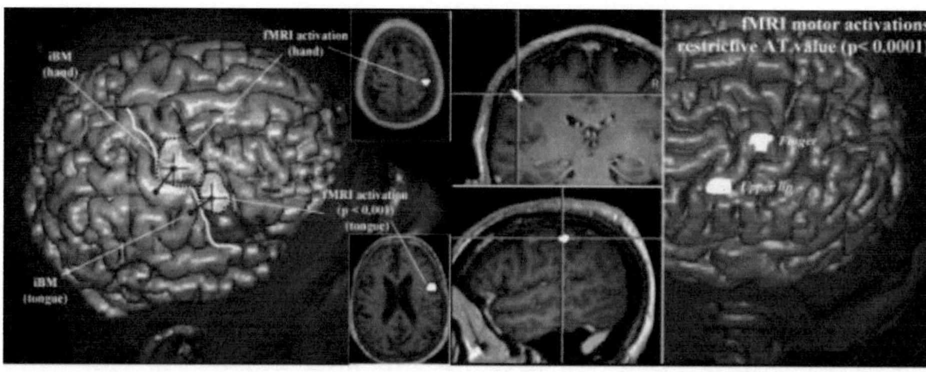

Fig. 1.9: Stereotactic planning in different views (3D) for targeting fMRI activation areas (images courtesy of Prof. B.Pirotte)

These structures can be visualized by oblique MRI sections parallel to a plane from the sylvian to the interhemispheric fissure in the axial views (the Rolandic fissure is the deepest mesiolateral sulcus extending from the sagittal to the Sylvian fissure), a feat not possible with conventional MRI views (Velasco et al 2002). By applying vitamin E capsules glued onto the skin overlying vertex, inion, nasion and pterion and superimposed on the oblique MRI sections, Velasco et al (2002) found that the Rolandic fissure begins mesially at a point 3.90-3.96 cm behind the vertex and with a postero-anterior trajectory over the convexity toward a point 0.3-0-9 cm above the angle formed by the zygomatic arch and the external orbital rim. The Rolandic fissure follows an angled trajectory of about 45° with respect to the sagittal plane (i.e. it is oblique to the cortical surface), its course being rather tortuous with two distinct and constant curves, one with an anterior concavity at the level of the superior frontal sulcus and another with an anterior convexity between the superior and the inferior frontal sulci. The oblique course may be relevant when the place of an extradural MI stimulator is decided on the basis of N20-P20 reversal. The vertex-pterion line invariably lies anterior to the upper two thirds of the motor strip, which may be critical when implanting stimulating paddles parallel to the Rolandic fissure in order to target arm, pelvis, leg and thorax territories. On the other hand, cerebral localization using the 10-20 EEG system is not adequate (Homan et al 1987), although some surgeons use it for localization purposes.

From a stereotactic perspective, the strikingly constant association of the CS with the midcallosal plane must be stressed. Lehman and colleagues (1992) demonstrated the reliability of a midcallosal line to intersect the inferior CS. Talairach et al (1993) recognized that most of the CS lies between two vertical planes extending from the AC and PC. The most superior aspect of the CS arises just behind the PC and the inferior sulcal limit just in front of the AC. The y coordinate (which determines the anteroposterior location) has the smallest range of values for face and tongue sensory activations consistent with the fixed position of the inferior CS in relation to midline commissural fiber bundles (Boling et al 2002).

A special reference should be made to the portion of the primary sensory cortex responsible for facial and buccal sensation in reference to cortical stimulation for facial pains. In open neurosurgical approaches, the tongue sensory area is easily recognized as a triangular gyral configuration in the most inferior aspect of the postcentral gyrus, just above the Sylvian fissure. The distance between the Sylvian fissure and the thumb-hand area is no more than 3 cm (Boling et al 2002). Anterior tongue sensory function is localizable to the superior aspect of the triangle. Lower face sensation is subserved by the narrow portion of the postcentral gyrus, which is situated immediately above the tongue area. The apex of the tongue sensory area thus narrows immediately into a thin segment of the postcentral gyrus, which is the substratum of low face sensation (Boling et al 2002). The tongue sensory area is the only area where the postcentral sensory gyrus is not thinner than the precentral motor cortex. When placing an extradural stimulating strip straddling the motor and sensory cortex, it is important to bear in mind this particular triangular anatomic configuration.

1.3 Conclusions

Individual variability causes the motor strip to lie anywhere from 4 to 5.4 cm behind the coronal suture, and landmark- based linear measurements may vary by up to 2 cm. This is mainly due to the natural individual variability and must be kept in mind when linear measurements based on anatomical landmarks from CT images are to be used to localize the precentral knob area.

Since neuronal populations in M1 active in movements of different fingers overlap extensively and control of a finger utilizes a network distributed throughout the hand area, this suggests that the position of the stimulating electrode is not critical as long as it is not close to the boundary of the hand representation. The average mediolateral span of the hand representation in M1 along the CS is 24-36mm, the vertical span being 36-56 mm.

One might think that the advent of frameless guidance system or neuronavigation has largely replaced localization relative to bony landmarks. Nonetheless, Reis et al (2008) concluded that the above-described classic craniocerebral topographic procedures are reliable methods for localizing CS and LS as well as associated landmarks and –most cogently- that modern imaging and neuronavigation have improved upon these methods by only 1 -3 mm! Velasco et al (2008) too found that rolandic fissure localization by external landmarks is satisfactory (mean error: 1.6 mm, range: 0-7 mm).

References

Boling W, Olivier A, Bittar RG: Localization of hand motor activation in Broca's pli de passage moyen. J Neurosurg 1999; 91: 903-910

Boling W, Reutens DC, Olivier A. Functional topography of the low postcentral area. J Neurosurg. 2002; 97:388-95

Broca A, Maubrac P. Traité de chirurgie cérébrale. Paris: Masson et Cie, 1896.

Broca P. Sur la topographie cranio-cérébrale ou sur les rapports anatomiques du crane et du cerveau. Rev d'Anthrop 1876;5:193-248.

Campero A, Ajler P, Martins C, et al. Usefulness of the contralateral Omega sign for the topographic location of lesions in and around the central sulcus. Surg Neurol Int 2011; 2: 164

Caulo M, Briganti C, Mattei PA, et al. New morphologic variants of the hand motor cortex as seen with MR imaging in a large study population. AJNR 2007; 28: 1480-1485

Charpy A, Poirier PJ. Traité d'anatomie humaine: système nerveux [in French]. Paris: Masson, 1899-1901.

Ebeling U, Steinmetz H, Huang YX, et al: Topography and identification of the inferior precentral sulcus in MR imaging. AJNR 1989; 10:937-942

Homan RW, Herman j, Purdy P. Cerebral location of international 10-20 system electrode placement. EEG Clin Neurophysiol 1987; 66: 376-382

Iwasaki S, Nakagawa H, Fukusumi A, et al. Identification of pre and postcentral gyri on CT and MRI images on the basis of the medullary pattern of cerebral white matter. Radiology 1991;179:207-213,

Kido DK, LeMay M, Levinson AW, Benson WE. Computed tomographic localization of the precentral gyrus. Radiology 1980;135:373-377.

Lehman RM, Olivier A, Moreau JJ: Use of the callosal grid system for the preoperative identification of the central sulcus. Stereotact Funct Neurosurg 1992; 58:179-188

Mogilner A.Y., Rezai A.R. Epidural motor cortex stimulation with functional imaging guidance. Neurosurg Focus 2001; 11, issue 3, p. E4

Naidich TP, Valavanis AG, Kubik S. Anatomic relationships along the low-middle convexity: Part I-Normal specimens and magnetic resonance imaging. Neurosurgery 36:517-532, 1995

Park MC, Goldman MA, Park MJ, et al.. Neuroanatomical localization of the 'precentral knob' with computed tomography imaging. Stereotact Funct Neurosurg 2007;85:158-161.

Park MC, Goldman MA, Friehs GM, et al. In: Canavero S (ed) Textbook of therapeutic cortical stimulation. New York: Nova Science, 2009, pp 3-16
Poirier PJ. La topographie cranio-encéphalique. Paris: Lescrosnier et Babè, 1891.
Reid RW. Observations on the relation of the principal fissures and convolutions of the cerebrum to the outer surface of the scalp. Lancet 1884;2:539-540.
Reis CV, Sankar T, Crusius M, et al. Comparative study of cranial topographic procedures: Broca's legacy toward practical brain surgery. Neurosurgery 2008;62:294-310.
Rhoton AL Jr. The cerebrum. Neurosurgery 2002;51:S1-S51.
Sobel DF, Gallen CC, Schwartz BJ, et al: Locating the central sulcus: comparison of MR anatomic and magnetoencephaloraphic functional methods. AJNR 14:915-925, 1993
Talairach J, Tournoux P, Missir O. Referentially Oriented Cerebral MRI Anatomy: An Atlas of Stereotaxic Anatomical Correlations for Gray and White Matter. pp 51-75, New York: Thieme Medical, 1993
Taylor AJ, Haughton VM, Syvertsen A, et al. Taylor-Haughton line revisited. AJNR Am J Neuroradiol 1980;1:55-56.
Taylor EH, Haughton WS. Some recent researches on the topography of the convolutions and fissures of the brain. Trans R Acad Med Ireland 1900;18:511-522.
Velasco M, Velasco F, Brito F, et al. Motor cortex stimulation in the treatment of deafferentation pain. I. Localization of the motor cortex. Stereotact Funct Neurosurg 2002; 79: 146-167
Velasco F, Arguelles C, Carrillo-Ruiz JD, et al. Efficacy of motor cortex stimulation in the treatment of neuropathic pain: a randomized double-blind trial. J Neurosurg 2008; 108: 698-706
Yasargil MG. Microneurosurgery, Vol. IV A CNS tumors. Stuttgart-New York: Thieme, 1994:1-114.
Yousry TA, Schmid UD, Alkadhi H, et al. Localization of the motor hand area to a knob on the precentral gyrus. A new landmark. Brain 1997;120:141-157.

Jean Paul Nguyen, Jean Pascal Lefaucheur

2 Neuroimaging Localization and Neuronavigation

The primary motor cortex (M1, Brodmann's area 4, BA4: Brodmann 1925) is currently the most frequently targeted area for extradural ICS (e.g. for neuropathic pain and Parkinson disease), but other areas have been stimulated, e.g. the primary somatosensory cortex (S1), the premotor cortex (PMC/BA6) and the dorsolateral prefrontal cortex (DLPFC/ BA9/46) (Canavero 2009). All can be localized anatomically on CT or preferably on MRI. This anatomical localization allows precise lead placement by using a neuronavigation system. In this chapter, we will describe neuroimaging localization techniques for cortical targets and the use of neuronavigation (Nguyen et al 1999, 2011). Although we focus on M1, a similar approach is employed elsewhere in the cortex.

M1 corresponds to the cortex situated just anteriorly to the CS and in the anterior bank of the CS. The existence of a somatotopic distribution in M1 has been known since the studies by Penfield (Penfield and Rasmussen 1950): the face is represented in the inferior part, the upper limb is represented in the middle part and the lower limb is represented in the superior part of M1 (Lefaucheur et al 2006). These various regions can be localized by identifying the CS, the superior frontal sulcus merging with the superior precentral sulcus and the inferior frontal sulcus merging with the inferior precentral sulcus (Fig.2.1). Anatomical examination of the brain surface and analysis of surface reconstructions do not always allow these structures to be clearly identified, as connections between the various sulci are often present on the brain surface. Classical CT or MRI slices are often able to localize the CS, but provide little information about the somatotopic distribution. However, when the most superficial layer of the brain is removed (Fig.2.1), the various sulci and fissures of the central region are more easily identified. Some image reconstruction software packages (e.g. Nexstim "peeling" function) provide analogous images that greatly facilitate recognition of M1 and cortical somatotopy (Fig.2.2). The CS is also easily recognized on oblique slices parallel to the cortical surface (Fig.2.3) that can be easily acquired with most image processing software. The same images can be obtained by using neuronavigation systems, corresponding to the "probe eye view" function, providing a view perpendicular to a trajectory that is itself perpendicular to the cortical surface.

Anatomically, the zone corresponding to representation of the upper limb is situated just anteriorly to the CS within the zone often presenting an Ω or hook shape situated just posteriorly to the posterior part of the superior frontal sulcus, and extending inferiorly to the zone corresponding to representation of the face (see Chapter 1). Similarly, the zone corresponding to representation of the face is located in the region situated flush with the posterior part of the inferior frontal sulcus and extends inferiorly to the lateral fissure (Fig.2.1, 2.2). By stimulating this region, Woolsey et al (1979) obtained motor responses in various parts of the face. The zone of representation of the lower limb, theoretically situated in the medial aspect of M1, very often extends onto the superior part of the convexity between the midline and the zone of representation of the upper limb (Fig.2.1-2.3). Anatomical localization may be corroborated by intraoperative electrophysiological testing (see Chapter 3). However, motor evoked potentials (MEPs) cannot be obtained in the presence of a motor deficit. Similarly, somatosensory evoked potentials (SEPs) are difficult to obtain in patients with a sensory deficit. Functional MRI may be useful in these cases (Fig.2.3, 2.4), but this procedure requires good patient cooperation.

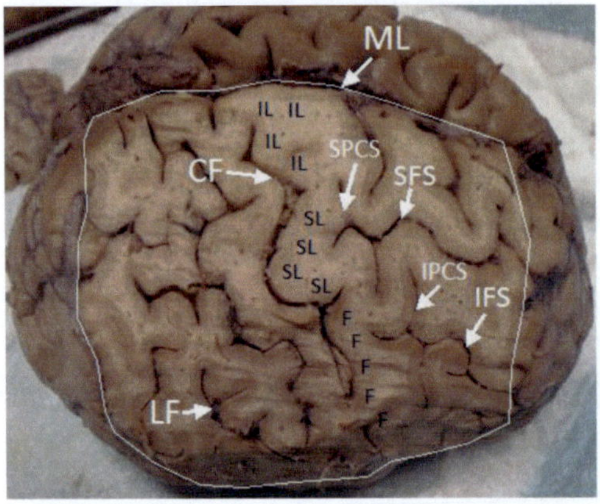

Fig. 2.1: Anatomy of the central region. The superficial layer of the brain has been removed (about 5 mm thick). The central sulcus (CS), lateral fissure (LF), superior frontal sulcus (SFS) and inferior frontal sulcus (IFS) and the superior precentral sulcus (SPCS) and inferior precentral sulcus (IPCS) are easily identified. Zones corresponding to representation of the face (F), upper limbs (UL) and lower limbs (LL) are delineated by the midline (ML), the lateral fissure (LF) and the level of the superior frontal sulcus (SFS) and inferior frontal sulcus (IFS).

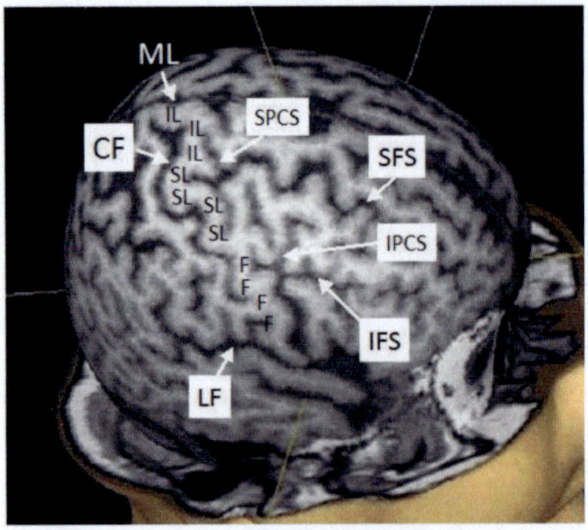

Fig. 2.2: Anatomy of the central region. The "peeling" function of Nexstim software can be used to virtually remove the superficial layer from all of the brain. The same structures as those observed on Figure 1 can be easily identified.

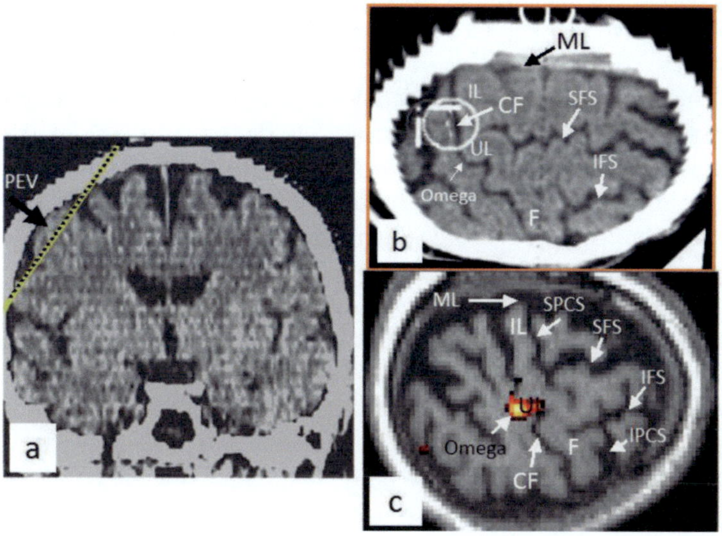

Fig. 2.3: Superficial oblique sections of the central region. a) Representation of a superficial oblique section through the central region (dotted line). The Probe Eye View (PEV) function of the neuronavigation software provides an equivalent view to this type of section. b) CT, c) MRI: The same structures as those observed in Figures 1 and 2 can be easily recognized. In the zone corresponding to the representation of the upper limb (UL), situated posteriorly to the posterior part of the superior frontal sulcus (SFS), the central sulcus often has an Omega shape. It is activated on functional MRI (Fig. c) when the patient performs movements of the contralateral hand.

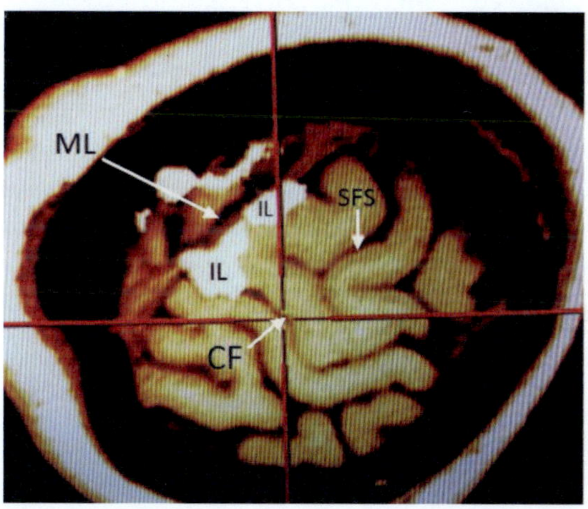

Fig. 2.4: Functional MRI. Activation of zones corresponding to the representation of the lower limbs (LL) was obtained by asking the patient to think that he was moving his lower limbs (paraplegic patient). In this case, the Medtronic workstation integrated functional MRI images in the neuronavigation planning. ML: Midline, CS: central sulcus, SFS: superior frontal sulcus.

2.1 Localization By rTMS

The development of transcranial magnetic stimulation (rTMS) has opened up new possibilities for localization of the stimulation target, as the use of rTMS for the treatment of chronic pain has made target selection according to cortical somatotopy somewhat irrelevant. Stimulation according to the somatotopic distribution is important in some cases, but not in others, in which it may be sufficient to stimulate the M1 of the zone corresponding to the upper limb (the easiest to recognize) to improve patients with diffuse or hemibody pain, or relieve parkinsonian symptoms. rTMS is already employed to predict response to extradural ICS in chronic pain conditions (Chapters 8-9), but it can also aid in more accurately defining the stimulation target.

In the absence of a motor deficit, it is relatively easy to locate M1 on the surface of the skull by moving the stimulation coil. M1 corresponds to the place at which stimulation induces a detectable motor response (MEP) (Fig.2.5). In the case of ICS for pain, we usually start by stimulating the zone of M1 corresponding to the representation of the upper limb on the side contralateral to the pain, irrespective of the localization of bodily pain. If pain is not improved, we test the cortical zone corresponding to the representation of the painful zone according to cortical somatotopy. As rTMS is a noninvasive stimulation technique, several stimulation targets can be tested successively. The zone at which stimulation is effective can be localized by using a neuronavigation system neuronavigated rTMS (Fig.2.5) (Ahdab et al 2014). This same zone could also be easily located by intraoperative neuronavigation (Fig.2.6). Under these conditions, intraoperative electrophysiological testing does not appear to be mandatory, as MEPs were previously obtained during rTMS (Fig.2.5).

We currently recommend extensive preoperative use of rTMS in order to select candidates for surgery, based on several effective sessions, as well as several placebo sessions in order to more reliably ensure a good response to rTMS. Several stimulation targets must be tested in order to be sure of selecting the best target. When all conditions are met, *the operation can be performed exclusively by neuronavigation, without intraoperative electrophysiological testing, hence the importance of good anatomical localization, the use of neuronavigated rTMS and intraoperative neuronavigation.*

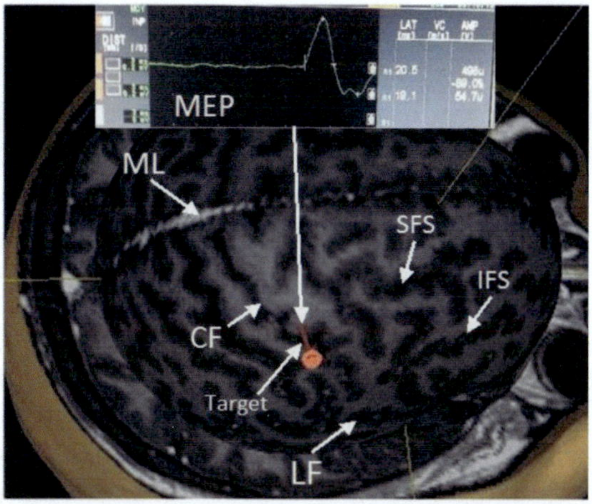

Fig. 2.5: Identification of the effective stimulation target by neuronavigated rTMS. The effective stimulation target on rTMS corresponds to the motor cortex (situated just anteriorly to the central sulcus (CS)) situated over the posterior part of the superior frontal sulcus (SFS). Stimulation of this target at about 70% of maximum power of the machine induced a motor evoked response (MEP) confirming that this target corresponded to the motor cortex corresponding to representation of the upper limb. SFS: superior frontal sulcus, IFS: inferior frontal sulcus, Target: target detected by neuronavigation corresponding to the zone of effective stimulation. IFS: inferior frontal sulcus, LF: lateral fissure, ML: midline.

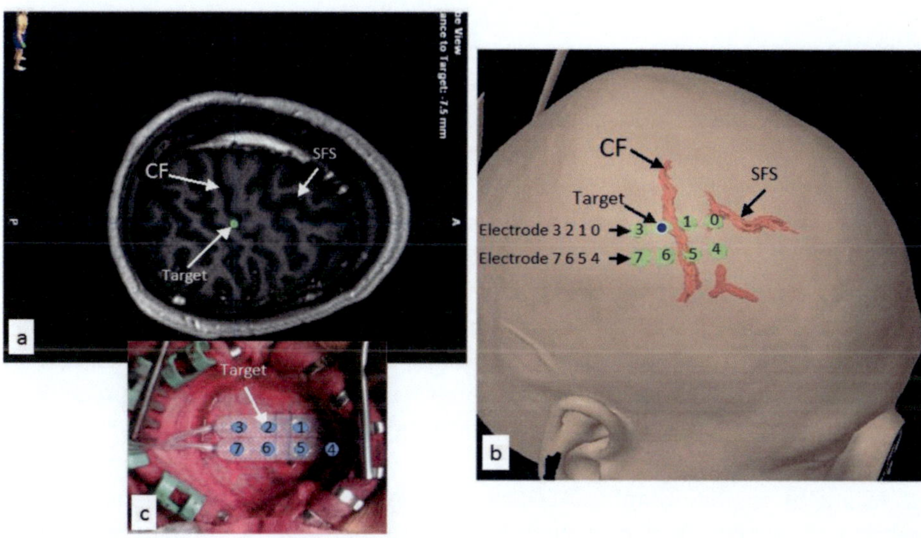

Fig. 2.6: Lead placement. We use two Resume 4-electrode leads, with electrodes numbered from 0 to 3 for the midline lead and 4 to 7 for the lateral lead (Figs b and c). We generally place electrode 2 on the target (target Fig. b) of the midline lead that is placed just posteriorly to the central sulcus (Fig. a), in the posterior part of the superior frontal sulcus (SFS). The optimal stimulation combination in this configuration should be 1-2+ and 5-6+. Electrode 0 is not shown on Figure c, as it placed underneath the bone edge.

2.2 Localization By Neuroimaging

Neuronavigation allows integration of different targeting methods, including 3-D MRI, fMRI, MEG and others (Mylius et al 2013).

fMRI guidance can provide independent and highly accurate targeting information for improving the surgical procedure. Blood oxygenation level-dependent (BOLD) fMRI data of motor functions of the tongue, arm or leg are obtained by using standardized paradigms, such as repetitive contraction of the lips, cyclic finger tapping of the contralateral hand or repetitive opposition of the thumb and each of the remaining fingers, or flexion-and-extension of the toes of the contralateral foot at a rate of 1 Hz after a training session before imaging is performed. These movements activate MI contralaterally (but also the ipsilateral MI, supplementary motor and premotor areas and the primary somatosensory areas bilaterally). Post-stroke motor deficits may hamper examination, but fMRI is particularly useful for amputees or plexus avulsion patients, since virtual movements of the phantom or paralytic limb easily induce contralateral precentral and postcentral gyri activations. Blocks of 30 seconds of alternating activation and rest are repeated a few times. Generally, a focal cortical activation area (diameter 5-10 mm) after hand motor tasks is localized to the contralateral precentral gyrus, but differences between the two sides in the surface and minor displacements of the precentral activation area are frequently observed (also due to cortical remapping). Concordance between the contours of fMRI activation areas and intraoperative electrical motor brain mapping (iBM) with SEPs and MEPs is found in a large majority of patients, and never exceeded 1 cm in a study (Bartos et al 2009). In a study (Pirotte et al 2009), correspondence between contours of fMRI activation area and iBM in the precentral gyrus was found in almost all (94%) patients. Moreover, fMRI was less altered by artifacts and provided data which were more constantly unambiguous than those from iBM. While in most cases fMRI data can be satisfactory matched with navigation data, in some cases, motion artifacts and low signal levels interfere with fMRI data analysis (see further discussion in Canavero 2009). Unfortunately, fMRI is a time consuming technique requiring training and engineering (statistical parametric mapping, spatial and functional validation) prior to its application to stereotactic conditions. Finally, fMRI can be combined with MR tractography and diffusion tensor imaging (DTI) for optimal brain damage assessment, especially in cases of stroke.

MagnetoEncephaloGraphy (MEG) has an excellent temporal resolution (1 second, real time acquisition) which is much better than that of fMRI (30 min, summation acquisition). Moreover, MEG records directly the magnetic field created by the electrical neuronal activity, while fMRI activation signals reflect indirectly transient changes in the rCBF secondary to the neuronal activity.

References

Ahdab R, Ayache SS, Farhat WH, et al. Reappraisal of the anatomical landmarks of motor and premotor cortical regions for image-guided brain navigation in TMS practice. Hum Brain Mapp 2014; 35: 2435-47

Bartos R, Jech R, Vymazal J, et al. Validity of primary motor area localization with fMRI versus electric cortical stimulation: a comparative study. Acta Neurochir (Wien). 2009;151:1071-80

Brodman K. In Vergleichende Lokalisationlehre der Grosshirnrinde in Prinzipien dargestellt auf Grund des Zellenbaues (ed. Barth JA), Leipzig, 1925.

Canavero S (ed) Textbook of therapeutic cortical stimulation. New York: Nova Science, 2009

Lefaucheur JP, Hatem S, Nineb A, et al. Somatotopic organization of the antalgic effects of motor cortex rTMS in neuropathic pain. Neurology 2006;67:1998-2004

Mylius V, Ayache SS, Ahdab R, et al. Definition of DLPFC and M1 according to anatomical landmarks for navigated brain stimulation: inter-rater reliability, accuracy, and influence of gender and age. Neuroimage. 2013;78:224-32.

Nguyen JP, Lefaucheur JP, Decq P, et al. Chronic motor cortex stimulation in the treatment of central and neuropathic pain. Correlations between clinical, electrophysiological and anatomical data. Pain 1999;82:245-251

Nguyen JP, Nizard J, Keravel Y and Lefaucheur JP. Invasive brain stimulation for the treatment of neuropathic pain. Nat Rev Neurol. 2011;7:699-709

Penfield W and Rasmussen T. The cerebral cortex of man. A clinical study of localization of function (Macmillan), New York, 1950.

Pirotte BJM, Voordecker P, Levivier M, Baleriaux D. Principles of surgical implantation and complications avoidance. In: Canavero S (ed) Textbook of therapeutic cortical stimulation. New York: Nova Science, 2009, pp 33-44

Woolsey CN, Erickson TC and Gilson WE. Localization in somatic sensory and motor areas of human cerebral cortex as determined by direct recording of evoked potentials and electrical stimulation. J Neurosurg. 1979;51:476-506

Jeffrey E. Arle, Jay L. Shils

3 Electrophysiological Localization

In this chapter, we describe our technique of electrophysiological mapping of M1 and the CS (Arle and Shils 2011, Shils and Arle 2011, Shils and Deletis 2013). The surgical entry point is determined by moving approximately 1-2 cm behind the midpoint between the nasion to inion toward the lateral canthus or anterior margin of the tragus using a curved scalp incision. This allows for a craniotomy –if elected- that measures roughly 5-6 cm in diameter and gives enough access for small adjustments either slightly superiorly or inferiorly along the convexity to map face or hand as desired. We do not use a Mayfield head holder since the head does not need to be rigidly held in place and if the patient has a seizure induced by mapping further injury can be avoided by not having them pinned in a rigid head-holder.

3.1 Somatosensory Mapping

This consists of placing the lead on the dura in a variety of directions, mostly perpendicular to the suspected pre-central gyrus. Median and/or ulnar nerve somatosensory evoked potential's (SSEP's) are then run using a 20 mA 200 μs monopolar square pulse at a rate of 4.32 Hz. SSEP stimulating electrodes are placed at the wrist overlying either the median or ulnar nerves with the anode placed distally to that cathode. SSEP's are recorded from the lead in both bipolar (contact 1-2, 2-3, ...) and monopolar (all referenced to the 10-20 location of Fz) recording montages. Otherwise, the median nerve is stimulated bipolarly at a frequency of 2-3 Hz and an intensity of 5-20 mA until slight twitches of the thumb are obtained. A ground electrode is placed around the forearm with a loop tape strap. Recordings are performed by using a filter band pass of 20-2000 Hz, a time base of 50 ms, and a grid of multiple contacts (12-24) or the epidural lead that is intended to be implanted and used for chronic stimulation. The main cortical components of the median nerve SSEPs include a positive response (downward peak) over the precentral (motor) gyrus with a mean latency of 20 milliseconds (P20) and a negative response (upward peak) over the postcentral (sensory) gyrus with a mean latency of 20 milliseconds (N20). The CS is determined as the point where the N20 response phase reverses (Fig.3.1) In order to get a complete picture of the CS, multiple mapping locations are needed.

This technique has *several limitations*. First, cortical SSEPs are absent in the case of severe or complete sensory deafferentation (e.g. amputation). Second, SEP phase reversal is not reliable for the stimulation of the face (trigeminal nerve) or the lower limb (tibial nerve). Third, the P20 component can be missing, even in awake or mildly sedated patients. Fourth, tortuosity of the CS, that in some parts becomes parallel to the midsagittal line, complicates the placement of the 4-contact strip on M1 by determining reversal only in a single point. Fifth, there may be a 1-2 cm discrepancy between SSEP maximum in SI and the hand motor area in M1, making SSEP targeting inaccurate (see Saitoh and Hosomi 2009 and Pirotte et al 2009 for full discussion). In practice, SSEP have been sidestepped by several authors.

According to Velasco et al (2002), recording corticocortical evoked responses (CCER) is simple, reliable, and superior to SSEPs. MI stimulation elicits negative CCER over the frontal scalp, whereas SI stimulation elicits positive responses over parietal and occipital scalp regions.

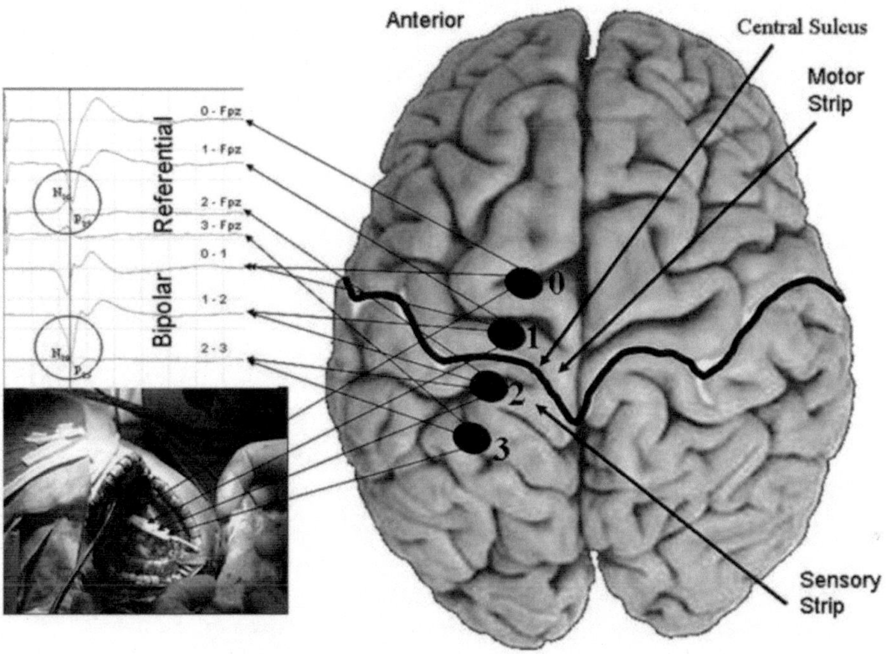

Fig. 3.1: Use of the SSEP reversal potential method to determine location of M1 extradurally. Contacts 0-3 of a typical 4-contact paddle-type electrode are shown in one example placement across the underlying central sulcus. The upper left waveforms show the SSEP in each contact. The reversal of phase occurs, in this example, between contacts 1 and 2. The inset picture at lower left is the intraoperative photo of this technique being used, revealing the relative size of the lead and the craniotomy opening. By moving the lead around in different locations, the path of the sulcus can be mapped out on the dura.

3.2 Motor Mapping

This is the most crucial step for optimizing M1 ICS electrode placement, i.e. performing intraoperative motor mapping (MM), which consists of activating M1 via electrical stimulation and recording the responses in specific muscle groups (Shils and Deletis 2011, Azabou et al 2013). Activation of M1 causes action potentials to travel down the corticospinal tract to alpha-motor neurons (αMN) in the ventral spinal cord. Once an αMN is activated actions potentials travel to muscle and generate a compound muscle action potential (CMAP). It goes without saying that *MM cannot be exploited in patients with total or severe motor deficits or with missing limbs.*

There are 3 important factors in mapping motor regions: (1) the strength of the stimulus; (2) the type of anesthesia; (3) and the type of stimulator probes used. First, when stimulating M1, the spread of the electric field will determine the resolution of the response. If the stimulus is too low, too few axons will be activated to generate a recordable CMAP. If the stimulus is too high, axons that are more distant (a few mm to 1 cm) may be activated and potentially falsely identify a region as M1. Additionally if there is excessive fluid in the surgical field the stimulus will be spread over a larger area, and therefore it is important to maintain a dry area for stimulation. Second, the αMN is very susceptible to the effects of anesthesia. The αMN is a highly modulated cell with many inputs that can adjust the firing threshold of the cell. When the patient is under anesthesia, the αMN's membrane is more inhibited due to the lack of basal background activity from its multiple inputs. Under such conditions it becomes difficult for a single axon to cause the αMN to fire. Different anesthetics have varying amounts of inhibitory effects on the αMN membrane. Thus it is highly recommended to use a total-intravenous anesthetic (TIVA) for these procedures (Sloan 1998), i.e. continuous dose of propofol (75 mcg/kg/min up to 150 mcg/kg/min) combined with either fentanyl or remifentanil (0.05 mcg/kg/min up to 0.5 mcg/kg/min) and no nitrous inhalational agent or muscle relaxants. Yet, even with TIVA, the membrane needs the help of temporal summation at the corticospinal axon input to counteract the relative loss of spatial summation. Historically this has been solved by using a low frequency (50 to 60Hz) long train (1 second or more) of stimuli. This technique, however, can incur up to 11% seizure rates (Yingling et al 1999). A second technique, known as high-frequency, involves using a train of 5-7 stimuli with a 2-4 ms inter stimulus interval (ISI) (Taniguchi et al 1993). This technique has demonstrated a much lower seizure frequency rate of 1.6% (Szeleny et al 2006) and significantly increases the 'on display' signal-to-noise ratio. Both bipolar stimulation (the anode and cathode are within 1 cm of each other) and monopolar stimulation (the cathode is placed at some far reference point on the body, usually the contralateral 10-20 system F1 or F2 position) can be employed. Although bipolar stimulation is supposed to offer a more focal stimulation response, if the field is kept dry and the stimulation is adjusted to the threshold response, monopolar stimulation fields remain focal. Furthermore, the location of the stimulus is directly under the electrode rather than at some arbitrary point between the two electrodes.

To record CMAP activity from the muscles, pairs of needles are placed in bipolar fashion (separated by 0.5 - 2 cm) in the orbicularis oculi, orbicularis oris, trapezius, deltoid, biceps, triceps, flexor carpi ulnaris, abductor pollicis brevis, first dorsal interosseous, quadriceps, anterior tibialis, and abductor hallucis muscles (MacDonald et al 2013). Surface electrodes can also be used, but we have found that they can easily be dislodged during the procedure and are more affected by noise. Stimulation consists of trains of 5-9 stimuli, each with an ISI of 250-500 ms, and a 500 μs pulse width. Once the probe is placed on the dura stimulation amplitudes are slowly increased starting at 5 mA (for subdural testing the amplitude is started at 3mA, though placement in the subdural space is rarely used) and increased to a maximum of 25 mA or until a response is found. Stimulation can be performed with any EMG system that allows for short low amplitude high frequency trains. When a CMAP response is generated (Fig.3.2), the location is marked on the dura with a sterile pen. Multiple areas are tested to map M1 to provide for optimal electrode placement. It is useful to have ice cold saline kept on the field with which to irrigate, should a seizure occur, as well as having lorazepam available in the OR. EEG can be monitored both during stimulation in order to identify seizure activity, as well as, more importantly, after discharge activity which is an indicator of *potential* seizure activity, allowing for a more timely cessation of stimulation in that area of the brain.

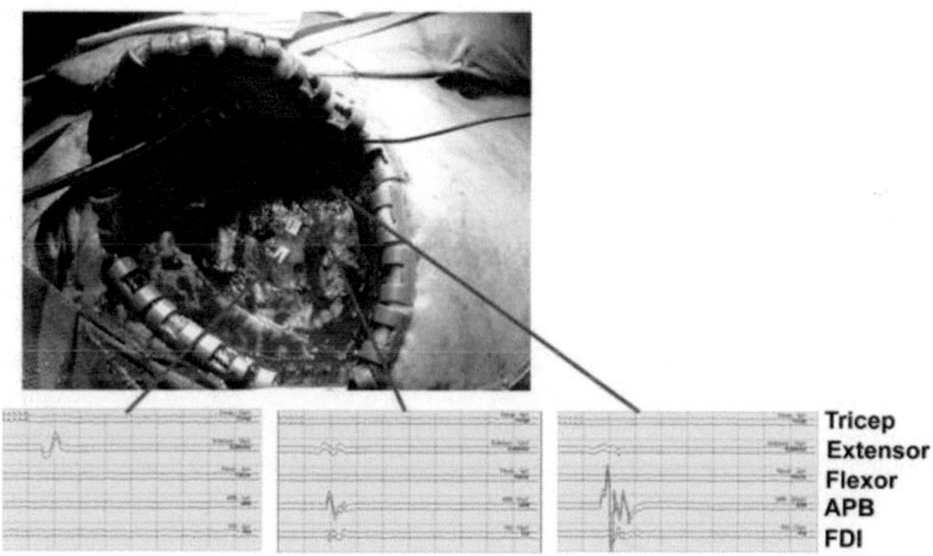

Fig. 3.2: Use of the cortical mapping technique for determing location of M1 regions. The EMG from muscles in the upper extremity are shown below following stimulation with a ball tip electrode in three locations on the dura. The far left shows activation of the extensor muscle in the forearm, the other two show activation of the APB muscle in the hand. This technique corroborates the SSEP method in figure 1 and helps determine more precisely the underlying thresholds for individual muscle groups.

Other protocols exist in the literature. Teixeira et al (2013) carry out transdural functional cortical mapping with the patient fully awake under local anesthesia. Transdural electrical stimulation exploit the following parameters: 4-6 mA, 30-60Hz, PW 1 ms. Lefaucheur and DeAndrade (2009) perform monopolar anodal stimulation (single square waves of 1 ms duration, delivered at an intensity range of 10-50 mA), each contact of the epidural grid or quadripolar lead being successively activated as the anode. The cathode (reference electrode) is a subcutaneous needle or a steel plate electrode placed in the occipital region, to avoid direct activation of face muscles by the stimulation; the ground electrode is placed around the forearm with a loop tape strap. EMG recordings detect motor responses at lower intensity thresholds than visual inspection. The MEPs are recorded using a filter band pass of 20-2000 Hz, a time base of 50-100 ms, and surface or subcutaneous needle electrodes placed over the target muscles. The infusion of anesthetic agents (propofol and remifentanil) is carefully monitored to maintain the bispectral index (BIS) around a value of 60. In rare cases, a single train of two or three stimuli (20 μs interpulse interval) may be required. They recorded intraoperative MEPs in any part of the body. The motor threshold is determined for evocation of a reproducible MEP of more than 100 mV in amplitude in the target territory. For this purpose, the contact of the epidural grid or quadripolar lead that theoretically corresponds to the optimal motor cortical representation of the painful region (according to image-guided navigation and intraoperative SEP mapping) is selected as the anode. With the use of this montage, stimulation intensity is gradually increased by increments of 2 mA to a maximum of 50 mA. Cortical mapping is then performed at a fixed intensity set at 20-30% above the motor threshold. The complete procedure includes MEP recordings to monopolar cortical stimulation, by using successively each contact of the epidural grid or quadripolar lead as an anode. From these recordings, the "best anode" is determined, i.e. the contact providing MEPs of maximal amplitude in the target territory when selected as an anode. Recordings using each contact as a cathode, with the occipital reference as the anode, are possible, but, in their experience, of little or no value. Recording MEPs in the target territory in response to bipolar cortical stimulation, using the "best anode" as the anode and successively each adjacent contact of the grid or quadripolar lead as the cathode, may be useful: the amplitude of the MEPs evoked by the various bipolar combinations can be compared with that produced by the optimal anodal stimulation to estimate how much the contacts adjacent to the "best anode" interfere with this electrode.

References

Arle JE and JL Shils (eds) Essential Neuromodulation. New York : Academic Press, 2011

Azabou E, Manel V, Andre-Obadia N, et al. Optimal parameters of transcranial electrical stimulation for intraoperative monitoring of motor evoked potentials of the tibialis anterior muscle during pediatric scoliosis surgery. Neurophysiol Clin. 2013; 43: 243-250

Henderson JM, Heit G, Fisher RS. Recurrent seizures related to motor cortex stimulator programming. Neuromodulation. 2010;13;37-43

Lefaucheur JP, de Andrade DC. Intraoperative neurophysiologic mapping of the central cortical region for epidural electrode placement in the treatment of neuropathic pain by motor cortex stimulation. Brain Stimul. 2009;2:138-48.

MacDonald DB, Skinner S, Shils J, et al. Intraoperative motor evoked potential monitoring – A position statement by the American Society of Neurophysiological Monitoring. Clinical Neurophysiology. 2013;124:2291-2316.

Pirotte BJM, Voordecker P, Levivier M, et al. Principles of surgical implantation and complication avoidance. In. Canavero S (ed) Textbook of therapeutic cortical stimulation. New York: Nova Science, 2009. pp 33-44

Saitoh Y, Hosomi K. From localization to surgical implantation. In: Canavero S (ed) Textbook of therapeutic cortical stimulation. New York: Nova Science, 2009. pp 17-32

Shils JL and Arle JE. Treatment Applications of Cortical Stimulation. In: Winn HR (ed) Youman's Neurological Surgery New York: Elsevier, NY, 2011, 6th ed.

Shils JL and Deletis V. Motor Evoked Potentials. In: Kaye AD and Davis SF (eds) Principles of neurophysiological assessment, mapping, and monitoring. New York: Springer, 2013.

Sloan T. Anesthetic effects on electrophysiologic recordings. J Clin Neurophysiol. 1998:15:217.

Szelényi A, Joksimovic B, Seifert V. Intraoperative risk of seizures associated with transient direct cortical stimulation in patients with symptomatic epilepsy. J Clin Neurophysiol. 2006;23:1-5.

Taniguchi M, Cedzich C, Schramm J. Modification of cortical stimulation for motor evoked potentials under general anesthesia: technical description.Neurosurgery 1993;32:219–26.

Teixeira MJ, Ciampi de Andrade D, Fonoff ET. Intra-operative transdural electric stimulation in awake patient: target refining for motor cortex stimulation. Acta Neurochir Suppl. 2013;117:73-8.

Velasco M, Velasco F, Brito F, et al. Motor cortex stimulation in the treatment of deafferentation pain. I. Localization of the motor cortex. Stereotact Funct Neurosurg. 2002;79:146-67.

Yingling CD, Ojemann S, Dodson B, et al. Identification of motor pathways during tumor surgery facilitated by multichannel electromyographic recording. J Neurosurg. 1999;91:922–927.

Dirk Rasche, Volker M. Tronnier

4 Implantation: Burr Holes

In this chapter, we illustrate the burr hole approach (Tsubokawa et al 1991, Meyerson et al 1993, Rasche et al 2006, Tronnier and Rasche 2013) and its advantages and disadvantages over the craniotomy approach. There is presently no consensus on which approach is best.

4.1 Single-Burr-Hole Technique

The use of a neuronavigation system is an accepted standard for this procedure. Preoperatively, either a CT- or MRI-scan of the patient´s brain with a 3-D-volume- or surface-reconstruction is performed. Although the primary orientation regarding the precentral gyrus is still following Penfield's homunculus, modern functional investigations and data like fMRI, DTI, PET and others are implemented in the neuronavigation system. These are useful tools for individual planning of the procedure and approach.

Before proceeding, informed consent needs to be signed by the patient and the experimental nature of the procedure explained and specifically approved, since the procedure is as yet not FDA/EMEA approved.

General anesthesia is preferred for craniotomies, but for burr hole techniques a mild neuroleptoanalgesia (intravenous metamizol 500-1000 mg, low-dose remifentanil or sufentanil or short-term inhalative isoflurane < 1 vol%) and local anesthesia (lidocaine 1% or bupivacaine 0.5%) are generally sufficient (see Box 4.1). The patient is lying in a comfortable dorsal position, has an intravenous infusion port, oxygen mask, electrocardiographic and oxygen saturation monitoring.

Anethesia is induced with a loading dose of Remifentanil 3–4 ng/ml in continuous infusion followed after 5–8 min by Propofol 5.5 µg/ml as induction dose. Endotracheal intubation is facilitated by vecuronium bromide 0.1 mg/kg; no further doses of muscle relaxants are administered throughout surgery. The lungs are mechanically ventilated with a 50% O_2 in air mixture, in order to maintain end tidal concentrations of CO_2 ($ETCO_2$) at 30–35 mmHg. Anesthesia is maintained with Remifentanil (5–6 ng/ml, up to 7-8 ng/ml if necessary) and Propofol (2.5-3.0 µg/ml). At the end of the surgical procedure, all patients are awakened within 15–30 min from cessation of TIVA.

Box 4.1: Total IntraVenous Anesthesia (TIVA).

Depending on the surgeon, fixation of the head, either in a clamp, pin-holder (Mayfield®) or with the use of vacuum cushions, may be carried out for accuracy and

Table 4.1: Procedural steps for the one-burr-hole approach.

Procedural steps	
Step 1	Neuronavigation
Step 2	Planning of the procedure/target identification
Step 3	Analgosedation
Step 4	Local anesthesia
Step 5	Fixation of the head
Step 6	Calibration of the neuronavigation system
Step 7	Identification of the target
Step 8	Planning of the approach/burr hole
Step 9	Antisepsis and sterile coverage
Step 10	Local anesthesia
Step 11	Wound incision
Step 12	Drilling of the burr hole
Step 13	Identification of the dura and hemostasis
Step 14	Epidural spacing
Step 15	Neuronavigation control
Step 16	Lead positioning
Step 17	Neuronavigation control
Step 18	Intraoperative stimulation, motor threshhold
Step 19	Intraoperative phase reversal
Step 20	Re-positioning of the leads
Step 21	Neuronavigation control
Step 22	in case of need, repeat Steps18-21
Step 23	Fixation of the leads
Step 24	Percutaneous extensions
Step 25	Identification of the leads
Step 26	Wound closure
Step 27	Remove head fixation
Step 28	Postoperative x-ray and CT scan
Step 29	Image fusion and matching
Step 30	Standardized test protocol incl. double-blinded and placebo stimulation

to avoid brain-shift; some, on the other hand, keep the patient's head loose. In case of fixation with pins, disinfection and local anesthesia is mandatory. Positioning of a cushion beneath the neck to stabilize the patient´s cervical spine is favorably received by many patients. Shaving of hair is only necessary in the area of the surgical approach and where the skin is pierced by the percutaneous extensions. After disinfection local anesthesia is administered, including the area of the expected skin perforation.

Registration of the neuronavigation system is performed after positioning of the head. Target identification of M1 or other cortical areas depends on the clinical symptoms and the focus of treatment.

The registration of the neuronavigation data set is followed by target identification and planning of the final position of the burr hole on the patient's skin. Therefore a skin marker is used; also the area of interest (e. g. M1) can be drawn on the skin for orientation. It is important to ensure that disinfection and sterile coverage of the operative field does not influence, mask or wash out these drawings.

After application of local anesthetic, a curved skin incision is performed and the calvaria exposed. Depending on the target, this is the frontal, temporal or parietal skull. A burr hole with a standard pneumatic drilling device and a drilling head with a diameter of 12-16 mm is placed (Fig.4.1). Bleeding from intraosseous vessels is treated with sterile wax. Bipolar coagulation is used for dural bleeding. The interior bony edge of the burr hole is prepared with bony cutters oriented according to the desired epidural localization of the leads. This is followed by separation of the dura from the skull, also taking into account the orientation of the desired position of the leads. Neuronavigation greatly facilitates orientation, direction, angle and length of the epidural separation.

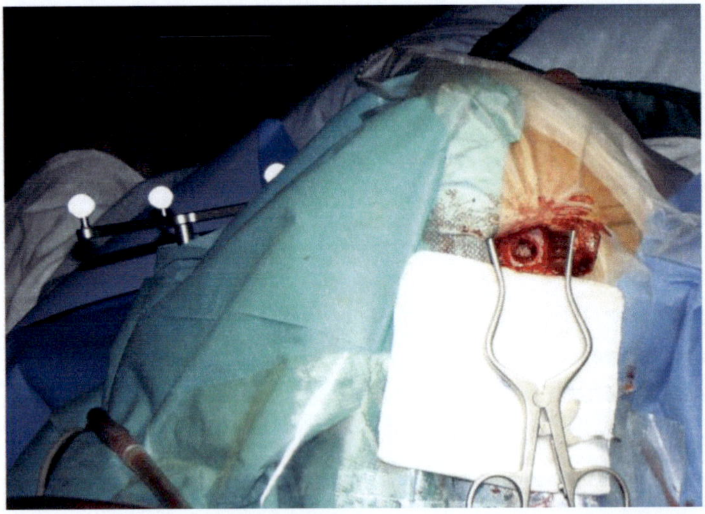

Fig. 4.1: Intraoperative photo demonstrating the one burr hole approach on the right hemisphere for left-sided BPA. Note that the patient is awake, the left hand and face can be seen and sterile neuronavigation markers are attached on the left side of the head clamp.

Intraoperatively, either temporary or permanent paddle leads can be implanted for testing. Different models of custom-made or commercially available leads are used. The quadripolar paddle lead is preferred for this procedure and permanent implantation (e.g. Resume® Model 3857, Medtronic Inc., Minneapolis, MN, USA). The size of this lead is 8 mm (width) by 45 mm (length). In cases of positioning of two leads, one has to take into account that enough space is prepared for both leads both in the epidural space and also the burr hole. Connecting the implanted lead with a test stimulation device allows intraoperative stimulation. A standard protocol for intraoperative testing is advised and different stimulation parameters and electrode combinations should be tested. In case of low-frequency stimulation (< 10 Hz) focal tics or muscle contractions can be evaluated corresponding to the stimulated M1 and in relation to the individual motor threshold. Suprathreshold stimulation with high frequencies (about 100 Hertz) leads to dystonic movements and contractions. This is seen also with lower amplitudes and the risk of focal seizures or general epileptic seizures is increased. The anesthesiologist must be prepared to administer an IV anticonvulsant (e.g. phenytoin). In the case of pain patients, many of them are already on drugs with antiepileptic acticity. The exact localization of the lead can be controlled by the neuronavigation system and correlation made with the preoperative imaging and target plan. If the surgeon elects to employ MEP or SSEP (see Chapter 3), connection of the implanted lead with the recording neurophysiology device is possible using an adapter cable.

Placing two leads in the epidural space allows a broader area of coverage of stimulation. The exact and optimal position is still a matter of debate. Different positions in relation to the precentral gyrus are possible. Either the lead contacts are placed to straddle the CS (i.e. horizontally) or parallel to CS running along the precentral gyrus. In the case of parallel positioning, one lead is directed over the CS and the second one covers the precentral gyrus. Identification of the two leads is advised by marking the connecting cable and also the percutaneous extensions by a ligature or suture.

Once the leads are implanted in the optimal position, fixation is advised. This can be done either by suture to the dura, fixation with plates and screws to the skull, or by use of cement pressed in the burr hole. Following the connection to extensions, these are externalized percutaneously in the ipsilateral temporal region.

Postoperatively a plain anterior-posterior and lateral x-ray of the skull is advised to document the position of the leads (Fig. 4.2). A CT scan is advised to rule out epidural bleedings. Image fusion and matching with the preoperative MRI and identification of the lead position can be performed.

A standardized test trial with an external stimulation device follows. Stimulation parameters vary regarding pulse width, frequency and amplitude: commonly used are a pulse width of 150-300 µsec and a frequency of 20-50 Hertz. Stimulation is always subthreshold. The test protocol includes a variety of different stimulation settings and also placebo or double-blinded testing. This is mandatory and allows the identification of false positive responders. Only patients with significant symptom reduction and concomitant withdrawal of medication should be considered for implantation of a permanent neurostimulation device. Patients receiving a full-system implantation with the above mentioned devices should be informed that the examination with MRI-scanners is neither allowed nor approved.

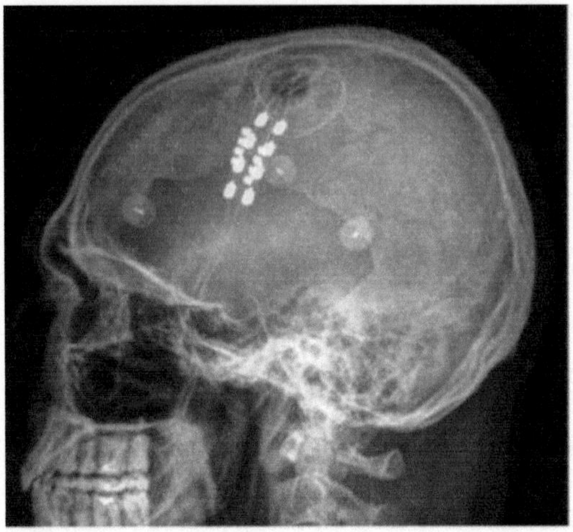

Fig. 4.2: Lateral x-ray of a patient's head with two implanted epidural leads via the one burr hole approach. The patient suffered from facial pain following surgery of a cranial base meningioma.

4.2 Two-Burr-Hole Technique

The surgeon makes an oblique linear skin incision (6-10cm) parallel to and 1 cm ahead of or behind the projection of the CS and then drills two burr holes at a distance of 2-4 cm (plus a bony groove parallel to the paddle to accommodate the connector between the looping lead and the extension) (Canavero et al 1999). A stimulating paddle is inserted epidurally from the edge of one burr hole overlying the targeted area; the bony bridge between the two holes will then hold the plate in place and simultaneously reduce the durocortical gap. For facial or leg targets, the paddle can be gently advanced caudally or rostrally by up to 2 cm. This technique entails no risk of epidural hematoma, and accidental displacement of the electrode has never been observed (Canavero 2009) (Fig.4.3). Uncooperative patients are infrequent and most patients find that having no screens in front of their eyes, including surgical cloths, makes the procedure much more tolerable (Canavero S, personal communication 2014: In this case, the surgical field is prepared by folding the surgical sterile cloth on the patient's forehead and hanging it to nearby posts providing unrestricted view of the surrounding environment.)

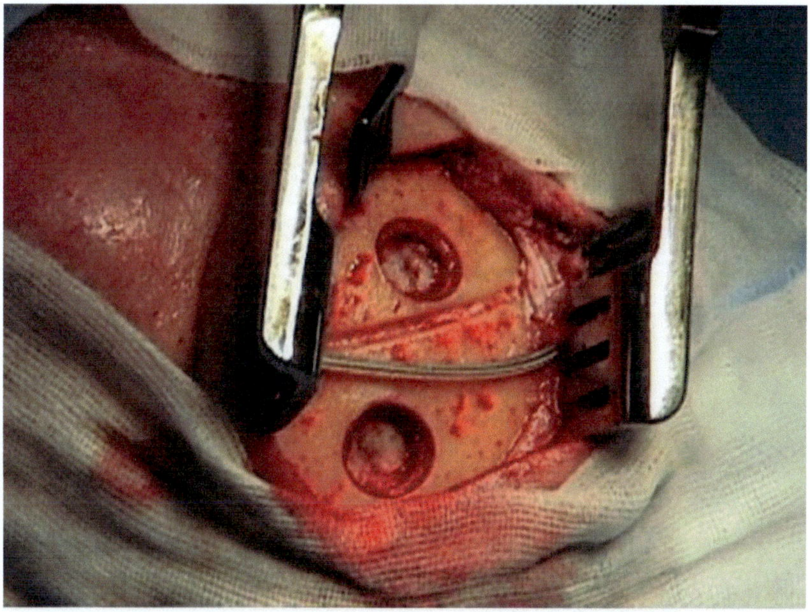

Fig. 4.3: Operative view of the two burr-hole technique. After drilling the holes (a), the electrode array is slipped underneath the bony bridge (b) which will keep the paddle in place; also, the dural-cerebral interface will be squeezed by the thickness of the strip, reducing the CSF thickness underneath. A bony cradle is fashioned for the cable joint (c) (courtesy of Sergio Canavero).

4.3 Commentary

One of the most frequent arguments for craniotomy is the reduced risk of epidural hematoma due to the open control of bleedings. Routine postoperative CT-scan of the skull showed no epidural hematoma in our series of 80 patients submitted to ICS using the one burr hole technique (Rasche et al 2006, Tronnier and Rasche 2013). The same applies to Canavero's series using the two-burr-hole technique (Canavero S, personal communication, 2014).

It is often assumed that positioning of the leads via craniotomy is more precise than via one or two burr holes, the larger exposure providing better electrophysiological mapping of the target area. Following this argumentation, one might rightfully expect that the results of the series using the burr hole technique be much worse than craniotomic series. A survey of the whole literature (this volume) proves this not to be the case. The primary goal of the procedure is the optimal position of the lead. This can be reached via all described techniques taking into account the different pro´s and con´s (Table 4.2) and the experience of the functional neurosurgeon.

Table 4.2: PROs and CONs of the one burr hole approach.

PRO´S	CON´S
small open wound	no control for epidural positioning or direction of the lead tip
minor trauma	limited access to target structures
shorter operating time	risk of epidural haematoma
leads easier to remove	risk of dislocation
leads easier to revise	risk of malpositioning
lesser risk of infection	electrophysiological monitoring only with adapter
reduced amount of local anesthetic	no direct visual control with neuronavigation pointer tip

Another aspect is the direction of the lead and contacts in relation to the CS. Many centers position the lead parallel to the CS, others perpendicular to it. Interestingly, the results of the series employing these two different approaches are wholly comparable, none being superior. This somewhat casts a pall on the "precision-of-placement" dogma and should be investigated properly in the future. Certainly, such noninvasive techniques as tDCS cover a much wider area and still obtain results. Perhaps what counts is simply the engagement of a widespread network in the brain rather than "pinpoint" precision as in DBS.

Finally, the risk of intraoperative seizures is said to be reduced by general anesthesia, but this advantage remains moot.

In sum, the burr hole technique is a safe and effective approach for the implantation of leads on the convexity of the brain. The dubious disadvantage of the limited access is offset by the lesser trauma and reduced risk for the patient. It also appears that lead migration is not an issue in this approach.

References

Canavero S, Bonicalzi V, Castellano G, et al. Painful supernumerary phantom arm following motor cortex stimulation for central poststroke pain. Case report. J Neurosurg 1999; 91: 121-123.

Meyerson BA, Lindblom U, Linderoth B, et al. Motor cortex stimulation as treatment of trigeminal neuropathic pain. Acta Neurochir (Wien) 1993; Suppl 58: 150-153.

Rasche D, Ruppolt M, Stippich C, et al. Motor cortex stimulation for long-term relief of chronic neuropathic pain: a ten year experience. Pain 2006; 121: 43-52.

Tronnier VM, Rasche D. Epidural and subdural stimulation. Handb Clin Neurol 2013; 116: 343-351.

Tsubokawa T, Katayama Y, Yamamoto T, et al. Chronic motor cortex stimulation for the treatment of central pain. Acta Neurochirur (Wien) 1991; Suppl 52: 137-139.

Jean Paul Nguyen, Jean Pascal Lefaucheur

5 Implantation: Flap and Subdural Lead Placement

Implanted electrodes used in reported studies have generally been Resume (Medtronic) or Lamitrode (ANS) stimulating strips, both quadripolar electrode arrays (each contact 5 mm in diameter; inter-contact distance center-to-center 1 cm); eight-contact paddles have been used in one failed trial(NCT00122915). Two strips can be positioned in parallel for wider coverage. The patient either lies down supine (Nguyen et al 1999, 2011) or in lateral decubitus (Park Bench) (Pirotte et al 2009) allowing horizontal orientation of the operative field and easy access to the contralateral limbs under the table.

5.1 Reference Technique

The first phase of the operation consists of identifying the CS on axial sections (Fig.5.1A-B), then plotting a trajectory starting at the CS in the zone corresponding to representation of the upper limb. This zone can be identified by the classical Ω shape (see Chapter 1) of the CS, or with reference to the posterior part of the superior frontal sulcus responsible for this particular shape of the CS. The trajectory entry point is defined so that the trajectory is *perpendicular* to the brain surface (Fig.5.1C); as explained elsewhere in this volume, many others opt for a *parallel* positioning and *results are similar with the two approaches*. A view perpendicular to the trajectory (*"probe eye view" mode*) is then selected to visualize all of the central region in order to more precisely choose the target according to cortical somatotopy. For example, in order to target the area of representation of the face, the target must be placed more laterally, in the posterior part of the inferior frontal sulcus (Fig.5.1D). Similarly, the area of representation of the lower limb is targeted by placing the target between the superior frontal sulcus and the midline.

The second phase of the operation consists of performing a circular craniotomy, about 4 cm (in other authors'experience up to 7 cm) in diameter (length of the quadripolar lead) centered around the target point chosen at the previous step. It is important to ensure at each step that the craniotomy is precisely centered around the target point (Fig.5.2).

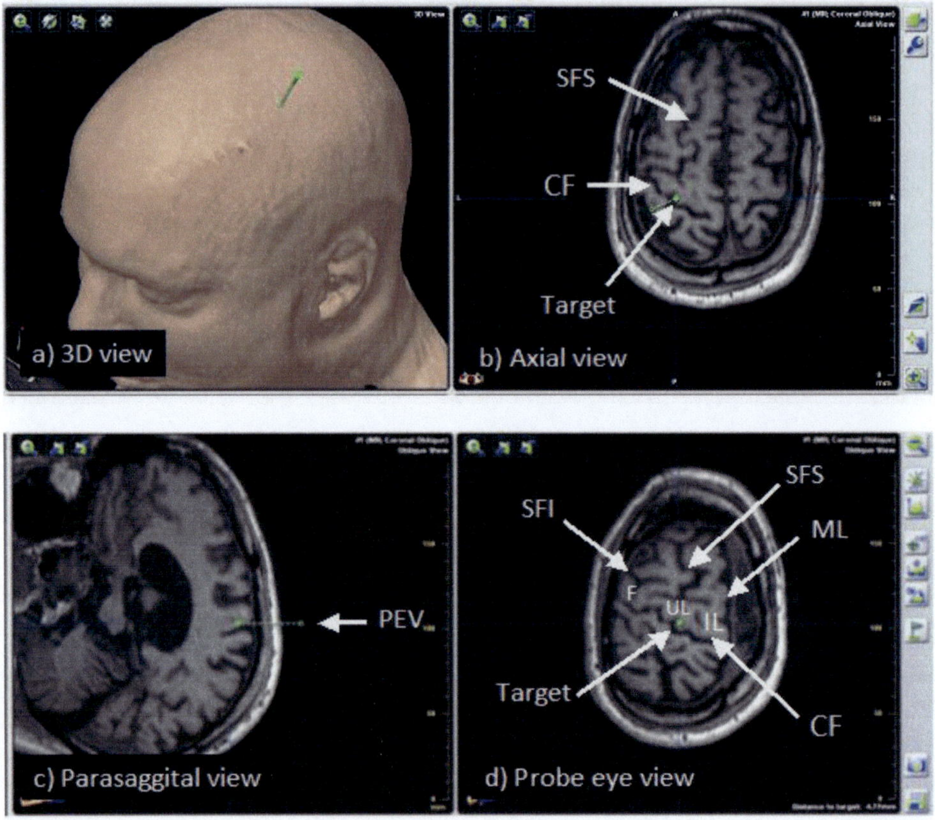

Fig. 5.1: Neuronavigation (Brainlab®). The first step consists of localizing the central sulcus (CS) on an axial scan (b). The first target consists of the zone of representation of the upper limb situated posteriorly to the posterior part of the superior frontal sulcus (SFS). The Probe Eye View (PEV fig. c and d) then allows easy identification of the various structures of the central region: CS: central sulcus, SFS: superior frontal sulcus, IFS: inferior frontal sulcus, ML: midline. The various functional zones of the motor cortex can be delineated in the axis of the trajectory (PEV). F: face, UL: upper limb, LL: lower limb.

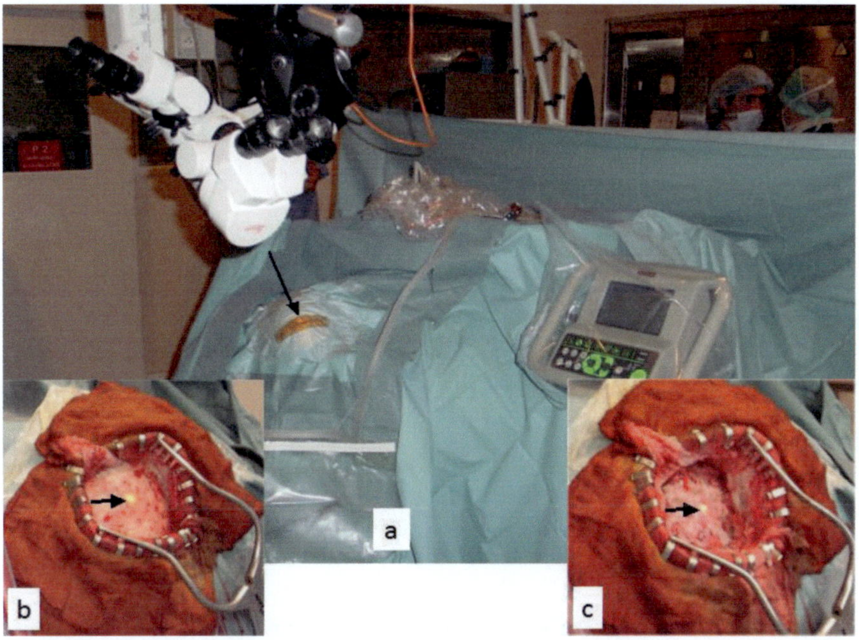

Fig. 5.2: Neuronavigation (Surgiscope®). The previously determined target (Fig. 1) is represented by a laser beam (black arrow Fig. a). After performing the skin incision (Fig. b) and craniotomy (Fig. c), it is important to check that the craniotomy remains centered around the target (black arrow).

The third phase corresponds to intraoperative electrophysiological testing. Electrophysiological testing can be performed with a grid (comprising 16 electrodes in this case) or a quadripolar lead, which will then be used for chronic stimulation (Fig.5.3). The disadvantage of this second option is that the electrodes must be moved to different positions to ensure electrophysiological testing of all of the zone exposed by the craniotomy. We use classical self-retaining retractors to temporarily maintain the electrodes on the dural surface. M1 can be localized indirectly by studying the SSEPs obtained after stimulation of the median nerve in the wrist. Inversion of the N20/P20 potential indicates the position of the CS (Fig.5.4). Motor evoked potentials (Chapter 3) can be used to localize the zone of M1 corresponding to representation of the upper limb or face, as responses to cortical stimulation are recorded in the first interosseous space of the hand (Fig.5.4A) or in the labial commissure. Localization of the zone corresponding to the lower limb is more difficult, but, in a fairly large number of cases, this zone sometimes largely overlaps the superior part of the hemispheric convexity and can be investigated as described above. We initially used repeated stimulation to obtain MEPs (Fig.5.5C), which had the advantage of evoking muscle contractions that are clearly visible (Fig.5.5A-B) or recordable under classical general anesthesia (Fig.5.5C). However, this approach was associated with a risk of inducing seizures, as the amplitude of the response progressively increased during stimulation (Fig.5.5C). We currently prefer single-impulse stimulation (Fig.5.4E). In order to reduce the intensity of stimulation required to obtain MEPs, anesthesia is lightened by using BIS monitoring (Conte et al 2013) (Fig.5.5D).

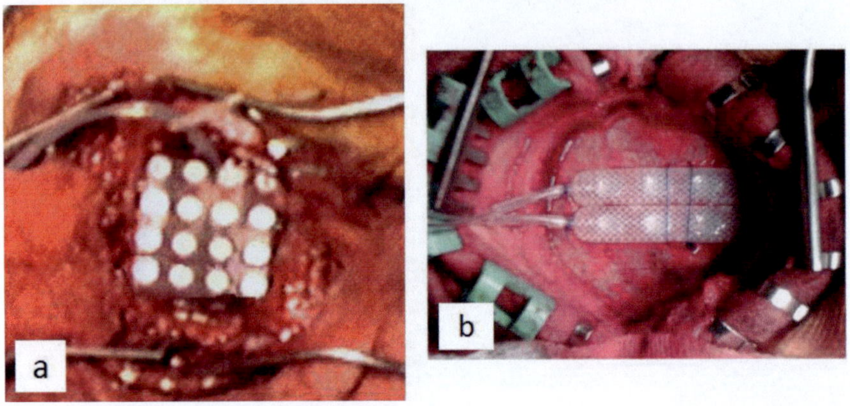

Fig. 5.3: Intraoperative electrophysiological testing. This study can be performed by using a grid (comprising 16 electrodes in this case) (Fig. a) placed on the dura mater or Resume leads, which will then be used for chronic stimulation (Fig. b). In this case, the electrode positions must be changed to test all of the exposed dural surface.

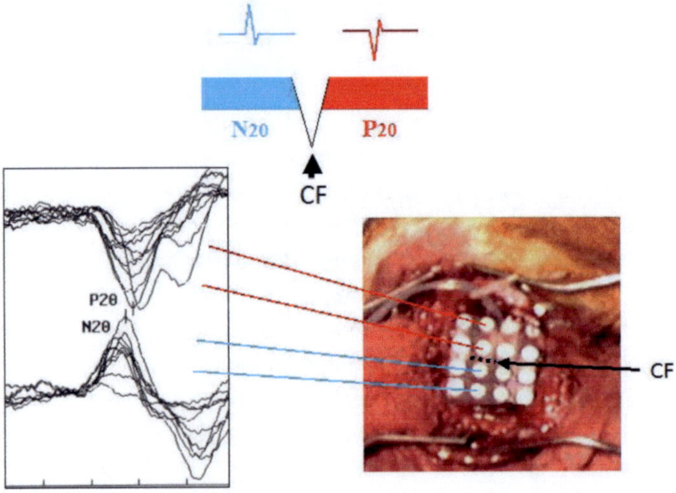

Fig. 5.4: Somatosensory evoked potentials. The signal evoked by stimulation of the median nerve in the wrist is recorded (after about 20 milliseconds) on all electrodes of the grid. The negative P20 potentials are recorded on electrodes placed anteriorly to the central sulcus (dotted line on the right-hand Fig.) and the positive N20 potentials are recorded on electrodes situated posteriorly to the central sulcus, which confirms the position of the central sulcus.

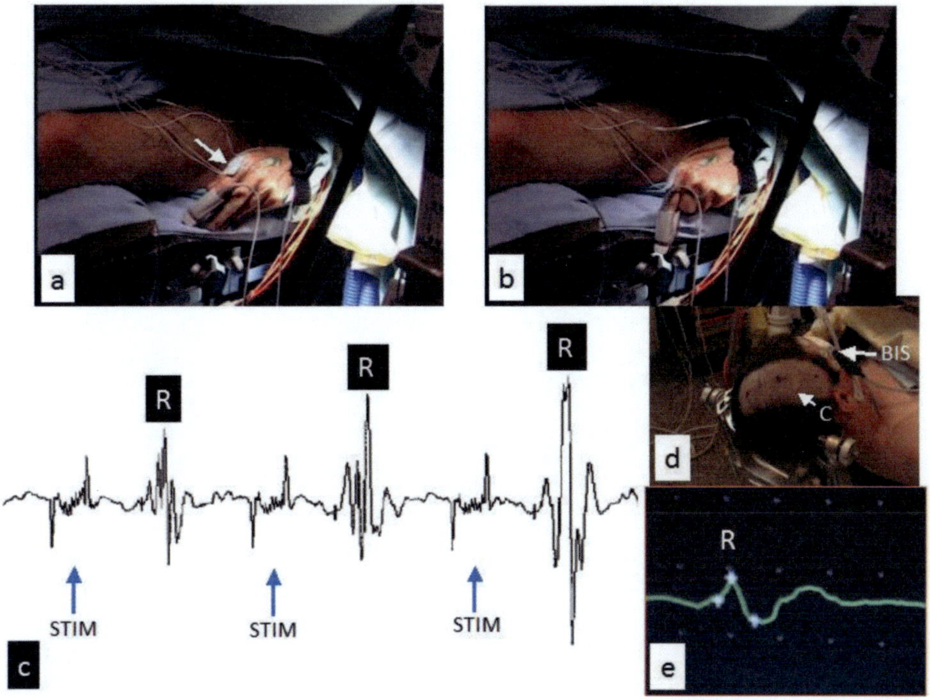

Fig. 5.5: Motor evoked potentials. Stimulation of electrodes placed anteriorly to the central sulcus induces motor responses, which confirm the position of the motor cortex. Motor responses can be observed clinically (Fig.s a and b) in response to repeated stimulation (Fig. c). In this case, stimulation at 16 Hertz (STIM) induces motor responses whose amplitude increases progressively with stimulation (R). A high stimulation intensity facilitates clinically visible motor responses (Fig. b), but is associated with a risk of seizures. We currently prefer to use single-impulse stimulation, which is not associated with any risk of seizures, but which usually does not induce a clinically visible response. The response must then be recorded (R Fig. e) and the depth of general anaesthesia must be lightened. Management of the depth of general anaesthesia is facilitated by the use of BIS monitoring. The EEG signal recording electrode is placed on the patient's forehead (B Fig.s d). Figure d also indicates the limits of the craniotomy (c).

No stimulation leads specifically designed for cortical stimulation are available at the present time. By analogy with spinal cord stimulation, which is also epidural, we use the same Resume leads (Medtronic, Minneapolis, USA) (Fig.5.3B). Other leads from other manufacturers are also adequate.

We decided to place stimulation leads perpendicularly to the CS, essentially to compensate for any placement errors that could be related to parallax error, as the sulci and fissures of the central region are easily recognized on relatively deep sections, but a parallax error may be observed on the surface (Nguyen et al 1999). On the other hand, by allowing stimulation on both sides of the CS, these leads can be used to stimulate the part of M1 situated in the anterior bank of the CS. The work by

Holsheimer et al (2007) suggested that the best combination consisted of placing the cathode (negative pole) just anteriorly to the CS and the anode (positive pole) just posteriorly to the CS (Fig.5.6A).

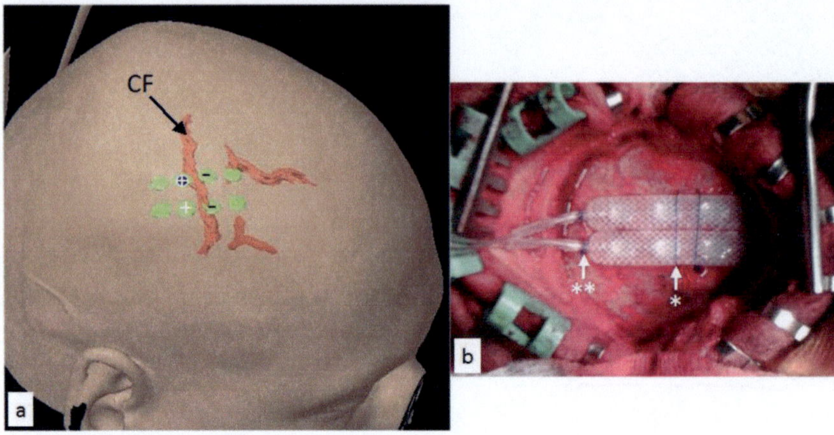

Fig. 5.6: Lead positions. We use two Resume 4-electrode leads placed in parallel and perpendicular to the axis of the central sulcus (CS). The optimal stimulation parameters consist of placing the cathodes (negative poles) anteriorly to the central sulcus (CS) and the anodes posteriorly to the central sulcus (Fig. a). Leads are sutured to the dura mater at 2 levels (Fig. b). A first suture comprises the two leads to limit lateral movements (*). The zone of connection of the lead with the extension is anchored by a second suture in order to limit anteroposterior movements (**).

The leads are then sutured to the dura mater (Fig.5.6B). We try to stabilize the anterior extremity of the leads by pushing them slightly underneath the edges of the craniotomy and the leads are anchored by a suture comprising the two leads, which limits the risk of lateral displacement. To avoid displacement along the long axis of the leads, the leads are sutured to the extension connector. Very careful hemostasis is highly recommended for avoiding epidural infectious or hemorrhagic complications. Full superficial denervation of the dura by bipolar coagulation of its surface may reduce the local (cranial) pain described by some patients when switching the stimulation on. The electrode must be fixed to the dura with very tight sutures to minimize the space between the electrode and the dura, in which scar tissue can develop and thereby increase the impedance of the stimulation and require higher voltage. One way to fix the electrode is by means of a single 3-0 silk suture every 5 mm, with 2 sutures bridging the electrode in order to maintain it against the dura. Some authors drill a groove at the posterior margin of the bone flap, to avoid crushing the wires after bone flat fixation to the skull. Extension wires are then tunneled under the skin, passing behind the ear and then in the neck and are then connected to the stimulator (Implanted Pulse Generator, IPG) placed subcutaneously in the pectoral region subclaveraly. A drain is occasionally inserted in the epidural space or in the subcutaneous space (Pirotte et al 2009). The skin is closed with separated 2-0 Dermalon sutures. Staples are used for skin closure, but attention must be lent not to damage the wires. It must be noted that, while for several applications (e.g. Parkinson's disease) a one-shot lead+IPG implantation is the norm, several authors only implant the IPG after a test period (few days to 2-4 weeks), e.g. in chronic pain conditions. In this case, the lead is connected subcutaneously in the retromastoid region (and not inferiorly in the soft tissues of the neck, as the connector may break or erode through the skin with time) to a temporary cable that exits through the skin behind the ear (by way of a small incision) and is then plugged into an external stimulator. Whatever the results of the test period, the temporary cable exiting through the skin is cut in order to allow the skin hole to heal properly (Pirotte et al 2009).

A postoperative CT scan is mandatory to check the exact lead position by fusing CT images with preoperative MRI images and evince postoperative hemorrhage.

5.2 Neuronavigated rTMS-guided Technique

rTMS can guide lead positioning by evincing the cortical area that affords the best clinical outcome. When rTMS induces e.g. marked pain relief, neuronavigated rTMS can be used to check the exact site of stimulation and MEPs can also be used to check that this site corresponds to M1 (Fig.5.5) and whether or not the target corresponds to the somatotopic distribution. The Nexstim neuronavigated rTMS system allows very precise localization (Ruohonen and Karhu 2010). The central region can be identified by using the "peeling" function. This function provides brain images corresponding to layers parallel to the cortical surface (Fig.5.7A-B), thereby minimizing parallax errors, while facilitating identification of the various sulci and fissures of the region (Fig.5.7B-D). Neuronavigated rTMS therefore allows precise localization of the effective target (the upper limb M1 area is shown in Fig.5.7A). This same target is easy to identify (Fig.5.7D), although the "peeling" function is not yet available on intraoperative neuronavigation systems. Intraoperative electrophysiological testing is no longer necessary, as MEPs have already been recorded during neuronavigated rTMS sessions (Fig.5.5). The procedure is therefore easier to perform and much more reliable, as the target has been precisely determined prior to the operation.

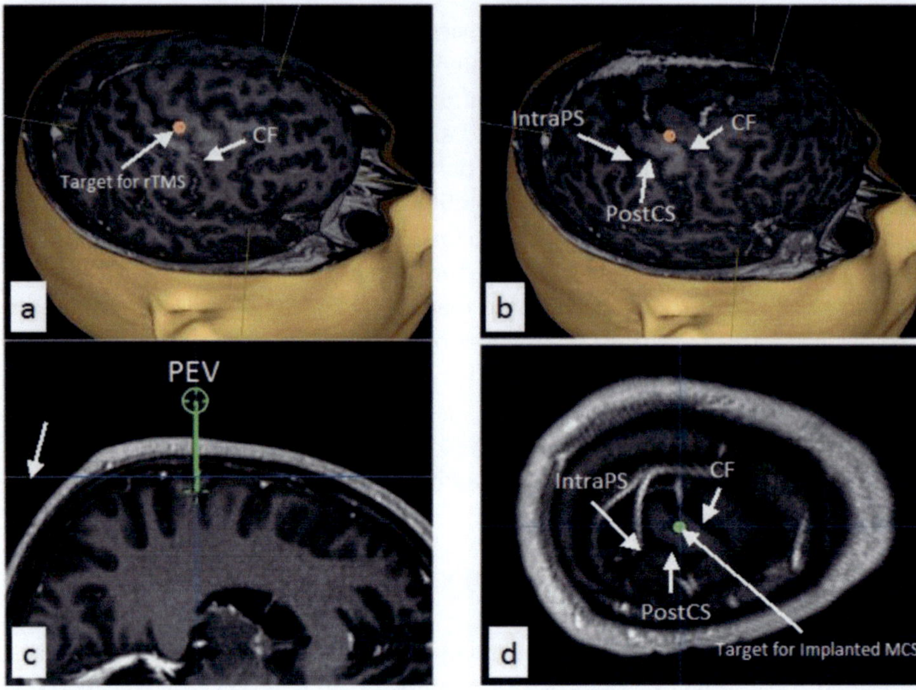

Fig. 5.7: Value of neuronavigated rTMS. Figures a and b show the position of the stimulation target shown to be effective on rTMS. It is situated just anteriorly to the central sulcus (CS Fig. a). Figure b: the same target is represented on the cortical surface. The postcentral sulcus (PostCS) and the intraparietal sulcus (Intra PS) can be easily identified. Figures c and d show the position of the target on neuronavigation. On Figure c, the arrow indicates the level of the section shown on Figure d. This Figure illustrates practically the same structures as those visible on Figure b. The target is placed slightly posteriorly to the central sulcus, just anteriorly to the intraparietal sulcus (Intra PS). Parallax errors can be minimized by carefully comparing neuronavigated rTMS data and intraoperative neuronavigation data.

5.3 Subdural Positioning

Some authors have proposed implanting leads in the subdural space, especially to treat pain in the lower limbs. The main disadvantage is that this is a relatively invasive technique with, in particular, a risk of injury to veins of the central region during positioning of leads on the medial surface of the hemisphere. It is also practically impossible to anchor the lead in a precisely determined position, which is associated with a risk of loss of efficacy due to lead displacement. The main publications describing this technique have reported disappointing results (e.g. Saitoh and Hosomi 2009). There may be a place for subdural lead placement in case of cerebral atrophy. However, results of ICS for Parkinson Disease and stroke rehabilitation clearly show that the lower limbs can be affected by stimulating the cortex outside the expected projection from Penfield's homunculus (see Chapters 10 and 12).

Some authors have recommended stimulating M1 directly by placing the electrode dead on the surface of the anterior bank of the CS. CS veins have been used as landmarks during subdural approaches, but, being sometimes located deep in the CS, cannot be identified by examining only the cortical surface. More relevant, large bridging veins sometimes interfere with implantation of the lead and adhesion may occur due to subarachnoid hemorrhage; dissection of the CS also involves the risk of developing new neurological deficits due to brain damage or vein obstruction. For upper limb and/or face pain, the arachnoid membrane of the CS must be carefully dissected and the vessels within it must be freed with a microsurgical procedure to expose the hidden lateral walls of the precentral and postcentral gyri. Since the paddle is too stiff to be placed within the CS, it must be trimmed off (Fig. 5.8). This approach is feasible only in patients with severe motor weakness or lack of function. Test stimulation of M1 within the CS is more effective in most cases than is subdural stimulation on the cerebral surface, but long-term clinical results are not on a par with extradural ICS. At the end of surgery, the lead extension is fixed to the dura or the border of the burr hole with a silk suture to prevent dislocation. However, migration of the electrodes seems to be more of a problem with a subdural than an extradural approach. A meticulous, watertight dural closure is mandatory to minimize the risk of cerebrospinal fluid leakage (Saitoh and Hosomi 2009). Stimulation by intradural electrodes is also associated with a high risk of seizures (Bezard et al 1999). Again, lead placement in the subdural space could be indicated in patients with cerebral atrophy who are markedly improved by rTMS.

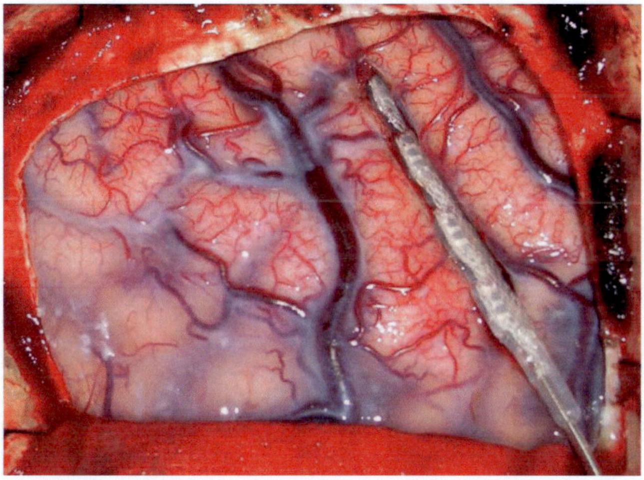

Fig. 5.8: Subdural lead placement. The quadripolar lead is inserted within the central sulcus after dissection of the arachnoid (From Saitoh and Hosomi 2009)

A so-called interdural approach has been proposed: one or two dural strips, similar in size and shape to the actual strip electrode(s) are resected overlying the targeted area. The strip electrodes are then positioned in place of the resected dural strips, in a patchlike fashion and sutured to the edges of the dura. Finally the entire dural flap is reversed to its original position and sutured with many stitches back to the edges of the surrounding dura (Sakas et al 2011). It is not clear what the (supposed) advantages should be.

In sum, lead implantation procedure has become simpler with the use of neuronavigated rTMS, as intraoperative electrophysiological testing is no longer required. It has also become more precise and more effective because the precise stimulation target can be predetermined by rTMS.

References

Bezard E, Boraud T, Nguyen JP, et al. Cortical stimulation and epileptic seizure: a study of the potential risk in primates. Neurosurgery 1999; 45: 364-350.

Conte V, L'Acqua C, Rotelli S, et al. Bispectral index during asleep-awake craniotomies. J Neurosurg Anesthesiol. 2013; 25: 279-284.

Holsheimer J, Nguyen JP, Lefaucheur JP, et al. Cathodal, anodal or bifocal stimulation of the motor cortex in the management of chronic pain ? Acta Neurochir Suppl. 2007 ; 97: 57-66.

Nguyen JP, Lefaucheur JP, Decq P, et al. Chronic motor cortex stimulation in the treatment of central and neuropathic pain. Correlations between clinical, electrophysiological and anatomical data. Pain 1999; 82: 245-251.

Nguyen JP, Nizard J, Keravel Y, et al. Invasive brain stimulation for the treatment of neuropathic pain. Nat Rev Neurol. 2011; 7: 699-709.

Pirotte BJM, Voordecker P, Levivier M, et al. Principles of surgical implantation and complications avoidance. In: Canavero S (ed) Textbook of therapeutic cortical stimulation. New York: Nova Science, 2009, pp 33-44

Ruohonen J and Karhu J. Navigated transcranial magnetic stimulation. Neurophysiol Clin. 2010; 40: 7-17.

Saitoh Y, Hosomi K. From localization to surgical implantation. In: Canavero S (ed) Textbook of therapeutic cortical stimulation. New York: Nova Science, 2009, pp 17-32

Sakas DE, Flaskas TN, Panourias IG, et al. Bifocal cortical electrical stimulation for pain by interdural implantation of the electrode. J Neurosurg 2011; 114:180-5.

Jeffrey E. Arle, Jay L. Shils

6 Programming

Various factors make ICS programming a very complex task: First, there are numerous possible combinations of parameters; Second, no sensory, motor, or other signs are generally produced during subthreshold stimulation; Third, for several conditions, clinical effects usually become noticeable several days beyond the time of stimulation parameter changes: benefit is delayed when the stimulator is switched "on" and plasticity-driven after-effects are prolonged when the stimulator is switched "off." This is the reason why it is impractical and inefficient to assess the possible effects that may be produced by the stimulation of the cortex intraoperatively. Conversely, in other neuromodulation techniques, programming can be guided by the clinical effects that are produced as soon as the stimulator is switched "on," like paresthesias in the painful limb after spinal cord stimulation or tremor arrest after thalamic or subthalamic nucleus stimulation (Arle and Shils 2011). Thus, it can take weeks to determine whether ICS is efficacious for the various conditions for which it is applied. Also in the case of pain, analgesia from intraoperative stimulation can sometimes be prolonged. A few rare cases of rapid clinical response (e.g. action tremor) are on record (Nguyen et al 1998).

Stimulation intensity appears to be the most difficult factor to determine. This parameter is all the more difficult to determine in that the only relevant value is the output current of the lead electrodes expressed in milliamperes (mA). According to our initial results, an intensity of about 2 mA was necessary and sufficient to effectively stimulate M1 and obtain a clinical effect. The first stimulators (Itrel 3, Synergy) did not directly indicate the values of the output current (I). Only the voltage (V) could be selected allowing deduction of the output current by calculating the impedance of the system (R) (V=RI). More recent stimulators (e.g. Prime Advanced, Restore) now directly indicate the output current. The output current values must be adjusted according to the distance between the electrode and the cortex. Higher intensity stimulation is obviously required in the presence of cerebral atrophy.

A trial period before permanent implantation may increase the risk of device infection at cortical level, so that, whenever possible, the whole ICS system is frequently implanted in a single session: this certainly applies to all conditions discussed in this volume, with the exception of pain, in which most authors test the results via temporary extensions. After implantation, the patient is kept in hospital for 1 week to ensure proper healing of the incision. During this time, several stimulation parameters are screened. At discharge, the stimulator can be switched "on."

Chronic stimulation parameters (pulse width: 60-180 µs; frequency: 20-60 Hz; voltage: 1-4 V) largely differ from those applied for intraoperative mapping. In particular, intensities used for bipolar chronic stimulation are far below motor threshold, whereas intraoperative motor mapping obviously requires suprathreshold intensities. Some authors believe that the contact that is the intraoperative "best anode"(+) should be selected as the negative electrode (cathode) for chronic stimulation (see chapter 5): this suggestion is based on a very small sample of patients, and as of yet there has been no independent replication. Although the stimulation of the nervous tissue generally occurs in the vicinity of the cathode, this is not true in M1 ICS: due to the large size of the electrode and different orientations of the cortical nerve fibers (parallel and perpendicular to the laminae), various populations of axons can be activated under the cathode and anode making bipolar stimulation bifocal, i.e. with simultaneous activation. Bifocal also means that the neural activity evoked near the cathode may affect activity near the anode and viceversa via intracortical connections. In other words, despite the large center-to-center distance of the cathode and the anode (=/>1 cm), some overlap of the corresponding stimulus-evoked fields is still present, which means that the electrical fields in the cortex below the cathode and the anode are different from real monopolar fields. Therefore, selecting more distant contacts for chronic stimulation does not increase the volume of cortical activation as previously suggested, but results in a more bifocal stimulation, activating more distinct neural pathways. Similarly, increasing stimulation intensity does not improve ICS efficacy that likely relates to fiber activation in superficial cortical layers, but recruits additional neural circuits that originate in deeper cortical layers.

Developments in stimulator and electrode designs have increased programming options. Instead of just 4 contacts and the ability to set a single contact configuration and electrical parameter configuration, new devices allow for a single program to contain multiple contact configurations with differing electrical parameters for each configuration.

While the program is running, each configuration is activated in a sequence specific to the manufacturer. These multiple configurations are extremely beneficial in allowing for the targeting of specific pain regions and even by adding multi-pulse patterns for a single region. Here we will focus on our experience with 23 patients with both pain and movement disorders using M1 ICS as treatment.

Programming of our pain patients includes a wide range of stimulation parameters with voltage varying from 2.2 volts up to 7.1V when using constant voltage devices and from 3 mA up to 17 mA when using constant current devices, pulse width varying from 120 µs up to 330 µs, and frequency varying from 50 Hz up to 130 Hz. This can be contrasted with other researcher groups who begin from 0.5V up to 10V, from 120 µs up to 450 µs and from 1Hz up to 130 Hz. All of our patients start with monopolar settings, but often bipolar settings are used with more anodal contacts. Most of the patients implanted with the newer constant current systems (Precisions Plus neural stimulator, Boston Scientific, Valencia, CA) have more than one program running. Prior to this all patients were implanted with the Medtronic quadripolar Resume lead and the Itrel II IPG (Medtronic, Minneapolis, MN). However, Itrel II and Synergy

(Medtronic) do not allow monopolar stimulation with the metal case of IPG as the distant indifferent electrode.

Initial patient programming typically begins within 24 hours of electrode implantation. Monopolar stimulation is used to evaluate all contacts using a stimulation rate of 210μs and a stimulation frequency of 130 Hz. The voltage is slowly raised to 4.0V or 8.0 mA (depending upon the device used) specifically looking for adverse motor movements and/or sensory changes. Additionally the patient state is evaluated with the primary concern being the possible generation of seizure activity during this evaluation (Henderson et al 2010). To date, we have had three seizures generated during the programming phase out of 23 patients, none of which occurred at the initial programming session. In the first patient, a focal motor seizure may have occurred 2 days after initial programming. This event was unwitnessed by medical personnel, yet the description fit well with the characteristics of this type of seizure. For this particular patient, a seizure was also generated during M1 mapping in the operating room. Since this time, all M1 ICS patients, where a seizure occurred during intraoperative mapping, are kept below 2.5 volts or 5 mA for the first two weeks post surgery. However, none of our patients were put on anti-epileptic medications, unlike other authors. The second programming seizure occurred at the 18 month follow-up in a post-stroke pain patient: a seizure was generated while raising the stimulator voltage from 4.0V up to 4.3V. Thereafter, voltage has been kept below 4.0V and no further seizure activity has been noted. The seizure lasted about 15 seconds. The patient was kept in the hospital overnight and no seizures have occurred since that time. In the third patient, a focal motor seizure, in the face region, was generated while increasing the amplitude of one of three configurations to 13 mA. This was at the 1 year follow-up. The seizure stopped within 3 seconds of reducing the stimulation. There was no electrographic recording during this particular event, yet the patient's description of a confused state after the event appeared to be more seizure-like than a pure motor event. The reason for the increase in this patient was due to a loss of benefit over time. Additionally this patient was programmed with three electrode combination and parameter sequences. Recently, we have had a patient develop what appeared to be a seizure disorder, with focal motor seizures and potentially more generalized events. However, despite multiple recording periods, no electrographic seizures have been recorded and this may turn out to be a unique development of pseudoseizures as the evaluation is ongoing.

In all cases of M1 ICS for pain, we have had to modify the programming settings. In some, the only modification was increasing the stimulation amplitude over time, while in other cases we have had to add multiple configurations. We initially choose new configurations based on the monopolar evaluation. Before adding multiple configurations, frequency and pulse width are adjusted for the single configuration. Pulse width is slowly increased looking for changes in effect. The most common change that we see is the recruitment of more "areas". Frequency changes tend to shift the location of the stimulation effect without causing an increased sensation over the initial stimulated region. This is very helpful if we are close to the area of pain, but also close to a point where the stimulation is painful. When adding new configurations, the goal is to either bring in new regions or to modulate the pulse pattern at a single region. Modulation of a region is done by keeping the same electrode combinations, but modifying the electrical parameters. Presently, no device allows the setting of the time interval between each configuration, so they all run sequentially with a very short interval between each configuration. This is ineffectual outside of cases concerning pain, since most other indication effects grow over time, and the rapid flipping of parameters runs the real risk of overlooking useful combinations.

For initial programming of movement disorder patients each contact is tested in a fashion similar to the pain cases, yet the lead center contacts are activated initially with an amplitude at 3mA. This is chosen based on the OR mapping which makes sure that the electrode is centered over the hand and arm region. If the patient feels for whatever reason that they cannot tolerate these settings, then more lateral contacts are added while removing the contacts furthest from the new lateral contact. In our experience two contacts are able to be activated at the initial programming session.

It is here useful to mention the approaches taken by other authors. According to Pirotte for example (Pirotte et al 2009), M1ICS induces pain relief within 10-15 minutes of the start of stimulation and lasting 15-120 minutes after the stimulation is switched off. Since in the first 3 days after implantation the pain often disappears or is strongly attenuated by general anesthesia, these authors usually wait for 3 days before starting the test run (i.e. patients are scheduled for surgery on Thursday, stay 24 hours in the intensive care unit and rest in their room during the weekend until Monday morning, when stimulation begins) or at least wait until the pain has returned to its disabling level. Some patients report that pain relief can remain stable for more than 24 hours, if the stimulation period is longer than 4 hours (so-called after-effect). Other patients describe that severe pain recurs when they switch the stimulation off for more than 2 days. The goal of the test period is to test all parameters during a short period of time, in order to decrease the risk of infection due to the presence of transcutaneous wires. Pain intensity is measured using a visual analog scale (VAS) by specially trained nurses or physicians; a pain diary has also to be completed by the patient. During the test, the bipolar combinations for which an analgesic effect has been observed must be re-tested many times in a single-blind (blinded patient) manner in order to exclude a placebo effect. This last step is crucial to consider the test as positive. Indeed, many combinations may appear as "good" only once, without being confirmed at further stimulations. Blinding is attained by covering and shielding the external stimulation device in the area of the lead combinations. Continuous stimulation is used during the test trial, but after IPG implantation, intermittent stimulation is programmed to avoid habituation, at least initially. In practice, a reproducible analgesic effect is often observed within the first 10 days of stimulation. In several cases, the coupling configuration is critical. Some patients mention a transient painful sensation (reported as a painful "click") centered on the craniotomy when stimulation is switched on, probably due to a direct stimulation of the dura. On occasion, stimulation may increase burning or tingling sensations.

A few caveats: 1) neurogenic pain can fluctuate significantly from one day to another; 2) patients tested in a hospital do not behave like at home. Furthermore, pain patients have large expectations that they strongly and very quickly jump to the conclusion that slight variations in pain levels can accurately predict successful outcomes.

Loss of effect after an initial excellent analgesia has been reported by many investigators. Switching from continuous to cyclical stimulation –or viceversa- may restore benefit in some cases within a few hours. Although pulse width and frequency may be increased as follow-up progresses, particularly in cases in which effects dwindle, the efficacy of stimulation changes very little with such incremental increases. On the other hand, some authors find that loss of efficacy may be due to keeping parameter settings constant, suggesting that perhaps longer-term plastic changes eventually catch up with ICS to limit its efficacy (see also Henderson et al 2004). Loss of effect can also be due to extensive fibrosis below and around the contacts: removal thereof may restore benefit (Canavero 2009).

References

Arle J, Shils J. Essential neuromodulation. San Diego : Academic Press, 2011

Canavero S (ed) Textbook of therapeutic cortical stimulation. New York: Nova Science, 2009

Henderson JM, Boongird A, Rosenow JM, et al. Recovery of pain control by intensive reprogramming after loss of benefit from motor cortex stimulation for neuropathic pain._Stereotact Funct Neurosurg. 2004;82(5-6):207-13.

Henderson JM, Heit G, Fisher RS. Recurrent seizures related to motor cortex stimulator programming. Neuromodulation. 2010;13:37-43.

Nguyen JP, Pollin B, Feve A, et al. Improvement of action tremor by chronic cortical stimulation. Mov Disord. 1998;13:84-88

Pirotte BJM, Voordecker P, Levivier M, et al. Principles of surgical implantation and complications avoidance. In: Canavero S (ed) Textbook of therapeutic cortical stimulation. New York: Nova Science, 2009, pp 33-44

Jeffrey E. Arle

7 Complications and Their Avoidance

Implantable cortical stimulation therapeutically is subject to the same risks as any typical surgical procedure, such as infection or other wound healing concerns and hematoma formation. Additional complications (such as seizures) may result, however, from cortical mapping necessary to place electrodes, from anchoring the electrodes (migration, hematoma, or CSF leak), tunneling wires (perforation, infection, erosion, significant tissue damage in the neck and or chest), longevity of the device (wire breakage, IPG fault, or lead migration), or in programming the device itself (seizures, sensory effects). Each of these potential pitfalls will be addressed here with advice as to how they may be avoided.

A comprehensive review of over 800 cases in the literature reveals that the extradural approach is not associated with mortality or disabling morbidity, whereas subdural implantation has been associated with significant subdural hemorrhage resulting in postoperative vegetative state (1 patient) and death (1 patient) (Saitoh and Hosomi 2009). Seizures (19 patients) were experienced, but epilepsy was never induced during follow-up, with 1 exception in the 1990's. Aphasia (1 patient) was also observed due to inadvertent overstimulation during the test period (see ahead). Post operatively, infection remains the most commonly reported reason for failure of a device, requiring either a reoperation or removal of the system. The most common significant programming side effect was seizures, occurring in a reported 17 patients. In particular, since 2008, there were 12 seizures and 11 infections.

In this chapter, I will cover basic complication avoidance and provide surgical management tips which may mitigate eventual complications.

7.1 Complications in Cortical Mapping

The most likely complication during the mapping phase of the surgical procedure is the generation of seizures. In our experience, seizures have occurred in approximately 25% of cases while attempting to delineate the M1 region, although all but one of these involved patients who had a history of seizures. Certain precautions may be taken to mitigate their occurrence and the method of mapping out cortical areas itself can significantly lower seizure risk. We have adopted both locating where the N20 somatosensory potential reverses polarity (the location of the CS) and direct cortical stimulation using a ball probe electrode on the surface of the dura and analyzing EMG responses in the face, arm and hand. The N20 potential may be appreciated and localized using either the implant electrode itself or, perhaps more easily adopted for the purpose, a 4 contact strip electrode typically used for intracranial epilepsy monitoring. Direct stimulation of the dura can be accomplished using a ball probe electrode with a diameter of 2-4mm, referenced to an electrode placed on the ipsilateral forehead. It is very helpful to work with a physiologist for these mapping techniques as the surgeon can concentrate on making sure the field stays clear of fluid and blood and can manipulate the electrodes and their location and contact stability to obtain the best signals. The physiology colleague may concentrate on making sure the system is working correctly, troubleshoot and fix technical problems should they arise in unsterile connections, and make continuous changes to amplitude or other parameters while the surgeon focuses more on localizing and moving the electrode to assess the appropriate orientation of the M1 gyrus and CS. In this way, the surgeon may move the electrode strip around after each N20 measurement while the physiologist calls out where the reversal of the potential polarity arises (i.e between which contacts on the strip the reversal occurs, if any). The surgeon may use a sterile marking pen on the dura to denote where this occurred and then move the strip to a different location and orientation for another measurement. Typically 6-8 assessments are made in this way and a reasonable mapping of the M1 region and CS can be found using the SSEP polarity reversal alone. We add direct stimulation mapping as well, because it can provide a second validation to the N20 map, but it also can clarify areas that may have been questionable with the reversal potential technique. The reversal potential is not always easily discerned and may be too broadly localized within the region making it difficult to place the final implanted electrode with assurance. The dipoles of the N20 and the geometry of the CS do not always correlate. Direct stimulation, however, is the most likely part of the technique to cause seizures. We have found that recording from the 4-contact strip electrode placed now over the dura but extending under the edge of the craniotomy opening and out of the way of the field for mapping can serve as a means of assessing cortical epileptiform activity during this stage. It is important not to leave the ball probe on any one area of stimulation too long as well. There is no single limit on this time-frame but more than 2-3 seconds is probably a good rule of thumb. It is better to use a train of 5 stimulus pattern if possible, because this has been shown to have a lower chance of causing seizures. Typical amplitudes to obtain EMG reliably are between 8 and 20 mA, though increasing up to 25 mA is not unreasonable if no EMG is found (i.e. just to establish that the system is delivering current, there are no technical or noise problems, and that the anesthetic technique is optimal). Consider also that one can stimulate exposed soft tissue such as the temporalis muscle to determine whether the system is delivering current. Mapping the hand region is the most reliable in this setting, having the highest density of representation, though reproducible responses to arm and face regions can usually be obtained with persistence. Finding flank, back, or lower extremities from an extra-dural approach is not reliable. It is useful to plan the craniotomy opening to account for the difference in face location on the M1 surface relative to hand or arm. It is usually significantly more latero-inferior and this can be difficult to reach if the craniotomy opening is not made appropriately, leading the surgeon to conclude erroneously that there is a technical problem or they simply cannot find the face region. Figure 7.1 shows representative cranial openings that can avoid these complicating hurdles. Using a functional MRI obtained pre-operatively (e.g. for hand localization) may help in craniotomy planning, or using historically tried-and-true scalp measurements (Fig.7.1) can be just as reliable in our experience. In line with this, the opening itself is best made to allow for the flat alignment and anchoring of the lead to the dura without compromise. Our experience suggests that a large craniotomy (>6cm in diameter) is not typically necessary, but that up to 5cm in diameter, located appropriately with forethought, is very reasonable for moving the electrode around for the N20 and mapping enough of the M1 orientation with the ball probe, as well as for aligning and anchoring the lead adequately (discussed further below). Of course, as outlined elsewhere (chapters 4-5), the electrophysiology part can be skipped and burr holes have proven equally effective; also, one can make a single bur hole and do some mapping with a strip electrode placed through the bur hole in various directions. Finally, should a seizure occur during mapping, it is helpful to have readily available a source of iced saline to irrigate the dura with. This cooling can be useful in terminating the seizure activity (recall that the patient is already under general anesthesia with a TIVA technique - usually Propofol). Avoiding the addition of medication which may compromise mapping is helpful, though if more than one seizure is generated during the mapping process, it is probably best to abort the mapping and decide either to place the electrode using the extant information, or simply to abort the entire procedure. One or two seizures during mapping under anesthesia is not associated with causing any future seizure disorder, within bounds of our accumulated current knowledge.

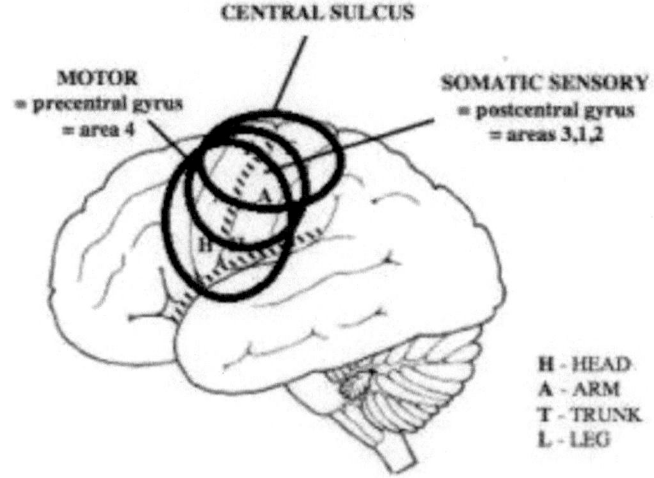

Fig. 7.1: Schema showing examples of craniotomy locations in order to map, for example, arm and flank (more superiorly) versus face (inferior). Pre-planning these adjustments will result in a smaller but adequate craniotomy opening, adequately allowing for manipulation of the electrode during mapping procedures and securing the electrode once final positioning is determined.

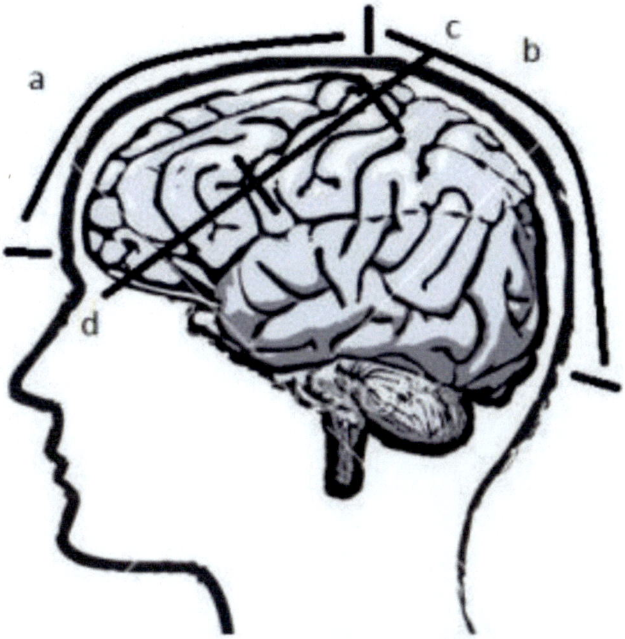

Fig. 7.2: Schema showing basic landmarks for reliably determining the general orientation of the central sulcus. One measures from the nasion to inion, finds the midpoint (vertical line at the top of the head in Figure so that a=b), and then follows a line extending from approximately two centimeters posterior from this midpoint (ie point c) to just posterior to the lateral canthus (point d). Making use of this information, with or without adjuvant functional imaging or physiology, is helpful and may be the only available means of planning the craniotomy if adjuvant procedures fail, which, of course, can happen.

7.2 Complications in Snchoring

As with most neuromodulation devices involving electrodes (Arle and Shils 2011), it is important to minimize the possibility of lead migration by using appropriate anchoring techniques and also perforating the tiny metallic contacts and wires into the electrode. The concepts of 'strain relief' and not kinking the insulation around the wires with sutures are both significant. Figure 7.3 shows typical orientations for our leads secured to the dura, the route of the proximal part of the wire on the dura providing strain relief, and the exit through the appropriately placed bur hole inferiorly and posteriorly, allowing the typical further route of the wire to the IPG to be relatively unimpeded. *All leads are surrounded by fibrosis entirely within weeks and the lead (a paddle-type lead) will not ever move once that happens.* As with epidural spinal cord stimulation lead placement, this scar formation is sufficient at about 6 weeks post-op.

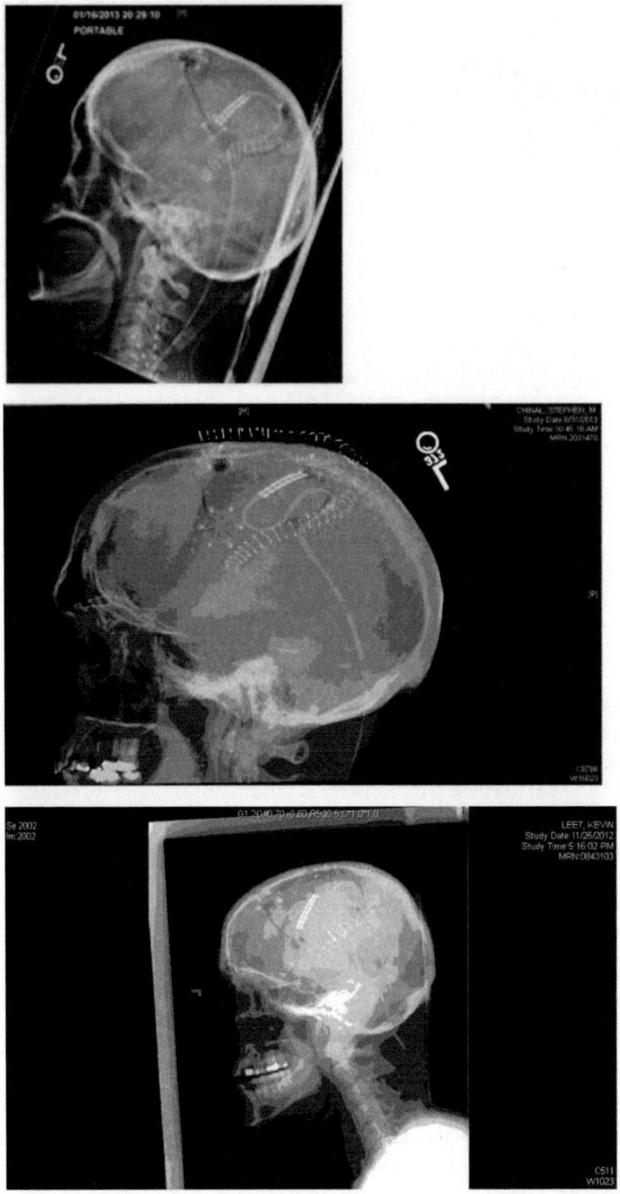

Fig. 7.3: Three representative MCS post-operative lateral skull films that show the size and location of the craniotomy, the lead orientation, the course of the wire as it makes its way to the bur hole and then the exiting of the wire from the bur hole toward the subclavicular region and IPG.

Until then, however, it is important to keep the lead as flat to the dural surface as possible to prevent significant fibrosis or highly non-linear fibrosis occurring between the lead and the dura. A few well-placed 4-0 Neurolon sutures, taking care not to damage the wires within the silicone are usually adequate to accomplish this. Damage to the wires within the lead should be carefully avoided when placing these sutures. Some electrodes have mesh within the silicone which makes them more resilient to anchoring; some leads have more room around their edges to accept a stitch. Where there is little room or no mesh, one must be particularly vigilant. Placing a piece of dry gelfoam between the bone flap and the lead during closure is useful as well, both to minimize bleeding, and thus fibrosis, and to hold the lead well against the dura. Migration of these leads early (within 6 weeks of surgery) has been non-existent in our experience if the lead is sutured to the dura and the wire is coiled around the dura before exiting the bur hole and tunneled. A suture or two may be helpful in directing the course of the wire as it coils on the dura before exiting the bur hole. All of these securing sutures should be made in the outer layer of dura only to avoid creating CSF leakage. The use of a larger grid or two paddle leads should be constrained in the same fashion and we have also had no migration or breakage issues in those cases. One or two wires may exit through the same bur hole.

7.3 Complications in Tunneling and IPG Placement

Although passing device components (shunt tubing, wires) from the skull region to the subclavicular space or elsewhere has been performed for decades with relative safety and reliability, there are potential pitfalls to be avoided. The main worry is that there will be inadvertent damage to tissues in the posterior or lateral neck, or that the tunneler will pass under the clavicle into the lung or subclavian vessels. Any and all of these complications have no doubt occurred somewhere, but they seem to be very rare. Such complications are unlikely to be reported in the literature. Several tips to keep in mind when tunneling are given below.

- Different tunnelers have different stiffness, sharpness, and ability to be manipulated by the way they are designed to be held. Be aware of these constraints before starting to tunnel. Some tunneler handles may loosen when they need to be secure and help create leverage.
- It is strongly advised to bend the tunneler, perhaps even more than seems appropriate, before tunneling. It is much easier to steer and manipulate the tip of the tunneler when under the skin if it is already bent (generally upwards relative to the direction of passage) than if one has to bend it after it is half or 3/4ths to its target.
- If the tunneler is bent (as suggested) it is then even more important to maintain vigilance in preventing the tip from piercing the skin before reaching the target.
- Keeping the tip bent up is helpful in avoiding other tissue damage and in avoiding allowing the tip to pass inadvertently below the clavicle potentially damaging the lung or subclavian vessels. However, it is also important to keep the tip from

turning too far right or left as it is being passed – a lack of attention in this regard may bring damage to nearby tissues in the neck.
- Finally, it is not too uncommon for there to be venous bleeding from passage of the tunneler, somewhere along the track. First, determine if it is from the edge of where the tunneler entered or is accessible to being cauterized with the bipolar. If not, then it is imperative that pressure be uniformly applied along the tunnel track, checking periodically to see if bleeding has stopped. Usually this takes at least 5 minutes of direct pressure. Avoiding potentially life-threatening hematoma formation in this manner is obviously very important. In our experience, this bleeding is always venous in origin and while sometimes brisk, always stops with adequate attention to pressure and time.

Most IPG's are going to be placed in the subclavicular region. Several important details should be kept in mind when using this area in order to minimize complications.
- The pocket should be made medial to the deltopectoral groove, approximately two finger-breadths below and parallel to the clavicle, and to a depth at or just anterior to the pectoralis fascia.
- A discussion should always take place pre-operatively, especially with female patients, as to whether placement in the axillary region or under the breast is at all desired. The paraumbilical region can be very convenient in fat persons, but sometimes painful in skinny patients because of frictions with trousers, belts or other clothes. Some young ladies may not accept subclavicular placement of the IPG for esthetic reasons: in these cases, the stimulator can be placed 5 cm lower and 10 cm more laterally with a vertical incision above the breast, just on the pectoral muscle (Pirotte et al 2009).
- A dissolving suture (such as a 4-0 monocryl) may be helpful cosmetically in this location but it is advisable to see the incision during healing anyway within 1-2 weeks post-operatively.

7.4 Complications in Device Hardware

We have devised or use several ways of assessing device hardware from outside the body (Shils et al 2008), but often the ultimate etiology of a problem can only be determined if the IPG and lead are directly accessed at surgery and tested. This is because *radiological evaluation cannot always visualize a wire breakage, especially if it is intermittent with certain positions or movements, impedance testing is unreliable in determining exactly which contacts or any contacts have failed, IPG assessments have limited ability to determine failure modes and recharging failures, and skin recordings, even with palpation and manipulation to determine a short, are not always successful.* The implanted pulse generator (IPG) can accidentally turn off due to electromagnetic interference from household devices in close (<10 cm) proximity, such as electric appliances of any kind, but also anti-theft devices and metal detectors or magnets in loudspeakers. The so-called radio test may be useful: IPGs emit a signal at 500-550 kHz which can be received as a continuous hum on a small battery operated AM radio receiver. Avoiding hardware complications, however, is more difficult. This is because some hardware complications are from intrinsic faults within the IPG and because some problems with hardware (painful IPG site, painful incision area near anchor, broken wires, disconnected wires, displaced lead location, or infection and erosion of wires or the IPG) are more related to patient comorbidities (diabetes, steroid use, thin and poorly perfused skin and soft tissues, and low pain thresholds) than anything else. Certainly, the surgeon can take pains to minimize some of these concerns, but it is likely that some will still occur despite taking every precaution. The old adage that if you don't have any of these complications occur, you probably haven't done enough cases (or you avoid the difficult cases) likely has a ring of truth to it. Below are some suggestions toward minimizing hardware risks for cortical stimulation procedures:

- Always mention to the patient pre-operatively that they may have discomfort from the IPG or that the wire may become tethered in the neck, and in some cases these may need to be revised and in rare cases it is problematic enough that the system may need removal. Managing expectations up front is helpful.
- Have patients generally avoid any significant movement (reaching, twisting, high-level activities) for the first 6 weeks after surgery.
- Avoid making the subclavicular incision too close to the clavicle – this error almost always leads to pain from the IPG pushing against the clavicle.
- Avoid leaving too little soft tissue coverage over the IPG, difficult in thin patients. This tissue shrinks away anyway following surgery and when the coverage is too thin, pain typically follows, or erosion in atypical cases.
- While it is often helpful to make a second incision in the retromastoid region to help with tunneling, this area can more likely become infected or eroded and open. This is because there is little coverage and the blood supply is often compromised. Try to have the wire pass under one side or the other rather than directly under the incision.
- Make sure there is some strain relief coiling under the IPG. Although this will also scar in place, it typically retains some ability to relieve tethering when the head is turned (personal observation under anesthesia).

7.5 Complications in Programming

This subtopic may seem unnecessary perhaps, but we have found that it is worth mentioning for a few reasons. First, in the USA, programming of cortical stimulation patients often falls to the company representatives (though we still often do it ourselves), and it is important to work with the same rep or reps often enough with these systems to avoid complications (or simply inadequate programming). Second, there is little feedback from patients during programming and little in the way of algorithms to help with programming, making most of the process one of hit-or-miss and guesswork. In general, we try to cover as much of the cortical region as possible and slowly increase the amplitude over a period of months until we see positive results, and then work our way back to minimize battery use while maintaining efficacy. Unfortunately, increasing amplitudes can inadvertently lead to seizures during the programming phase and that becomes the boundary or ceiling for programming. Seizures tend to occur when amplitudes are set above approximately 7mA – but our own data shows we have caused seizures when amplitudes have been set (in different patients) at: 3.4V, 14mA, 7mA, between 4 and 8mA, and 9mA. Seizures tend to be focal motor seizures and can be stopped quickly by turning off the stimulator immediately in the clinic. However, they can generalize and they can occur after the patient has left the programming session with the typical unpredictability that seizures have. We recommend the following guidelines in programming to minimize the likelihood of seizure generation.

- Start at 2V or 5-6 mA and leave at that level for the first two weeks.
- Increase amplitude only in 0.1 mA or volt steps and make no adjustments at less than 4 week intervals.
- Do not exceed amplitudes wherein there is likely driving of the motor system itself (causing speech slurring, contractions, or other strange feelings) – if no benefit occurs at this 'motor threshold' for approximately 6 months, then it is worth informing the patient that they are unlikely going to reap any benefit with the device. However, it is still worth making some changes in PW and frequency anyway to see if there are benefits. Importantly, cycling on/off to preserve battery power may be imperative to keep the patient from having to recharge too often, and switching between several programs may keep the system from 'habituating' to one setting (there seems to be a benefit in some patients to the 'novelty' of a program and the circuitry responds for a short period of time before failing). Also, the patient may not realize they have some benefit until the device is turned off entirely for several days at which point the patient may appreciate that there was benefit. This technique is always worth pursuing when benefit is questionable.

A couple of caveats. Too many of these patients, who do not 'feel' any of the stimulation, are all too aware of when their IPG battery runs down and needs to be replaced without any prompting to be coincidence. Significant others too often notice appreciable improvements in interaction, mood, and activity levels, even when patients themselves may not notice, to dismiss the therapy out of hand.

7.6 Other Complications

Some patients report painful sensations either at the scalp – around the bone flap - or at the supramastoid region – where the connection is located - or around the neurostimulator. Visual inspection, as well as CT, X-rays or MRI usually do not show anything wrong. Pirotte et al (2009) experienced two patients reporting a painful sensation along the subcutaneous trajectory of the extension cable in the neck as if it was stretched like a rope in rotatory movements of the head. Indeed, a fibrous reaction can occur around the extension cable, so that it is best not to tunnel it too superficially in the neck in order for the platysma muscle to cover it completely. It should be borne in mind that normal sensory perception is generally disturbed in neurogenic pain patients, even in places located far from the painful limb or segment. This may cause minor – but chronic and sometimes disabling – complaints centered on the sites of implantation of the electrodes, cables or stimulators.

As classically observed in all surgical disciplines, the risk of *infection* is increased by the presence of implanted materials. Infection can occur as a primary process, directly related to the electrode implantation and rapidly presents as epidural or subdural (if the dura has been opened – see above) empyema. Infection can also start at the cutaneous exit of the electrode. Finally, infection of the electrode may occur secondarily to incomplete healing of the skin at the level of the scar on the vertex (wound dehiscence). Erosion of the connector through the skin is possible. Placement of the connector in the soft tissues of the neck should be avoided, given the stress related to cervical motion and the connectors' tendency to erode through the skin or break. In practice, the infection rate is not high. Pirotte et al (2009) experienced infections in 3 cases only (1 primary epidural empyema 15 days after surgery, 1 subdural empyema 10 days after surgery and 1 epidural empyema with cortical abscess secondary to incomplete healing of the scar 6 weeks after surgery): all 3 cases required surgical removal of the entire stimulating system, followed by 4 weeks of intravenous antibiotics. In order to avoid primary infection of the electrodes, aseptic measures must be carefully enacted throughout the procedure. Double gloving, avoiding implants manipulations, as well as systematic use of 24-hour-prophylactic intravenous antibiotics are mandatory. If epidural or subdural infection occurs, a cycle of intravenous antibiotics can be attempted, but, in almost all cases, explantation of the whole system is the only effective way to achieve remission. Local cutaneous infection at the exit of the temporary cables behind the ear is benign and rather infrequent, in spite of the cables lying externally for weeks (several centers keep the patients on antibiotics as long as the connection cables are externalized, though). Daily application of an antiseptic (e.g. Betadine) at the local site is usually sufficient to control local inflammation and impede progression of the infection to the epidural space. Secondary infection of the scar due to incomplete healing of the wound at the convexity should not be underestimated. It represents a major source of electrode infection that can lead to forced explantation. Indeed, an incomplete healing of the wound can contaminate the subcutaneous space, where the electrode wires can be affected. Pirotte et al (2009) experienced one case of secondary epidural infection of the electrodes complicated by a cortical abscess; another patient developed an epidural empyema secondary to suboptimal wound healing and a cortical abscess just below the electrode. This abscess was visible on CT and MRI and lasted for 6 months before disappearing. A good solution is to draw a large skin incision on the convexity so that the wound would not overlie any bone fixation or any wire or material, the skin incision being far away from the edge of the craniotomy. Finally, skin closure must be technically perfect.

Montes et al (2002) analyzed event-related potentials (ERPs) and behavioral performance during an auditory target-detection task in 11 consecutive patients obtained during MI ECS and 10 minutes after switching off stimulation. While sensory responses remained unaffected by MCS, there was a significant delay of brain potentials reflecting target detection in the older patients (N2 and P3), rapidly reversible after MI ECS discontinuation. No effect was observed in patients younger than 50 years. Individually, the effect was highly variable from no effect to a delay of tens of milliseconds. Cognitive effects of MCS appeared as mild and non-specific, directly related to the stimulation period (i.e. with no post-effect), in a manner reminding of cognitive effects reported during MI rTMS. Thus, MCS may interfere with relatively simple cognitive processes such as those underlying target detection, notably in the elderly and in the presence of preexistent cerebral lesions.

References

Arle JE, Shils JL. Essential Neuromodulation. San Diego : Academic Press, 2011

Montes C, Mertens P, Convers P, et al. Cognitive effects of precentral cortical stimulation for pain control: an ERP study. Neurophysiol Clin. 2002;32:313-25.

Pirotte BJM, Voordecker P, Levivier M, et al. Principles of surgical implantation and complications avoidance. In: Canavero S (ed) Textbook of therapeutic cortical stimulation. New York: Nova Science, 2009, pp 33-44

Saitoh Y, Hosomi K. From localization to surgical implantation. In: Canavero S (ed) Textbook of therapeutic cortical stimulation. New York: Nova Science, 2009, pp 17-32

Shils JL, Alterman R, and Arle JE. DBS Fault Testing. In: Tarsy D, Okun M, Vitek J, and Starr P (eds) Deep Brain Stimulation in Neurological and Psychiatric Disorders. Humana Press, 2008, pp 473-95

PART II: **Conditions**

Sergio Canavero, Walter Fagundes-Pereyra

8 Central Pain

Central pain has been defined as "*spontaneous and/or evoked, anomalous, painful or non-painful, sensations projected in a body area congruent with a clearly imaged lesion impairing –transitorily or permanently- the function of the spinothalamoparietal pathway*" (Canavero and Bonicalzi 2011). It follows cerebrovascular accidents, spinal cord injury, multiple sclerosis and other neurologic conditions affecting the CNS. There are approximately 7 million patients worldwide.

In 1991, Tsubokawa et al introduced Motor Cortex Stimulation as a treatment of central pain. In 1995, Canavero and Bonicalzi reported the first case of effective somatosensory cortex stimulation. Since then, the most positive results have been seen when the stimulating poles overlie parts of cortex corresponding to painful body parts (generally face, arm, chest, leg singly or in combination), although data suggest that precise, "millimetric," somatotopic localization of the electrode may not be required. In addition, the leg area often extends, at least partially, on the convexity.

8.1 Efficacy

Globally, more than half of all reported patients with CP originating from the brain were relieved more than 40% on a VAS scale during the long term. Pain in patients with CCP was also relieved, although the number of treated cases (about 20) is too small for any definite conclusions to be drawn (Table 8.1). Concurrent drugs can be reduced or even stopped in many cases. A suggestion of greater response of evoked versus spontaneous pains is not confirmed in most series and M1 ICS does not relieve nonpainful paresthesias.

What is rather puzzling is the observation that some groups report both good short- and long-term results, some have excellent initial results with a loss of benefit within weeks or months, and that some have scarce or no results at all. In practically all papers, there failure rates have ranged between 12% and 84%. However, the majority of these reports list as treatment failures cases improving by <30-40%, but there are several patients who are actually satisfied with 20-40% relief, at least for a time, due to improved functional ability and quality of life. Conversely, other patients may report high levels of pain reduction, yet fail to demonstrate any functional improvement. Accordingly, changes in VAS scores alone do not always accurately reflect the true effectiveness of a particular therapy, and clearly are inadequate for determining benefits with regard to functional capacity, quality of life, and so on. Nonetheless, explaining such variable results is not easy. Localization of stimulation target can be ruled out. Groups that meticulously explored the whole target cortex with intraoperative stimulation and used sophisticated localization technology (neuro-navigation, evoked potentials...) achieved either excellent or poor results in the same proportion. Inadequate (too short or too few contact combinations tried) neurostimulator programming is certainly a reason in some cases, and so is a team's lack of experience with neuromodulatory techniques and, above all, chronic pain management. A few groups ascribe their success to elimination of nonresponders to subacute therapeutic stimulation from those receiving long-term stimulation, which amounts to a sizable population. Accordingly, some neurosurgeons are enthusiastic about the technique, whereas others are rather cold or downright negative. It may be that ICS is performed at many more centers than those which publish and most of the failures go unreported, with only series with good results being published. This spurred the search for prognostic markers. Some have been proposed:

1. An intact or nearly-intact corticospinal motor function has been touted as a favorable prognostic sign, with about 75% of patients without major motor deficits getting benefit, but several exceptions are on record (Table 8.1).
2. Severe sensory changes not modified by M1 ICS represent a predictor of unfavorable outcome, whereas improvement in sensory deficits that appears during the subacute therapeutic trial is followed by a favorable outcome (Drouot et al 2002, Velasco et al 2008). Exceptions to the rule exist, and at least 3 cases of CP improved by ICS in spite of almost total lack of sensory cortex are on record (e.g. Peyron et al 1995; Nguyen et al 1999). Normal or near-normal sensory thresholds are not necessarily predictive of favorable outcome.
3. Response to noninvasive stimulation (e.g. rTMS) may identify patients who will get successful stimulation, but this is not an iron-cast criterion (see Box 8.1).
4. Drug dissection protocols may help identify responders. The first was proposed by Tsubokawa's group (Table 1): doses of 3 mg of morphine are injected every 5' up to 18 mg followed by naloxone 0.2 mg bid, followed by thiopental 50 mg IV bolus every 5' up to 250 mg and ketamine 5 mg IV bolus up to 25 mg. Canavero and Bonicalzi (2002, 2007, 2007b) developed the subhypnotic propofol test, in which the patient is injected in a single blind fashion with 1.5 mg of Intralipid or similar white fat solution and after 20' with 0.2 mg/Kg IV bolus of propofol.
5. Canavero and Bonicalzi (1995) introduced parietal cortex stimulation on the basis of neuroimaging data, the first report of neuroimaging-directed brain stimulation. However, functional neuroimaging has not yet been evaluated in a clinically meaningful fashion.
6. Successful ICS may be impossible in patients with a large surface of the cortex destroyed (e.g. stroke) and in those with a cortex distant from the dural surface (subdural hygroma, post-stroke atrophy...). However, Canavero has made a strong case for ipsilateral (to pain) ICS (Canavero 2009).

Table 8.1: Invasive cortical stimulation

Author(s)	Type of pain (no. of patients)	Results (follow-up) Parameters	Notes
Tsubokawa's group *Pain 1990; Suppl 5:S491 (abs.952)*	CP (thalamic) (7 pts)	Excellent (5: no drugs needed) or good (2: some drugs needed) pain relief *(abstract: effective in 75% of cases (>7 mos)*	First report of MCS for CP (1988) MCS vs. thalamic stimulation. MCS is more effective than thalamic stimulation. Improvement of motor function in some pts MCS improved movements of the painful limbs. Pain subsided within a few minutes. 5'–10' ON, 4–5 h relief 5–6 times daily, then 2–3 times daily
Tsubokawa *et al.* (1991) *Also see : Acta Neurochir Suppl (Wien) 1991; 52:137–9*	CPSP (12 pts; thalamic lesion: 6 pts; putaminal lesion: 3 pts; pontine hemorrhage: 1 pt; other lesions: 2 pts)	Complete pain relief in 5/12 pts (1 yr), considerable pain reduction in 3/12 pts (1 yr). Long-term benefit in 8/12 pts (>1 yr)	Intermittent stimulation effective in 5/12 pts. No seizures; pain relief at stimulus intensities below movements threshold. Paresis improvement. Pain improvement in barbiturate-sensitive, morphine-resistant pts. Disappearance of the analgesic effect in 3 pts, with reappearance after revision of electrode placement
Tsubokawa *et al.* (1993) *Also see : Tsubokawa et al. Pain 1993; 58 (Suppl.):150*	CPSP (11 pts; thalamic stroke: 8 pts; putaminal hemorrhage (+ small lesion in the posterior limb of the internal capsule): 3 pts)	Pain relief: Immediate: Excellent (>80%): 6/11 (54%) Good (60–79%): 2/11 (18%) Fair (40–59%): 1/11 (9%) Poor (<40%): 2/11 (18%) Long-lasting: Excellent (>80%): 5/11 (45%) Good (60–79%): 0/8 Fair (40–59%): 0/8 Poor (<40%): 3/8 (37%) (2 yrs)	Barbiturate-sensitive pts: 5 (+3?)/11; morphine-resistant pts: 10 (+1?)/11. Stimulation of area 4 ipsilateral to the inciting lesion. One week test period. Fair and poor responders not implanted. Satisfactory immediate pain relief in 8/11 pts (73%). Gradual effect reduction over several months in 3/8 pts. Long-term response in barbiturate-sensitive and morphine-resistant pts (also for Vc DBS). No pain-relieving effect by high-frequency postcentral stimulation (11/11 pts): in 2, worsening of pain, similar to their spontaneous ones. In 3 pts, areas rostral to MI stimulated without relief. Nonpainful paresthesias unrelieved. 5'-10' 'ON' at a time – no stimulation at night 50 – 120 Hz 100-500 μs
Katayama *et al.* (1994) *Stereotact Funct Neurosurg 1994; 62:295–9*	CPSP (6 pts; lateral medullary infarct)	MCS in 3 pts. Pain relief: 2/3 > 60%; 1/3 > 40% (4 mos)	Pain relief > 40% in 1 pt previously unsuccessfully treated by Vc DBS. No satisfactory pain control by thalamic stimulation in any pts

continued **Table 8.1:** Invasive cortical stimulation

Author(s)	Type of pain (no. of patients)	Results (follow-up) Parameters	Notes
Yamamoto *et al.* (1997)	CPSP (39 pts; thalamic stroke: 25 cases; suprathalamic stroke: 14 pts)	28 MCS. Excellent/good (50–100%) pain relief: Thalamic pts: 10/19 (53%) Suprathal. pts: 3/9 (33%) (difference not significant) T+ or K+ & M+: 2/4 (50%) T+ or K+ & M-: 10/14 (71%) T- & K- & M+: 0/2 (0%) T- & K- & M-: 1/8 (13%) Overall: 13/28 (46%) (12 mos)	Suprathalamic stroke = infarct or hemorrhage of the posterior limb of internal capsule, or parietal lobe, sparing the thalamus. No pts with midbrain or medullary lesions. MCS test period: 1 wk. 8/39: morphine responsive 22/39: thiamylal responsive 11/23: ketamine responsive Thiamylal+ketamine sensitivity + morphine resistance may predict a positive effect of MCS
Katayama *et al.* (1998) *(Also includes: Katayama et al. Stereotact Funct Neurosurg 1997; 69:73–9 & Tsubokawa et al. In: Abst. 3rd Int Congress INS. Orlando, 1996, p. 123) includes all pts from previous publications!*	CPSP (31 pts. Thalamic stroke: 20 pts; putaminal hemorrhage: 8 pts; lateral medullary infarction: 3 pts)	Early satisfactory (>60%) pain relief: 23/31 pts (74%). Long-term efficacy (≥2 yrs): 15/31 pts (48%)	Damage of the posterior limb of the internal capsule in pts with putaminal hemorrhage. Previous ineffective SCS. Pain relief >60%: 13/18 pts (73%) with no or mild motor weakness (70% of pts with inducible muscle contraction); 2/13 pts (15%) with moderate or severe motor weakness (difference statistically significant). Satisfactory pain control in 14/20 pts (70%) with inducible muscle contraction but in only 1/11 pts (9%) without inducible motor contractions ($p < 0.01$). No relationship between pain control and presence of hypesthesia, dysesthesia, hyperpathia, allodynia or disappearance of SSEP N20 wave plus stimulation-induced paresthesias, or motor performance improvement. 3 pts with MCS or DBS became pain-free without stimulation for years (all 3 getting initial excellent relief at progressively longer stimulation intervals during intermittent stimulation). 1 subcutaneous infection, 3 seizures during testing at intensities higher than muscle threshold. 10'-20'ON at a time 20-50 Hz 100-500, most at 200 μs 2-8 V

continued **Table 8.1:** Invasive cortical stimulation

Author(s)	Type of pain (no. of patients)	Results (follow-up) Parameters	Notes
Yamamoto *et al.* (2000)	Small thalamic stroke, then action tremor, then Vim DBS, then cardioversion, then CPSP	50% relief over 2 years	Thiamylal/ketamine responsive, morphine resistant
Katayama *et al.* (2001)	CPSP (45 pts)	Satisfactory pain control: SCS: 7% of pts; DBS: 25% of pts; MCS: 48% of pts	DBS and MCS in 4 pts: better result: MCS 1/4 pts; DBS 2/4
Fukaya *et al.* (2003) *Also includes: Katayama et al. Acta Neurochir Suppl. 2003; 87:121–3*	CPSP (31 pts)	Unsuccessful MCS in 2 CPSP pts reporting abnormal pain sensation after stimulation of the motor cortex (see text)	Experimental study on conscious somatosensory response during surgery for electrode placement
Paris group : Nguyen et al (2009) Also includes : *Nguyen et al 1997 Acta Neurochir Suppl. 1997; 68:54–60 Nguyen et al (1999) Nguyen et al. Arch Med Res 2000; 31:263–5 Nguyen et al. Neurochirurgie 2000; 46:483–91* Drouot et al 2002	CPSP (32 pts) BCP (thalamic abscess) (1 pt) BCP (head injury) (2 pts) SCI (9 pts) 1993-2004	>60% relief: 13 40-60% relief: 15 <40% relief: 7 mean improvement on VAS: 53%, on MPQ: 56.7%, on WBPQ: 62.7%, on MQS: 32.9% NA (in a previous series of 4: <40% in a paraplegic pt (18 mos); 100% (visceral pain + substantial reduction of diffuse pain) in a tetraplegic pt (22 mos), another improved >40%, one failure) f-up (global): 29-170 mos	Progressive loss of effect in some pts reversed in most by correct repositioning of paddle. 3 hours 'ON' and 3 hours 'OFF' (12 h die) 40 Hz (25 Hz – 55 Hz) 82.5 (60 –180) μs

continued Table 8.1: Invasive cortical stimulation

Author(s)	Type of pain (no. of patients)	Results (follow-up) Parameters	Notes
Nguyen *et al* (2008) (with Velasco's group in Mexico)	3 CPSP	Pt 1: -16% Pt 2: -38% (both hemisoma CP) Pt3 (face CP): -80% f-up: 1 year (stable benefit)	Benefit NOT due to placebo effect. MCS decreased MPQ affective subscore Drugs down 55% (pt 3) Improved QoL
Lyon group: Nuti et al. (2005) *Includes all previous publications: Peyron et al. Pain 1995; 62:275–86 Garcia-Larrea et al. Stereotact Funct Neurosurg 1997; 68:141–8 Garcia-Larrea et al. (1999) Mertens et al. Stereotact Funct Neurosurg 1999; 73:122 Sindou et al. 9th World Congress on Pain, Book of abstracts, IASP Press, 1999 Montes et al. Neurophysiol Clin 2002; 32:313–25*	CP (27 pts) -Ischemic lesions 11 pts (3 thalamic (Vc), 4 medulla, 2 cortical parietal, 1 parietal/insula/ ACC, 1 parietal/ insula) -Haemorragic lesions 11 pts (1 thalamic (Vc), 1 thalamus/ midbrain, 5 capsulothalamic, 1 capsulolenticular/insula, 3 cortical parietal) -Frontoparietal trauma, 1 pt SCI (discal hernia-associated myelopathy): 3 pts Spinal conus AVM: 1 pt 1992-2003	Follow-up: 2-104 mos (mean 49 mos). Pain relief: BCP: Excellent (>70%): 3 Good (40-69%): 8 Poor (10-39%): 8 Negligible (0-9%): 4 CCP: Excellent: 0 Good: 3 Poor: 1 Negligible: 0 Decreased analgesic intake: 52% of pts (complete withdrawal 36%); unchanged: 45% of pts, unavaible data: 3%. Decrease/withdrawal of analgesic in 10/11 poor responders (!: Contradictory results as noted by Authors) Favour re-intervention: 70% of pts	Parameters: 0.5-5V (mean 1.5V), 30-80 Hz (mean 45.5 Hz), 60-330 μs (mean 140 μs), ON 30-120 min, OFF 15min-24 hours. 5 – 6 hours of stimulation each day Prospective evaluation of MCS. Long-term outcome evaluated by means of: 1) %pain relief 2) VAS 3) postoperative VAS decrease 4) reduction in drugs intake 5) yes/no response for being operated again. MCS efficacy not predictable by motor status, pain characteristics, lesion type, QST, SSEP/LEPs, pain duration, BCP vs CCP, presence of evoked pain. No subjective sensations during active stimulation. Partial epileptic seizures in 3 pts in the early postoperative stage or during trials for increasing intensity. 1 speech disorders and 1 motor deficit resoved spontaneously Long term relief predictable from early pain relief. 1-2 paddles. 3 subdural MCS may have adverse cognitive effects. The risk may increase with age (>50 yrs)

continued **Table 8.1:** Invasive cortical stimulation

Author(s)	Type of pain (no. of patients)	Results (follow-up) Parameters	Notes
Maarrawi *et* al. (2013)	CPSP 10 pts (capsular/thalamic/lenticular: 6 pts; brainstem: 3 pts; insular: 1 pt) SCI (1 pt) 2002-2009	Pain relief: Excellent (>70%): 2 Good (40-69%): 6 Poor (10-39%): 2 SCI pt: 20% relief	Drug therapy: clonazepam (2.5-3 mg/d); Gabapentin (2400-3200 mg/die); Paracetamol (1500 mg/d) (!!!), Oxcarbazepine (1200 mg/d), Carbamazepine (1000 mg/d), Clomipramine (125-150 mg/d), All patients either unresponsive/intolerant to oral opioids (7 pts) or only mild relief (8 pts). 0.5-5V, 180μs,35-45Hz, cyclic (30'-60'ON, 2 Hrs OFF)
Turin Advanced Neuromodulation Group (TANG) Canavero and Bonicalzi. (1995)	CP (2 pts; CPSP: 1 pt; syringomyelia: 1 pt)	Pain relief: 30–50% in syringomyelia pt (2 yrs); no relief in CPSP	Syringomyelia pt: parietal somatosensory stimulation. Spreading of pain to contralateral side and vanishing of analgesia at 2 yrs. Modest propofol response CPSP pt: propofol unresponsive
Canavero *et al.* (1999)	CPSP (1 pt; thalamocapsular stroke)	Effective short-term pain relief (allodynia disappearance and 50% reduction of burning pain) (5 wks)	Propofol-responsive pt. Painful supernumerary phantom arm during MCS and lasting 6 mos after stimulator switch-off. Pain relapse after 5 wks
Canavero and Bonicalzi (2002, 2007) Includes: *Canavero et al.: In: Proc 4th Int Congress of INS, Luzern, 1998* Canavero *et al. Neurol Res 2003; 25:118–22*	CP (CPSP 5 pts; SC pain: 2 pts) + 1 (algodystonia) 1993–2003	Effective (30–100%) pain relief with MCS/PCS in 2/7 pts. Long-term efficacy (4 yrs) in 2 pt (BCP and MS CP). Ineffective MCS in 4/7	Effective SI stimulation in 1, then resubmitted to MCS with same benefit plus 50% opioid reduction (however, patient unsatisfied and explanted). Overall efficacy: 3/7 CP pts, all propofol-responsive. Ineffective MCS in 4/7 CP pts, all propofol-unresponsive, but 1 who could not be assessed due to intermittent nature of pain. Algodystonia: temporary benefit

continued **Table 8.1:** Invasive cortical stimulation

Author(s)	Type of pain (no. of patients)	Results (follow-up) Parameters	Notes
Saitoh's group: Hosomi et al (2008) Includes all previous publications including Tani et al JNS 2004 ; 101 :687-689 *Saitoh et al. Neurosurg Focus 11(3), article 1, 2001 Includes Saitoh et al. J Neurosurg 2000; 92:150–5 Tani et al. J Neurosurg 2004; 101:687–9*	CPSP (thalamic) (10 pts) [+1 pt relieved without stimulation] CPSP (putaminal) (3 pts) CP (brainstem: stroke 3pts, injury 1pt) CPSP (temporo-parietal) (1 pt) CCP (SCI) (2 pts) 1996–2005	4: no initial relief 6: 21-90% initial relief (mean: 55.6%) [late relief at 14-75 mos: 10-80% (mean: 31.6%)]; 1 explant due to enduring benefit from CS manipulation -all 3 relieved initially 60-75% (mean: 65.3%) [late relief at 13-88 mos: 15-60% (mean: 41.6%)]; 1 explant (15% relief pt) 1: no relief 3: 25-63% initial relief (mean : 42.6%) [late relief at 33-73 mos: 15-50% (mean: 35%) 30% initial relief, then 10% at 72 mos 50-89% initial pain relief (60-65% late relief at 27-75 months); 1 explant	Pharmacological test with phentolamine, lidocaine, ketamine, thiopental, morphine, placebo. Ketamine-sensitive pts seem to be good candidates for MCS Some pain reduction by SI stimulation. Ineffective prefrontal stimulation. First report of bilateral cortical stimulation for SCI pain. 4 mos interval between implants. 2 serious ICH, with 1 vegetative. 2 infections subdural approach, 1-2 plate electrodes within central sulcus, in 9 pts 1 plate in interhemispheric fissure, extradural ECS in only 2 pts. MCS within central sulcus more effective than surface MCS. Globally: initial VAS score reduction in BCP: 42%; late relief: 26% at 1+ year 3–4 periods ON (30' each) a day, followed by 5–6 h benefit in OFF. 25-50 Hz 200 µs 0.9 to 5 volts
Other groups:			
Tasker et al (1994)	CPSP (1 pt, large suprathalamic infarct) CPSP (2 pts) (1 pt with AVM)	Substantial pain relief with *ipsilateral to pain MCS*; gradual abatement over 6 yrs; relief with subdural stimulation over a few months. 1 relief, 1 failure	Contralateral MCS due to a lack of sufficient MI on the affected side. Stimulation-induced ipsilateral paresthesias

continued **Table 8.1:** Invasive cortical stimulation

Author(s)	Type of pain (no. of patients)	Results (follow-up) Parameters	Notes
Hosobuchi (1993) Also includes: *Stereotact Funct Neurosurg 1992; 59:76–83 Abstr. IASP congress 1993*	CPSP (5 pts; post-removal of parietal cortical AVM: 1 pt; brainstem infarction: 1 pt; thalamic lesion: 3 pts)	Pain relief: Initial: 5/5 excellent. At 2–3 mos: 4/5 excellent (>50%); 1 fair. At 9–30 mos: 3/5 excellent (thalamic, parietal, brainstem)	Efficacy dramatically reduced in 2 thalamic pain pts, to 0% in 1 pt and 30% in 1 pt 2–6 mos after implantation 1h ON/6h OFF 20-30 Hz, 180-260 μs, 3-5V
Meyerson *et al.* (1993) *Acta Neurochir Suppl (Wien) 1993; 58:150–3*	CPSP (3 pts; thalamic hemorrhage: 2 pts; brainstem infarction: 1 pt)	Pain relief: CPSP: none: 3/3	In spite of multipolar electrode grid in 1 and relocation of paddle in another. Most patients had one or two seizures during test stimulation. Painful sensations at the electrode site in 2 pts. 1 epidural clot leading to aphasia. 20'-30' ON 5 times a day; 50 Hz, 300 μs, amplitude 20 to 30% below motor threshold
Dario *et al.* Long-term results of chronic MCS for CP. *Abstr. 9th World Congress on Pain, IASP Press, 1999, A185. Also includes Dario et al. Riv Neurobiol 1997; 43:625–9*	CPSP (thal. stroke: 2 pts; brainstem stroke: 1 pt)	70% pain relief in 1 thal. pt. (3 yrs) Gradual abatement of pain relief over 2 yrs. 60–90% relief. Then 50–70%, then 20–30% at 3–41 mos (ave: 27 mos)	All pts propofol-responsive. 2–2.5 V, 50–75 Hz, 120–210 ms, continuous mode.

continued **Table 8.1:** Invasive cortical stimulation

Author(s)	Type of pain (no. of patients)	Results (follow-up) Parameters	Notes
Franzini *et al.* (2003) Also includes: *Franzini et al. In: Abstr. XLVIII Congresso SINCH, Copanello, 1999 Franzini et al. J Neurosurg 2000; 93:873–5*	CPSP (3 pts, A, B, C)	Satisfactory (30–50%) pain relief: Pts A (>4 yrs) and B (>2yrs). Short-term pain relief (6 mos): pt C	2 responders propofol-sensitive. Pain abolition after a second stroke in pt B. Unsatisfactory pain relief (30%) by further stimulation in pt C. Complete abolition of thalamic hand
Herregodts *et al.* (1995)	CP (thalamic) (2 pts)	Immediate pain relief: >50% in both pts Long-lasting: 1/2 (full relapse in one at 4 mos). 1h ON every 6 hrs	
Migita *et al.* (1995)	CPSP (2 pts; putaminal hemorrhage: pt A; post-20 mos stereotactic thalamotomy; pt B)	Pain relief: 70–80% in pt A (1 yr) No relief in pt B	Pt A: morphine and barbiturate unresponsive. 30% pain relief with TMS Pt B: previous 6 month effective Vc DBS. Barbiturate responsive, morphine and TMS unresponsive
Fuji *et al.* (1997)	CPSP (thal. infarction: 2 pts; thal. hemorrhage: 5 pts)	Satisfactory pain relief: 6/7 pts (1 mo) Unsatisfactory pain relief: 5/7 pts (3 mos).	Lesions included internal caspule, Vc and pulvinar (MRI confirmed, 5 pts). Early electrode removal in 1 pt after unsatisfactory test stimulation. 30' ON 10 – 100 Hz 200 µs 3-8V
Barraquer-Bordas *et al.* (1999)	CPSP (1 pt: capsuloinsular hemorrhage)	MCS trial ineffective (motor response elicited)	Hemisoma burning pain, + evoked pains. DBS reduced CP for 5 mos and evoked pains, until glioma displaced electrode with relapse and death
Roux *et al.* (2001)	CPSP (2 pt) SCI (1 pt) Myelopathic pain (1 pt)	-both >80% relief -60% relief -90% relief f-up: 6-14 months	

continued **Table 8.1:** Invasive cortical stimulation

Author(s)	Type of pain (no. of patients)	Results (follow-up) Parameters	Notes
Mogilner and Rezai (2001)	SCI (1 pt)	Relief (not broken down) (mean follow-up 6 mos)	30'-2h ON 5-10 times die, 110 Hz, 210 μs 2-8V
Rodriguez and Contreras (2002)	SCI (post-cervical ependymoma removal) CP (1 pt)	Evoked pain dramatically improved. Steady burning pain moderately relieved (2 mos)	3rd party analysis of results. Tremor improvement. No reduction of analgesic intake after MCS. 7.1 V, 5 Hz, 450 ms, ON 2 h, OFF 3 h, 0-/2+
Nandi *et al.* (2002) *Includes all pts reported in Carroll et al. Pain 2000; 84:431–7 Smith et al. Neurosurg Focus 2001; 11(3):article 2*	CPSP 7 pts (cortic. stroke 1 pt; thal. stroke: 3 pts; brainstem stroke: 2 pts). Gunshot brainstem injury (1 pt)	Appreciable pain relief: 1 pt, cortical (4 yrs); 2 pts (weeks to months) No relief: 4 pts (thalamic, brainstem) Brainstem injury: 50–60% (31 mos): 1 pt	The only pt where it was tried: propofol-sensitive. Pain disappearance for 5 mos after stimulator switched off in the responder. Enduring benefit in 1 pt only
Frighetto *et al.* (2004)	CPSP (1 pt)	Relief (no details given)	Previous ineffective thalamotomy
Henderson *et al.* (2004)	CPSP (1 pt)	Relief, then loss, then new relief (?) after intensive reprogramming	

continued **Table 8.1:** Invasive cortical stimulation

Author(s)	Type of pain (no. of patients)	Results (follow-up) Parameters	Notes
Brown and Pilitsis (2005)	CPSP, Wallenberg (1 pt) CPSP, thalamic (1 pt)	0% VAS 10 to 8; McGill Quest. Index from 65 to 32 (both sensory and affective scores)	Follow-up max. in whole series (PNP and CP): 10 months. Contrary to Nguyen, they conclude that precise, somatotopic localization of the electrode may not be required, because the optimal inter-electrode distance determined during cortical mapping and afterwards with subjective patient evaluation of pain control was fully 3 cm. Intraoperative neuronavigation and cortical mapping for stimulation site targeting. Strength and discriminative sensation improvement from MCS in 3 pts with facial weakness and sensory loss. Dysarthria improvement in 1 pt More than 50% reduction in pain medication dose. Continuous stimulation 40 Hz, 90-240 µs 2-8V
Slawek *et al.* (2005)	CPSP, brainstem (1 pt)	20% VAS reduction; withdrawal of narcotic and decrease of non-narcotic medications, ability to introduce rehabilitation and improvement of sleep	Follow-up: 4 mos. No side effects
Savas and Kanpolat (2005)	CP (1 pt)	0% relief during test stimulation	
Gharabaghi *et al.* (2005) *Also includes Tirakotai et al. Min. Invas. Neurosurg 2004; 47:273–7*	CPSP (hemorrhage) (3 pts) CP, insular (1 pt)	70–100% relief (follow-up: 6–18 mos) 90% relief (follow-up: 24 mos)	Frameless neuronavigation. Single burr hole and vacuum headrest. Awake patient. No complications 3rd party evaluation Volumetric 3-D MR with superimposed fMR data plus intraoperative electrical stimulation

continued **Table 8.1:** Invasive cortical stimulation

Author(s)	Type of pain (no. of patients)	Results (follow-up) Parameters	Notes
Pirotte *et al.* (2005) *Also includes Pirotte et al. Neurosurg Focus 2001; 11(3)*	CPSP : subcortical: 3 pts; capsular: 2 pts; brainstem: 1 pt; MS pain: 1 pt; cervical syrinx: 1 pt; SC ependymoma: 1 pt 1998–2003	Pain relief (%) 100%/50%/worsening 83%/failure (both plegic) 87.5% 100% 70% Failure	50–75% drug dosage reduction among responders 3rd party evaluation. Plegia not an unfavorable prognostic factor. 1h ON every 4 hrs 40 Hz, 100 μs 1-5V
Rasche *et al.*(2006) *Includes : Tronnier VM. Schmerz 2001; 15 : 278-279*	CPSP (thalamic): 7 pts 1994-2005	3 responders (-31%,-41%, -62%) 2/7 pts placebo responder. Duration of positive effect: 2, 4, 1.5 years Relief of dysesthesia, allodynia and hyperpathy in 2 CPSP pts (pts were able to touch the painful area without having painful sensations).	4.5-6.0 V, 50–85 Hz 210–250 μs, continuous stimulation, then intermittent. Double-blind test trial. VAS evaluation. Single burr hole, neuronavigation. Paddle parallel to central sulcus No sensation evoked by stimulation. Minor changes of parameters during f-up. Immediate or almost immediate (30'-60') pain reduction after turning the MCS on. After-effect: 30'-hours
Tronnier and Rasche (2009)	CPSP (11 pts)	4 pts:>50% relief f-up: up to 15 years	
Son *et al* (2006)	BCP (traumatic): 1 pt	90-95% relief of spontaneous burning pain in arm and lower trunk, 70-80% relief of burning pain, heaviness and deep pressure-like pain in leg, 50% relief of heaviness and deep pressure allodynia in foot follow-up: 1 year	Severe motor deficit in distal arm and leg. Subdural electrode for arm pain; extradural paddle for leg pain parallel to the course of the superior sagittal sulcus 21 Hz, 210 μs, 0.8-2.5V 0-/3+, continuous stimulation (arm electrode) 30Hz, 210 μs, 2-2.5V 0-/2+ continuous stimulation (leg electrode) After-effect: 5'
Sokal *et al* (2006)	CP (thalamic) (1 pt)	Decrease of pain	

continued Table 8.1: Invasive cortical stimulation

Author(s)	Type of pain (no. of patients)	Results (follow-up) Parameters	Notes
Cioni *et al* (2007)	CPSP (4 pts, thalamic) SCI (2 pts)	Pain relief (50–60%): 1/4 pts, but unsatisfactory relief at 1 yr 1 >40% relief, 1 failure	Extradural multipolar (16–20) grid in all plus electrophysiologic mapping; several combinations assessed over 12 h
Molet *et al* (2007)	CPSP (thalamic) (3 pts) CCP(paraplegia) (1 pt)	Benefit in some	CP and PNP series: results not broken down
Arle *et al* (2008) Arle (2014, personal communication)	2 poststroke pain (PSP) pts (P5, 58 yrs; P7, 64 yrs) 3 mixed pain and movement disorders (PSM) pts (but according to their table 2: P1 64 yrs, P2 61 yrs, P4 64 yrs, P6 49 yrs = 4 pts) CPSP (8 pts)	1 CPSP < 20% at 17 mos 1 CPSP >60% at 30 mos PSM: good result: P2, 36 mos follow-up; fair results: P1, 39 mos follow up, P4, 34 mos follow-up; poor result: P6, 23 mos follow-up P5: good pain control in her upper extremities and face, but less pain control in her leg region, minimal control of a third-limb sensation. 5 benefits >50% (f-up: up to 9 years)	2 intraoperative seizures 1 post-operative programming seizure. No further seizure with voltage <4.0 V. Continuous stimulation 60-130 Hz, 60-400 µs, 2-7 V
Velasco *et al* (2008)	CPSP (thalamic) (1 pt)	60% relief (allodynia disappeared; hyperalgesia decreased) at 1 year follow-up	Double-blind randomized trial Hypesthesia unchanged. 40-130 Hz, 2-3.5V, 90 µs
Shabalov *et al* (2008)	SCI (cervical) (1 pt)	VAS reduced >50%	V 1-5.5 ; 20-50 Hz, 60-210 µs (whole group)
Mondani *et al* (2008)	CPSP (2 pts) MS (2 pts)	50-80% benefit at 3 months.	Subdural strips

continued **Table 8.1:** Invasive cortical stimulation

Author(s)	**Type of pain (no. of patients)**	**Results (follow-up) Parameters**	**Notes**
Delavallee *et al* (2008)	CPSP (3 pts) 1 thalamic ischemia 1 MCA hemo. 1 MCA ischemia	Poor result (pain relief <40%): P2 (VAS 9 vs 6) Excellent result (pain relief 100-80%): P4: (VAS 8 vs 1), P6: (VAS 9 vs 1) F-up: mean 54 mos (range, 19–69 mos) for whole group (CP + PNP)	Subdural strips. Octopolar electrode. One severe motor deficit was satisfactorily relieved P2: Initial satisfactory pain relief, rapidly diminished to poor relief. System dysfunction/lead mobilization ruled out Parameters of stimulation: P2: 3.0 V, 210 μs, 80 Hz, 30 min, several times/d; P4: 2.1 V, 210 μs, 50 Hz 60 min, 1 time/d; P6: 2.0 V, 210 μs, 60 Hz 30 min, 1 time/d.
Finet and Raftopoulos (2009)	CPSP (1 pt)	Initial satisfactory analgesia, rapid loss of effect (poor result).	Subdural octrode in interhemispheric fissure in front of CS.
Vesper (2010)	CPSP (1 pt) CP (post AVM irradiation) (1 pt)	>50% relief 100% relief f-up: 1-4 years	rTMS predictive
Tanei *et al* (2010)	MS CP (1 pt)	Test: >50% VAS relief 60% relief f-up: 6 mos	ON 1 h OFF 2 h 0/1+ 2/3- 6.5V >100Hz Reduction of pre-op drugs (+ketamine stopped)
Fagundes-Pereyra et al (2010)	(1) CPSP (5) (2) Traumatic BCP (2) (3) MS (1) (4) Tumoral BCP (1) (5) SCI (1) 1994-2002	(1) Relief 30%, 35%, 50%. 50%, 70% (2) Relief: 50%, 80% (3) Relief: 32% (4) Relief: 50% (S) Not available Follow-up: 12 months	First 7 patients: single burr hole; 3 later patients: craniotomy and Robotic Neuro-navigation with 3D MRI reconstruction Paddle perpendicular to central sulcus. Presence of motor deficitor duration of pain: insignificant factors Better results with robotic neuronavigation. Decrease of effects in some patients. CP group; VAS preop, 7.8, postop.: 3.82 (p < 0.00001) 45-130 HZ. 45-210 μs. 2-5.3V, monopolar or bipolar stimulation. Pts with <40% relief intolerant of MCS interruption!

continued **Table 8.1:** Invasive cortical stimulation

Author(s)	Type of pain (no. of patients)	Results (follow-up) Parameters	Notes
Tanei *et al.* (2011)	CPSP(8) CCP (tumor) (1) brainstem CP (MS, Chiari I) (2) 1999-2009	CPSP: 80-100% relief (2 patients) 60-79% relief (4 patients) < 40% relief (2 patients) other CP: 60-79% relief (3 patients)	Single burr hole. 1 week trial. VAS assessment. ON 1 h, OFF 2 h Statisticaly significant Thalamic (55 Hz) and brainstem-cord CP (106 Hz) (3.04 vs. 6.68 V; 180 vs. 308 µs) DBS + MCS in 2 cord CP patients: additive effect
Lefaucheur *et al.* (2011)	CPSP (6)	VAS scores were 0,0,0,2,4.5,and 8 (Initial: all > 7) at 1 year	Postoperative stimulation OFF for 1 month followed by a single-blind randomised phase (1 month) with stim OFF (3 patients) or ON (3 patients), then 10 months of open label. No crossover. Safety, not efficacy study. Octopolar round paddle (surgery: average length 320 minutes!). 2 pts had IPG explanted for infection and then reimplanted 6 months later. Assessment: VAS, BPI, MPQ, SIP, MQS, PGIC Final parameters: 40-50Hz, 60 µs, 2-6V. Continuous in 4 patients, cyclic in 2, in the randomized, blinded arm, only 1/3 patients with stim ON reported > 50% VAS relief. Open label: improvement increased over time but significant only after 6 months.
Sakas *et al* (2011)	CPSP, thalamic (1 pt)	MI CS : 40% VAS reduction SI CS: 0% MI+SI: 90% VAS relief (face) 70% (arm) <10% (leg) f-up : 2 yrs	2 eight-polar paddles in direct contact with MI and SI. Interdural positioning, subdural interface
Ito *et al.* (2011) *Also includes :* *Ito et al (2006)* Kuroda *et al* (2000)	CPSP (thalamo-capsular/basal ganglia) (6 pts) 2005-2008 CPSP (evacuated putaminal hematoma) (1 pt)	100%, 100%, 54%, 50%, 2 failures during test period MCS ineffective. Later SI/SII CS effective for 4 yrs	Follow-up: 46-60 mos 25-50Hz, 2.5-6V, 210-450 µs, 3+/1-,0+/3-,1+/4-,0+/3-, cyclical (15-30' ON, OFF?) Paddle parallel to MI Minimal motor deficit in 4 responders

continued **Table 8.1:** Invasive cortical stimulation

Author(s)	Type of pain (no. of patients)	Results (follow-up) Parameters	Notes
Mandat *et al* (2012)	? (possibly 8 with hemibody pain, others possible) in a group of 23 patients with neuropathic/deafferentation pain	Improvement in the whole group of patients (p < 0.001). Best results in the neuropathic facial pain group (p < 0.001) while the worst ones were noted in the deafferentation pain group (p = 0.04).	16 out of 23 patients treated with rTMS with a positive response in 10 cases. VAS assessment 1 month before and 3 months after MCS. Pain duration positively correlated with outcome. 1 post- nfection explantation.
Reyns et al (2013)	CPSP (thalamocapsular/basal ganglia) (4 pts) CPSP (insula) (1 pt) CPSP (brainstem) (1 pt) CCP (syrinx) (1 pt)	-0%, 15%,25%, 40% -80% -15% -75%	45Hz, 60µs, 1.5-3V, bipolar, continuous stimulation
Vargas-Lopes *et al* (2014)	SCI (1)	VAS reduction from 10 to 4	Use of neuronavigation. Subdural, interhemispheric. 50Hz, 200 µs, 5V

Noninvasive cortical stimulation (rTMS, tDCS) is known to offer less pain relief that ICS, and for a short time only. A review of all studies shows that several patients did not deviate from baseline Visual Analog Scale (VAS) ratings. In some TMS studies, reductions in pain ratings were also noted among patients in the sham conditions, and, in some trials, did not differ significantly from pain-rating reductions noted with active treatment (Canavero and Bonicalzi 2011). There is no uniformly effective frequency of stimulation, and both high (10-20 Hz) and low (0.2-0.5Hz) frequencies can be effective. The effect of TMS may start within minutes, but the duration of analgesia after a single session is usually brief (5'-8 days). Some authors emphasize how repeated sessions on consecutive days may lead to cumulative effects lasting beyond the time of stimulation, which might be exploited clinically in patients awaiting surgical implantation. Unfortunately, differences in mean VAS ratings reported in all studies before and after treatment can be misleading, influenced by a large change in only a small subset of patients. Furthermore, significant differences were obtained even with small reductions in the VAS after rTMS treatment. In a sample series, Ohn et al (2012) found rTMS only modestly analgesic for CP in 64% of the patients for two weeks. Thus, noninvasive cortical stimulation cannot be recommended for chronic treatment at the present time, except in an unpredictable fashion in some highly responsive patients. TDCS does not appear to offer superior efficacy over rTMS.
The first to suggest that a trial of TMS could predict analgesia following ECS were Migita et al (1995). Canavero et al (1998, 2002, 2002b, 2003) first confirmed this finding. Other reports followed (Saitoh et al 2007, Lefaucheur et al 2011, Andrè-Obadia et al 2006, 2014). While there is a consensus on the relation between a positive effect after TMS and subsequent analgesia with ECS, a negative TMS trial should not necessarily rule it out. We found a relation between TMS and propofol, and suggested that the propofol test may predict analgesia with ICS (Canavero et al 1998, 2002, 2002b, 2003, Canavero and Bonicalzi 2005, 2011).

Box 8.1: Can TMS help select patients for Invasive Stimulation?

There is no significant statistical difference between results obtained in thalamic or cortico-subcortical brain CP patients. Coverage of restricted painful territories (e.g. chest) should not be taken as contraindicating ECS, even though no sensori-motor phenomena are elicited during test stimulation. Paddles have been placed parallel to the rolandic fissure or perpendicular, with similar results. What is clear is that, despite some claims to the contrary, subdural implantation does not seem to improve results and may actually be less effective than extradural implantation: for CP, benefit at 1 year was 26% only in the largest series (Hosomi et al 2008). Pain relief is not associated with age, sex, presence or absence of cerebral lesion, treated painful region or pain laterality. Some authors offer ICS if the mean VAS score is 6 or more, but this is moot.

Therapeutic ICS does not generally induce any motor activation, even at a high voltage, or any sensory phenomena in a majority of patients. Thus blinded controlled studies are feasible. All studies performed up to now (e.g. Rasche et al 2006, Velasco et al 2008, Nguyen et al 2008) exclude a placebo effect as the primary basis of analgesia.

Absolute exclusion criteria from ICS include: suicidal thoughts or gestures, major psychosocial stressors (job dissatisfaction, marital problems...), major personality disorders, alcoholism and drug addiction. Hemisoma pains do not represent a contraindication, as these can be managed with two strip electrodes combined.

Programming includes a wide range of stimulation parameters (each patient is different and no indications are possible) with voltage varying from 0.5 volts to 6V up to 10.5V (mean 3.8V), pulse width varying from 60 μs up to 500 μs (mean: 251.2 μs), and frequency varying from 5 Hz to 60Hz (often 25-50Hz, mean: 51.1Hz) up to 80Hz and 130 Hz. Chronic stimulation can be cyclical (battery sparing) or continuous. When cyclical, the duration of each stimulating session varies anywhere from 5' to 9 hours 1-to-10 times a day. The choice of stimulation parameters also depends on the presence of the so-called post-effect. Many, but not all patients, have their pain relieved or improved immediately or within 5'-60' during intra-operative stimulation for periods ranging from several minutes to hours or several days without further stimulation. This effect has a tendency to abate over time and by the second month may stabilize at several minutes to a few hours.

Analgesia also can fade over time. Repositioning of the electrode or intensive reprogramming may restore benefit in some cases, although at a lower level than before. Tolerance and fatigue are proposed mechanisms of such effects. Granulations and fibrosis around the contacts have been found in some failures (e.g. Hosomi et al 2008, Canavero and Bonicalzi 2002): surgical curettage may restore benefit.

8.2 Adverse and unusual effect

Permanent disabling morbidity (including epilepsy and intracerebral hemorrhage) and mortality have not been reported for the extradural approach, while there is a small such risk for the subdural approach. The most common adverse effect reported in the literature consists of short generalized seizures, all of which were observed during the initial testing phases. The literature does not reveal cases of epileptic seizures during chronic treatment for CP (Canavero and Bonicalzi 2002). Anti-epileptic medications are -or are not- administered for 1 to 6 months. Caution is however to be exercised when adjusting parameters even long after stimulation has been instituted. Infections are possible (but not meningitis/ encephalitis) and so are hardware failures. Extradural hematomas in need of evacuation are possible, but very rare. Worsening of original pain via ipsi- or contralateral stimulation of MI/ SI has been observed sporadically and one of our CP patients developed a painful supernumerary phantom arm after MCS (see Canavero et al 1999).

Analgesia via ipsilateral stimulation is on record. No major modification of cortical somatotopy is seen in these patients, but bilateral benefit from unilateral stimulation is possible and focal stimulation of the hand area also relieved hemisoma pain in one case (see in Canavero 2009).

A handful of patients with excellent initial analgesia and increasing periods of post-effect have not relapsed for years after switching off the stimulating apparatus, a sign of neuroplastic phenomena induced by M1 ICS in SI.

References

Andrè-Obadia N, Peyron R, Mertens P, et al. Transcranial magnetic stimulation for pain control. Double-blind study of different frequencies against placebo, and correlation with motor cortex stimulation efficacy. Clin. Neurophysiol. 2006; 117, 1536-1544.

Andre-Obadia, N, Mertens, MP, et al.. Is Life Better After Motor Cortex Stimulation for Pain Control? Results at Long-Term and their Prediction by Preoperative rTMS. Prospective Evaluation. Pain Physician 2014;17:53-62

Antal A, Terney D, Kuehnk S, Paulus W. Anodal transcranial direct current stimulation ameliorates chronic pain and reduces short intracortical inhibition. J Pain Symptom Manage 2010; 39: 890-903

Arle JE, Shils JL. Motor cortex stimulation for pain and movement disorders. Neurotherapeutics 2008; 5: 37-49.

Arle JE, Mei LZ, Shils JL. Modeling parkinsonian circuitry and the DBS electrode: I. Biophysical background and software. Stereotact Funct Neurosurg 2008;134:1-15.

Barraquer-Bordas L, Molet J, Pascual-sedano B, et al. Dolor central retardado asociado a hematoma subinsular seguido por tumor parietooccipital. Efecto favorable de la estimulacion cronica del nucleo VPL talamico. Rev Neurologia 1999; 29, 1044–1048.

Binder A, Schattschneider J, Wolff S, et al. Inhibition of human motor cortex by tonic cutaneous pain. A fMRI study. IASP Congress 2002, 1125-P41

Boggio PS, Amancio EJ, Correa CF, et al. Transcranial DC stimulation coupled with TENS for the treatment of chronic pain. A preliminary study. Clin J Pain 2009; 25: 691-695

Brodie EE, Kane FMA, Gijsbers K, et al. Contralateral limb movement modulates cold pressor pain. Acute Pain 2009; 11: 121-128

Brown JA, Pilitsis JG. Motor cortex stimulation for central and neuropathic facial pain: a prospective study of 10 patients and observations of enhanced sensory and motor function during stimulation. Neurosurgery 2005; 56, 290–297.

Canavero S, Bonicalzi V. Cortical stimulation for central pain. J Neurosurg 1995; 83, 1117.

Canavero S, Bonicalzi V. Review article. The neurochemistry of central pain: evidence from clinical studies, hypothesis and therapeutic implications. Pain 1998; 74: 109-114.

Canavero S, Bonicalzi V, Paolotti R, Cerutti A. Extradural cortical stimulation for neurogenic pain and Parkinson's disease: the Turin experience. Proceedings of the 4th International Congress of the International Neuromodulation Society, Luzern, August 20-26, 1998.

Canavero S, Bonicalzi V, Castellano G, et al. Painful supernumerary phantom arm following motor cortex stimulation for central post-stroke pain. J Neurosurg 1999; 91, 121–123.

Canavero S, Bonicalzi V, Dotta M, et al. Transcranial magnetic cortical stimulation relieves central pain. Stereotact Funct Neurosurg 2002; 78:192-196 (duplicate in: Neurol Res 2003; 25: 151-152)

Canavero S, Bonicalzi V. Therapeutic extradural cortical stimulation for central and neuropathic pain: a review. Clin J Pain 2002; 18, 48–55.

Canavero S, Bonicalzi V. Neuromodulation for central pain. Expert Rev Neurotherapeutics 2003; 3, 591–607.

Canavero S, Bonicalzi V. Transcranial magnetic stimulation for central pain. Curr Pain Headache Rep 2005; 9, 87–89.

Canavero S, Bonicalzi V, Intonti S, et al. Effects of bilateral extradural cortical stimulation for plegic stroke rehabilitation. Neuromodulation 2006; 9: 28-33

Canavero S, Bonicalzi V. Extradural cortical stimulation for central pain. In: D Sakas, B Simpson, E Krames, eds. Operative Neuromodulation. Vol.2. Wien: Springer-Verlag, 2007, 27-36.

Canavero S (Editor). Textbook of therapeutic cortical stimulation. New York: Nova Science, 2009

Canavero S. Surface stimulation. In Arle JE, Shils JL. Essential Neuromodulation. Elsevier-Academic Press, 2011, 19-42

Canavero S, Bonicalzi V. Central pain syndrome. Pathophysiology, diagnosis and management. 2nd ed. Cambridge: Cambridge University Press, 2011

Capel ID, Dorrell HM, Spencer EP, Davis MW. The amelioration of the suffering associated with spinal cord injury with subperception transcranial electrical stimulation. Spinal Cord 2003; 41: 109-117

Carroll D, Joint C, Maartens N, et al. Motor cortex stimulation for chronic neuropathic pain: a preliminary study of 10 cases. Pain 2000; 84: 431-437.

Cioni B, Meglio M. Motor cortex stimulation for chronic non-malignant pain: current state and future prospects. Acta Neurochir Suppl 97: 45-49.

Defrin R, Grunhaus L, Zamir D, et al. The effect of a series of repetitive transcranial magnetic stimulations of the motor cortex on central pain after spinal cord injury. Arch. Phys. Med. Rehabil. 2007; 88, 1574-1580.

Delavallée M, Abu-Serieh B, de Tourchaninoff M, et al. Subdural motor cortex stimulation for central and peripheral neuropathic pain: a long-term follow-up study in a series of eight patients. Neurosurgery. 2008;63:101-5.

De Ridder D, De Mulder G, Verstraeten E, et al. Somatosensory cortex stimulation for deafferentation pain. Acta Neurochir. Suppl. 2007; 97: 67-74.

Drouot X, Nguyen J-P, Peschanski M, et al. The antalgic efficacy of chronic motor cortex stimulation is related to sensory changes in the painful area. Brain 2002; 125, 1660–1664.

Fields HL, Adams JE. Pain after cortical injury relieved by electrical stimulation of the internal capsule. Brain 1974; 97, 169–178.

Finet P, Raftopoulos C. Interhemispheric subdural motor cortex stimulation : two cases. Surg Neurol 2009; 72: 522-523

Franzini A, Ferroli P, Dones I, et al. Chronic motor cortex stimulation for movement disorders: a promising perspective. Neurol Res 2003; 25, 123–126.

Fregni F, Boggio PS, Lima MC, et al. A sham-controlled, phase II trial of transcranial direct current stimulation for the treatment of central pain in traumatic spinal cord injury. Pain 2006; 122,197-209

Frighetto L, De Salles A, Wallace R et al. Linear accelerator thalamotomy. Surg Neurol 2004; 62, 106–113.

Fujii M, Ohmoto Y, Kitahara T et al. [Motor cortex stimulation therapy in patients with thalamic pain]. No Shinkei Geka 1997; 25, 315–319.

Fukaya C, Katayama Y, Yamamoto T et al. Motor cortex stimulation in patients with post-stroke pain: conscious somatosensory response and pain control. Neurol Res 2003; 25 : 153-156.

Garcia-Larrea L, Peyron R, Mertens P et al. Positron emission tomography during motor cortex stimulation for pain control. Stereotact Funct Neurosurg 1997; 68, 141–148.

Garcia-Larrea L, Peyron R, Mertens P et al. Electrical stimulation of motor cortex for pain control: a combined PET-scan and electrophysiological study. Pain 1999; 83, 259–273.

Garcia-Larrea L, Maarrawi J, Peyron et al. On the relation between sensory deafferentation, pain and thalamic activity in wallenberg's syndrome: a PET-scan study before and after motor cortex stimulation. Eur J Pain 2006; 10: 677-688

Gharabaghi A, Hellwig D, Rosahl SK et al. Volumetric image guidance for motor cortex stimulation: integration of three-dimensional cortical anatomy and functional imaging. Neurosurgery 2005; 57(ONS Suppl. 1), 114–120.

Goto T, Saitoh Y, Hashimoto N, et al. Diffusion tensor fiber tracking in patients with central post-stroke pain; correlation with efficacy of repetitive transcranial magnetic stimulation. Pain 2008; 140: 509-518

Henderson JM, Boongird A, Rosenow JM, et al Recovery of pain control by intensive reprogramming after loss of benefit from motor cortex stimulation for neuropathic pain. Stereotact Funct Neurosurg 2004; 82, 207–213.

Herregodts P, Stadnik T, Deridder F, et al. Cortical stimulation for central neuropathic pain: 3-D surface MRI for easy determination of the motor cortex. Acta Neurochir (Wien) 1995; Suppl 64, 132–135.

Hirayama A, Saitoh Y, Kishima H, et al. Reduction of intractable deafferentation pain by navigation-guided repetitive transcranial magnetic stimulation of the primary motor cortex. Pain 2006; 122:22 27

Holsheimer J, Lefaucheur J-P, Buitenweg JR, et al The role of intra-operative motor evoked potentials in the optimization of chronic cortical stimulation for the treatment of neuropathic pain. Clin Neurophysiol 2007 ; 118 : 2287-2296

Hosomi K, Saitoh Y, Kishima H, et al. Electrical stimulation of primary motor cortex within central sulcus for intractable neuropathic pain. Clin Neurophysiol 2008; 119: 993-1001.

Hosobuchi Y (1993) Motor cortical stimulation for control of central deafferentation pain. In Devinsky O, Beric A, Dogari M, eds., Electrical and Magnetic Stimulation of the Brain and Spinal Cord, Advances in Neurology Series. New York: Raven Press, pp. 215–217.

Ikeda A, Ohara S, Matsumoto R, et al.: Role of primary somatosensory corticies in generating inhibitory motor response in humans. Brain 2000;123:1710-1721.

Irlbacher K, Kuhnert J, Roericht S, et al. Zentrale und periphere Deafferenzierungsschmerzen: Therapie mit der repetitiven transkraniellen Magnetstimulation? Nervenarzt 2006; 77: 1196-1203.

Ito M, Kuroda S, Takano K, et al. [Motor cortex stimulation for post-stroke pain using neuronavigation and evoked potentials: report of 3 cases] No Shinkei Geka 2006; 34: 919-934.

Ito M, Kuroda S, Shiga T, et al. Motor cortex stimulation improves local cerebral glucose metabolism in the ipsilateral thalamus in patients with poststroke pain: case report. Neurosurgery. 2011;69:E462-9.

Johnson S, Summers J, Pridmore S. Changes to somatosensory detection and pain thresholds following high frequency repetitive TMS of the motor cortex in individuals suffering from chronic pain. Pain 2006; 123, 187-192.

Kang BS, Shin HI, Bang MS. Effect of repetitive transcranial magnetic stimulation over the hand motor cortical area on central pain after spinal cord injury. Arch Phys Med Rehabil 2009; 90: 1766-1771

Katayama Y, Tsubokawa T, Yamamoto T. Chronic motor cortex stimulation for central deafferentation pain: experience with bulbar pain secondary to Wallenberg syndrome. Stereotact Funct Neurosurg 1994;62:295-299.

Katayama Y, Fukaya C, Yamamoto T, Poststroke pain control by chronic motor cortex stimulation: neurological characteristics predicting a favorable response. J Neurosurg 1998; 89, 585–591.

Katayama Y, Yamamoto T, Kobayashi K et al. (2001) Motor cortex stimulation for post-stroke pain: comparison of spinal cord and thalamic stimulation. Stereotact Funct Neurosurg 2001; 77, 183–186.

Khedr EM, Korb L, Kamel NF, et al. Long-lasting antalgic effects of daily sessions of repetitive transcranial magnetic stimulation in central and peripheral neuropathic pain. J Neurol. Neurosurg. Psychiatr. 2005; 76, 833-838.

Kishima H, Saitoh Y, Osaki Y, et al. Motor cortex stimulation in patients with deafferentation pain : activation of the posterior insula and thalamus. J Neurosurg 2007; 107: 43-48

Kuroda R, Yamada Y, Kondo S et al. Electrical stimulation of the second somatosensory cortex for intractable pain: a case report and experimental study. Stereotact Funct Neurosurg 2000; 74, 226.

Lefaucheur JP, Drouot X, Menard-Lefaucheur L,et al. Neurogenic pain relief by repetitive transcranial magnetic cortical stimulation depends on the origin and the site of pain. J Neurol Neurosurg Psychiatry 2004; 75:612-616.
Lefaucheur JP, Ménard-Lefaucheur I, Goujon C, et al. Predictive value of rTMS in the identification of responders to epidural motor cortex stimulation therapy for pain. J Pain. 2011;12:1102-11.
Leo RJ, Latif T. Repetitive Transcranial Magnetic Stimulation (rTMS) in Experimentally Induced and Chronic Neuropathic Pain: A Review. J Pain 2007; 8, 453-459.
Liepert J, Restemeyer C, Muenchau A, Weiller C. Motor cortex excitability after thalamic infarction. Clin Neurophysiol 2005; 116, 1621–1627.
Lima MC, Fregni F. Motor cortex stimulation for chronic pain. Systematic review and meta-analysis of the literature. Neurology 2008; 70: 2329-2337.
Maarrawi J, Peyron R, Mertens P, et al. Motor cortex stimulation for pain control induces changes in the endogenous opioid system. Neurology 2007; 69: 827-834
Maarrawi J, Peyron R, Mertens P, et al. Brain opioid receptor density predicts motor cortex stimulation efficacy for chronic pain. Pain. 2013;154:2563-8.
Mandat T, Koziara H, Barszcz S, et al. Motor cortex stimulation in the treatment of neuropathic pain. Neurol Neurochir Pol 2012; 46:428-35
Meyerson BA, Lindblom U, Linderoth B, Lind B, Herregodts P. Motor cortex stimulation as treatment of trigeminal neuropathic pain. Acta Neurochir Suppl. 1993;58:150-153.
Migita K, Uozumi T, Arita K, Monden S. Transcranial magnetic coil stimulation of motor cortex in patients with central pain. Neurosurgery 1995; 36, 1037–1040.
Mogilner AY, Rezai AR. Epidural motor cortex stimulation with functional imaging guidance. Neurosurg Focus 2001; 11, article 4.
Molet J, Rodriguez R, Munoz F, et al. Estimulacion cortical para el tratamiento del dolor cronico neuropatico. Abstracts, Spanish Neurosurgical Society 2007 Congress, Zaragoza, 2007, p20.
Mondani M, D'Auria S, Ius T, et al. Refractory pain in patients with thalamic involvement. Results obtained by motor cortex stimulation. Acta Neurochir (Wien) 2008; 150: 968 (A09)
Montes C, Mertens P, Convers P et al. Cognitive effects of precentral cortical stimulation for pain control: an ERP study. Neurophysiol Clin 2002; 32, 313–325.
Montgomery EB Jr. Deep brain stimulation programming. Principles and practice. New York: Oxford University Press, 2010
Mori F, Codecà C, Kusayanagi H, et al. Effects of anodal transcranial direct current stimulation on chronic neuropathic pain in patients with multiple sclerosis. J Pain 2010; 11: 436-442
Nahmias F, Debes C, Ciampi De Andreade D, et al. Diffuse analgesic effects of unilateral repetitive transcranial magnetic stimulation (rTMS) in healthy volunteers. Pain 2009; 147; 224-232
Nandi D, Smith H, Owens S, et al. Periventricular gray stimulation versus motor cortex stimulation for poststroke neuropathic pain. J Clin Neurosci 2002; 9: 557-561.
Nguyen JP, Lefacheur JP, Decq P et al. Chronic motor cortex stimulation in the treatment of central and neuropathic pain: correlations between clinical, electrophysiological and anatomical data. Pain 1999; 82, 245–251.
Nguyen JP, Velasco F, Brugieres P, et al. Treatment of chronic neuropathic pain by motor cortex stimulation: results of a bicentric controlled crossover trial. Brain Stimulation 2008; 1: 89-96
Nguyen JP, Lefaucheur JP, Raoul S, et al. Motor cortex stimulation for the treatment of neuropathic pain. In: Krames E, Peckham PH, Rezai AR (eds) Neuromodulation. London: Academic Press, 2009, pp 515-526
Nuti C, Peyron R, Garcia-Larrea L, et al. Motor cortex stimulation for refractory neuropathic pain: four year outcome and predictors of efficacy. Pain 2005; 118, 43-52
O'Connell NE, Wand BM, Marston L, et al. Non-invasive brain stimulation techniques for chronic pain. Cochrane Database Syst Rev 2010; 9: CD008208

Ohn SH, Chang WH, Park CH, et al. Neural correlates of the antinociceptive effects of repetitive transcranial magnetic stimulation on central pain after stroke. Neurorehabil Neural Repair. 2012;26:344-52

Pagni CA, Canavero S. Functional thalamic depression in a case of reversibile central pain due to a spinal intramedullary cyst. J Neurosurg 1995; 83: 163-165

Peyron R, Garcia -Larrea L, Deiber MP et al. Electrical stimulation of precentral cortical area in the treatment of central pain: electrophysiological and PET study. Pain 1995; 62, 275–286.

Peyron R, Faillenot I, Mertens P, et al. Motor cortex stimulation in neuropathic pain. Correlations between analgesic effect and hemodynamic changes in the brain. A PET study. Neuroimage 2007; 34: 310-321

Pirotte B, Voordecker P, Neugroschl C et al. Combination of functional magnetic resonance imaging-guided neuronavigation and intraoperative cortical brain mapping improves targeting of motor cortex stimulation in neuropathic pain. Neurosurgery 2005; 56(ONS Suppl. 2), 344–359.

Rasche D, Ruppolt M, Stippich C, et al.Motor cortex stimulation for long-term relief of chronic neuropathic pain: a 10 year experience. Pain 2006; 121, 43-52

Reyns N, Houdayer E, Bourriez JL, et al. Motor cortex stimulation-induced modulation of central beta rhythms and somatosensory evoked potentials. A correlation with its analgesic effect. Acta Neurochir (Wien) 2008; 150: 970-971

Reyns N, Derambure P, Duhamel A, et al. Motor cortex stimulation modulates defective central beta rhythms in patients with neuropathic pain. Clin Neurophysiol. 2013;124:761-9

Rodriguez RF, Contreras N. Bilateral motor cortex stimulation for the relief of central dysesthetic pain and intentional tremor secondary to spinal cord surgery: a case report. Neuromodulation 2002; 5: 189–195.

Rollnik JD, Wustefeld S, Dauper J, et al. Repetitive transcranial magnetic stimulation for the treatment of chronic pain: A pilot study. Eur Neurol 2002; 48:6-10.

Roux FE, Ibarrola D, Lazorthes Y, Berry I. Chronic motor cortex stimulation for phantom limb pain: a functional magnetic resonance imaging study: technical case report. Neurosurgery. 2001; 48:681-7.

Saitoh Y, Kato A, Ninomiya H et al. Primary motor cortex stimulation within the central sulcus for treating deafferentation pain. Acta Neurochir Suppl 2000; 87: 149–152.

Saitoh Y, Kato A, Ninomiya H, al.: Primary motor cortex stimulation within the central sulcus for treating deafferentation pain. Acta Neurochir Suppl 2003;87:149-152.

Saitoh Y, Osaki Y, Nishimura H et al. Increased regional cerebral blood flow in the contralateral thalamus after successful motor cortex stimulation in a patient with poststroke pain. J Neurosurg 2004; 100: 935–939.

Saitoh Y, Hirayama A, Kishima H et al. Reduction of intractable cleafferentation pain due to spinal cord or peripheral lesion by high-frequency repetitive transcranial magnetic stimulation of the primary motor cortex. J Neurosurg. 2007; 107, 555-559.

Sakas DE, Flaskas TN, Panourias IG, et al. Bifocal cortical electrical stimulation for pain by interdural implantation of the electrodes. J Neurosurg 2011 ;114(1):180-5

Savas A, Kanpolat Y. Comment. Neurosurgery 2005; 56, 296.

Schoenen J, Grant G. Spinal cord: connections. In Paxinos G, Mai JK, eds., The Human Nervous System, 2nd edn. Amsterdam: Elsevier Academic Press 2004; pp. 233–250.

Seyal M, Shatzel AJ, Richardson SP. Crossed inhibition of sensory cortex by 0.3Hz transcranial magnetic stimulation of motor cortex. J Clin Neurophysiol 2005; 22: 418-421.

Shabalov VA, Isagulyan ED, Tomskiy AA. Motor cortex stimulation in the treatment of central pain syndromes. Acta Neurochir (Wien) 2008; 150: 968 A11

Slawek J, Reclowicz D, Zielinski P, et al. [Motor cortex stimulation in the central pain syndrome] Neurol Neurochir Pol 2005; 39: 237-240.

Smith E, Joint C, Nandi D, Stein JF, et al. Motor cortex stimulation for neuropathic pain. Neurosurg Focus 2000;11: E2.
Sokal P, Harat M, Gryz J, et al. [Motor cortex stimulation in the treatment of the central pain: a case report] Neurol Neurochir Pol 2006; 40: 253-257.
Sol JC, Casaux J, Roux FE, et al. Chronic motor cortex stimulation for phantom limb pain: correlations between pain relief and functional imaging studies. Stereotact Funct Neurosurg 2001; 77: 172-176.
Soler D, Kumru H, Vidal J, et al. Transcranial direct current stimulation (tDCS) and virtual reality (VR) techniques for treatment of neuropathic central pain in spinal cord injury (NP-SCI). Eur J Pain 2010; Suppl.4 p105 A370
Soler MD, Kumru H, Pelayo R, et al. Effectiveness of transcranial direct current stimulation and visual illusion on neuropathic pain in spianl cord injury. Brain 2010; 133: 2565-77
Son BC, Lee SW, Choi ES, et al.: Motor cortex stimulation for central pain following a traumatic brain injury. Pain 2006;123:210-216.
Tan G, Rintala DH, Thornby JI, et al. Using cranial electrotherapy stimulation to treat pain associated with spinal cord injury. J Rehabil Res Dev 2006; 43: 461-474
Tanei T, Kajita Y, Wakabayashi T. Motor cortex stimulation for intractable neuropathic facial pain related to multiple sclerosis. Neurol Med Chir (Tokyo) 2010; 50: 604-607
Tani N, Saitoh Y, Hirata M, et al.: Bilateral cortical stimulation for deafferentation pain after spinal cord injury, J Neurosurg 2004;101:687–689.
Tasker RR, Parrent AG, Kiss Z, et al. Surgical treatment of stroke-induced pain. Stereotact Funct Neurosurg 1994; 62, 311-312.
Terney D, Bergmann I, Poreisz C, et al. Pergolide increases the efficacy of cathodal direct current stimulation to reduce the amplitude of laser-evoked potential in humans. J Pain Symptom Man 2008; 36: 79-91.
Tirakotai W, Riegel T, Sure U, et al. Image-guided motor cortex stimulation in patients with central pain. Minim Invas Neurosurg 2004;47:273-277.
Tronnier V, Rasche D. Precentral stimulation for different neuropathic pain syndromes.clinical experience of 15 years. Eur J Pain 2009; 13: S48 A138
Tsubokawa T, Katayama Y, Yamamoto T, et al.: Chronic motor cortex stimulation for the treatment of central pain. Acta Neurochirurgica Suppl 1991;52:137-139.
Tsubokawa T., Katayama Y., Yamamoto T., et al. Treatment of thalamic pain by chronic motor cortex stimulation. PACE - Pacing Clin. Electrophysiol 1991; 14: 131—134
Tsubokawa T, Katayama Y, Yamamoto T, et al. Chronic motor cortex stimulation in patients with thalamic pain. J Neurosurg 1993;78:393-401.
Tsubokawa T., Katayama Y., Yamamoto T., et al. Treatment of deafferentation pain with thalamic and motor cortex stimulation: possible role of reorganization of neural circuits, VIIth World Congress on Pain. Book of Abstracts, 1993b, IASP Publications, Seattle. pp. 504-505.
Turk DC, Dworkin RH, McDermott MP, et al. Analyzing multiple endpoints in clinical trials of pain treatment: IMMPACT recommendations. Pain 2008; 139: 485-493
Vargas Lópes AJ, Carballal C, González Quaranta LH, et al. Motor cortex stimulation in the interhemispheric subdural space as treatment of neuropathic pain in the lower limbs. Neurologia 2014; 29: 310-1
Velasco M, Velasco F, Brito F, et al. Motor cortex stimulation in the treatment of deafferentation pain. I. Localisation of the motor cortex. Stereotact Funct Neurosurg 2002; 79: 146-167.
Velasco F, Arguelles C, Carrillo-Ruiz JD, et al. Efficacy of motor cortex stimulation in the treatment of neuropathic pain: a randomized double-blind trial. J Neurosurg 2008; 108: 698-706.
Vesper J. Chronic motor cortex stimulation and predictive value of rTMS. Eur J Pain 2010 suppl.4 p.135 A476

Wongsarnpigoon A, Grill WM. Optimization of parameter selection and electrical targeting. In: Canavero S (Editor). Textbook of therapeutic cortical stimulation. New York: Nova Science, 2009, pp 69-90

Yamamoto T, Katayama Y, Hirayama T, et al. Pharmacological classification of central post-stroke pain: comparison with the results of chronic motor cortex stimulation therapy. Pain 1997; 72, 5–12.

Yamamoto T. Katayama Y, Fukaya C, et al.Thalamotomy caused by cardioversion in a patient treated with deep brain stimulation. Stereotact Funct Neurosurg 2000; 74: 73-82

Walter Fagundes, Sergio Dantas

9 Peripheral Neuropathic Pain

Peripheral Neuropathic Pain (PNP) is defined as a pain initiated or caused by a primary lesion or dysfunction of the peripheral nervous system. It is a common disorder that can severely impact physical and psychological health with detrimental effects on individual quality of life, employment, and economic well-being. PNP is a significant health problem and one of the most difficult conditions to treat in clinical practice. Patients suffering of chronic PNP are twice as likely to commit suicide (lifetime prevalence of attempted suicide: about 10%). Chronic PNP may be due to trauma, inflammation, metabolic diseases, tumors and iatrogenic causes, among others. The extracerebral part of the cranial nerves is considered peripheral. In this chapter, the use of ICS (generally M1 ICS) is reviewed as regards PNP in its several permutations.

9.1 Results

A review of the world literature since 1993 allows us to break down results according to the types of PNP. It is more than likely that many more patients have been treated by this technique than have been included in published data. In order to reduce duplications, we considered only the latest work by the same group. However, problems exist in the relevant literature. A lack of consistency exists across studies in outcome reporting methods: some authors refer to VAS scale variations, others rate outcomes as “excellent”, ”good”, ”fair”, ”poor”. In this latter instance, 40% relief is considered a good outcome in some series, whereas others consider a good result a >50% pain abatement. Reports vary considerably in terms of surgical technique, too (e.g. subdural vs epidural ICS). Last, but not least, most studies reported in the literature thus far are observational cohorts or retrospective analyses. Fortunately, controlled trials exist that prove that ICS has effects above placebo (Rasche et al 2006: 1-week test trial; Nguyen et al 2008 and Velasco et al 2008,2009: ICS randomized to ON or OFF condition at 2 or 3 months postoperatively for 2 weeks or 1 month; Lefaucheur et al 2009).

9.1.1 Trigeminal PNP

Undoubtedly, M1 ICS appears to be the treatment of choice for this condition, given the high number of long-term responders (Table 9.1). It is both superior and safer than DBS.

Table 9.1: Trigeminal Neuropathic Pain (TNP)* and allied conditions (all M1 ICS)

Authors	Type of Facial pain (number of patients treated)	Results (follow-up)	Notes/Parameters
Meyerson et al (1993)	TNP (5)	Pain relief 5/5 60 – 90% (8 - 28 mos)	Epidural Lead Quadripolar, parallel to CS, 70-80% MT, 300μs, 50 Hz Intermittent
Herregodts et al (1995)	TNP (5)	Pain relief 4/5 > 50% VAS (10-22 mos)	Epidural Lead Quadripolar, parallel to CS, 4-8V; 50-75Hz 3D MRI reconstruction
Ebel et al (1996)	Anesthesia Dolorosa (6)	Pain relief 5/6 5 pts: > 80% 2 pts: < 40% (5 - 24 mos)	Epidural Lead Quadripolar, parallel to CS, 3.5-10.5V; 180-350 μs; 60-130 Hz Postictal speech arrest duiring testing – IPG not implanted
Gonzáles-Martinez et al (2002) Includes: Mogilner and Rezai (2001)	Atypical facial pain (8)	Pain relief 8/8 7 > 50-60% 1 = 30% (13.8 m)	Epidural Lead, neuronavigation 1 quadripolar electrode (4) 2 quadripolar electrodes (4) 2-8V; 210-250μs; 50-110 Hz Cycling Seizure episode
Rainov et al (2003) Includes : Rainov et al (1997)	Trigeminal Neuralgia (1) Glossopharyngeal Neuralgia (1)	Pain relief: 2/2 VAS from 7 to 3 (TN) (f-up: 69-72 mos)	Epidural Lead 5-9.5V, 300-400μs,100-120 Hz Intermittent use (6-9h daily)
Canavero e Bonicalzi (2002)	- trigeminal neuropathic pain (5) (after trigeminal nerve procedures, anesthesia dolorosa)	Pain relief 2/5 All lost pain relief between 3 and 6 mos postop	Epidural Lead, quadripolar, parallel to CS
Henderson et al (2004)	Facial Pain (1)	Pain Relief 1/1 (F-up: ?)	Epidural Lead, parallel to CS 1.7-9.5V; 240-390μs; 50-110Hz
Brown and Pilitisis (2005)	TNP (5)	Pain relief 4/5 implanted Drug intake reduction (3 – 24 mos)	Epidural Lead, parallel to CS 2-10A; 90-240μs - 40Hz

continued **Table 9.1:** Trigeminal Neuropathic Pain (TNP)* and allied conditions (all M1 ICS)

Authors	**Type of Facial pain (number of patients treated)**	**Results (follow-up)**	**Notes/Parameters**
Pirotte et al (2005)	TNP (5)	Pain relief 4/5 (VAS reduced >70%) (6 – 60 mos)	Lead epidural, cross 1-5V; 100μs; 40Hz
Gharabaghi et al. (2005)	TNP (2)	Pain relief 2/2 (14-40 mos)	Epidural Lead 75% MT; 200μs; 20-70Hz
Maarrawi et al (2007)	TNP (trauma) (1)	30% VAS pain relief FU (ns)	Epidural Lead, Quadripolar Parameters ns
Cioni and Meglio (2007)	TNP (5)	Pain relief 1/5 (another successful, then failure, then recaptured, then failure again) (FU ns)	Epidural Lead Parameters ns
Hosomi et al. (2008) *(Saitoh Osaka Group)* Includes: Saitoh et al (2000) Saitoh et al (2001) Saitoh et al (2003) Saitoh et al (2006)	TNP (1)	Pain relief 1/1 93% VAS reduction during test stimulation (< 6 mos)	Subdural Lead, Quadripolar, 0.9-5V; 200μs, 25-50 Hz
Delavallée et al (2008) Delavallee et al (2011)	TNP (3) TNP (1) (child)	Pain relief 3/3 2 = 80-100% 1=40-59% (19-69 mos) 100% relief and drugs reduction (then infection, explantation, full relape, reimplantation with full analgesia)	Subdural Lead, Octopolar, neuronavigation Oblique, intermittent, 1.5-4V; 210μs; 45-80Hz Wound infection, seizures. Subdural Lead, Octopolar (Specify), continuous, bipolar, 90Hz, 50μs, 2.5V

continued Table 9.1: Trigeminal Neuropathic Pain (TNP)* and allied conditions (all M1 ICS)

Authors	Type of Facial pain (number of patients treated)	Results (follow-up)	Notes/Parameters
Rasche and Tronnier (2009) Includes: Rasche et al (2006)	TNP & other facial pains (e.g. trigeminal neuralgia) (17)	Test passed: 10/17 Long-term relief 7/10 >50% VAS reduction (f-up: >3 years)	Epidural Lead, Quadripolar 2-7mA, 30-85Hz, 210-300 μs, continuous/cycling, quadri/octopolar, parallel/cross to CS
Nguyen et al (2009) Includes: Nguyen et al (1997, 1999, 2000, 2004, 2008, 2009a) Drout et al (2002)	TNP (31)	Pain relief in 25pts (29-170 mos)	Epidural Lead, Quadripolar, cross, Neuronavigation 1.0-3.5V; 60-150μs; 25-60Hz, cycling
Lefaucheur et al (2009)	Treated idiopathic trigeminal neuralgia (3) Secondary trigeminal neuralgia (1) Atypical Orofacial pain (1)	-Pain relief 2/3 (VAS reduced 66% and 86%) -Failure 1/1 -Pain relief 1/1(45% VAS reduction) (ns)	Epidural Lead, Quadripolar, perpendicular to CS, 2-3V; 60μs; 40-50Hz
Fontaine et al (2009)	TNP (trauma) (1)	Pain relief 1/1 VAS from 8 to 2 (drugs reduced),both constant an paroxysmal (f-up: 18 mos)	Epidural leads (2), perpendicular to CS, 3V, 40Hz, 210μs <u>Renormalization of thermal & tactile thresholds (i.e. M1 ICS modulates sensory processing)</u>
Anderson et al (2009)	TNP (1)	VAS 10 to 6-8, relapse 5 weeks later, reprogramming: pain (and dysphagia) controlled, battery depletion with full relapse, IPG replaced with analgesia	Perpendicular to CS, iBS 5Hz/250μs, cyclical (36hrs ON, 12hrs OFF), 2V, 5Hz, then 7.8V, 60Hz, 5.8mA

continued **Table 9.1:** Trigeminal Neuropathic Pain (TNP)* and allied conditions (all M1 ICS)

Authors	Type of Facial pain (number of patients treated)	Results (follow-up)	Notes/Parameters
Vesper (2010)	TNP (1)	Pain relief 1/1 (>50%) Drugs reduction (f-up: >1 year)	RTMS +
Sakas et al (2010)	TNP (2)	Pain relief 2/2 100% and 80% VAS reduction with combined M1+S1 ICS (f-up: 12-15 mos)	Interdural Lead 2 octopolar, perpendicular to CS, 3D MRI reconstruction, Neuronavigation Pt1 : 4-5mA, 120Hz, 150μs, cyclical (15'ON,60'OFF) Pt 2 : 3mA,66Hz,350μs, cyclical (30' ON, 60'OFF) NB: M1+S1 ICS>>M1 ICS>>S1 ICS
Fagundes-Pereyra et al (2010) Includes: Fagundes-Pereyra et al (2007)	TNP (1)	Pain relief 1/1 VAS 50% (21 mos)	Epidural Lead, Quadripolar, parallel to CS 2.6-4.5V; 100-500μs;45-60 Hz
Raslan et al (2011) (Burchiel's group)	TNP (10)	Pain relief 5/8 pts (6-72 mos); Unsatisfactory relief after 6.5/36 mos in 3/8 (+2 initial test failures)	Epidural Lead, quadri- or octopolar (Specify), parallel to CS, 2-5V; 120-450μs; 30-50Hz, Neuronavigation Average programming sessions were 1.55/year (5 patients who sustained long-term pain control) and 3.33 for short-term responders (3: 6 mos,6mos, 36 mos). 1-9 (mean 4) reprogramming sessions. Patients with anesthesia dolorosa or trigeminal deafferentation pain who had previously undergone ablative trigeminal procedures responded poorly to MCS.
Esfahani et al (2011)	TNP (2)	Pain relief 2/2 VAS from 8-10 to 1-2 (78 mos) and 9-10 to 1-2 (60 mos)	Subdural Lead, 5-6-5 polar SPECIFY grid, Resore Ultra, parallel to CS, Neuronavigation 3-T fMRI, 0.2-3V (mean1.6V), 93μs; 43Hz

continued Table 9.1: Trigeminal Neuropathic Pain (TNP)* and allied conditions (all M1 ICS)

Authors	Type of Facial pain (number of patients treated)	Results (follow-up)	Notes/Parameters
Mandat et al (2012)	TNP (11)	Pain relief (nr:?) (3 mos)	RTMS+
André-Obadia et al (2014)	TNP (4)	Pain relief 4/4 (6.1± 2.6 y) Improved QoL	Epidural Lead, Quadripolar (1 or 2), 3D MRI and neuronavigation 1.5 – 4.5V; 60µs; 25-50Hz
TOTAL	140	97	-

*After dental surgery, ENT surgery, trigeminal nerve injury e.g. after tumor (e.g. cavernous sinus) surgery/fibrous dysplasia surgery, percutaneous/intracranial/radiosurgical procedures for trigeminal neuralgia, trauma, etc...

9.1.2 Plexopathies

ICS can only be considered after failed attempts at spinal cord stimulation or intrathecal drug infusion. The efficacy (Table 9.2) appears to be equivalent to DBS, but no technique has so far proved better than DREZ lesions. However, this latter is an ablative technique and should thus be reserved to patients who failed neuromodulation or understand the risks of neuroablation.

Table 9.2: Brachial Plexus Avulsion (all M1 ICS)

Authors	Brachial Plexus Avulsion (number of patients)	Results (follow-up)	Notes/Parameters
Smith et al (2001)	1	0% relief	Epidural Lead, Quadripolar, parallel to CS, 2.5-7V;450µs; 25-75 Hz
Mogilner and Rezai (2001)	1	55% pain relief (6 mos)	Epidural Lead, Functional imaging guidance 2-8V; 210µs,110 Hz cycling

continued **Table 9.2:** Brachial Plexus Avulsion (all M1 ICS)

Authors	Brachial Plexus Avulsion (number of patients)	Results (follow-up)	Notes/Parameters
Nuti et al (2005) *(Lyon Group)* Includes: García-Larrea et al (1997) García-Larrea et al (1999) Mertens et al (1999) Sindou et al. (1999) Montes et al (2002)	2	Pain relief 1/2 > 40% VAS (1 pt refused to discontinue M1 ICS) (2 – 6 mos)	Epidural Lead, Quadripolar, parallel to CS, 1.3-4V; 60-330µs ;30-80 Hz cycling
Pirotte et al. (2005)	2	Failures (4-60 mos)	Epidural Lead, Quadripolar 1-5V; 100µs,40 Hz
Nuti et al. (2005) Includes: Mertens et al (1999)	4	Pain relief 1/4 (VAS –43%) (60 mos) (at 1 mo, all 4 had >30% VAS relief)	Lead epidural, Quadripolar 1-5V; 100 s,40 Hz
Kishima et al (2007) *(Saitoh's Group)*	3	Pain relief 3/3 Median VAS from 8.2 to 3.9 (FU ns)	Subdural Lead, quadripolar 0.6-3.5V; 210µs, 25-40 Hz cycling
Hosomi et al. (2008) *(Saitoh Osaka Group)* Includes: Saitoh et al (2000) Saitoh et al (2001) Saitoh et al (2003) Saitoh et al (2006)	7	Pain relief 3/7 1 = 80% 1 = 50%) 1 = 57% (19-112 mos)	Subdural intrasulcal lead, Pharmacological tests, 0.9-5V; 200µs, 25-50 Hz 1 repositioning of an electrode from epidural to subdural, 2 removals after 9 and 76 mo 1 death after 36 mo (ICH)
Delavallée et al (2008)	1	Pain relief VAS from 9 to 4 (54.2 mos)	Subdural Lead, Octopolar Oblique, Intermittent, neuronavigation 2.5V; 210µs; 60Hz
Velasco et al. 2008	1	Pain relief <40% (12 mos)	Epidural Lead, Quadripolar, parallel to CS, 2.0-7.0V; 90µs; 40 Hz

continued Table 9.2: Brachial Plexus Avulsion (all M1 ICS)

Authors	Brachial Plexus Avulsion (number of patients)	Results (follow-up)	Notes/Parameters
Teixeira et al (2008)	8	Pain relief : 5 good/excel-lent 1 fair 2 bad/none (f-up: 12 mos)	RTMS + (suggested better response if wider area on scalp evoking contralat.limb paresthesias during rTMS, statistically insignificant association)
Rasche and Tronnier (2009)	3	Pain relief 2/3 at long term (3/3 at test) VAS reduced >50% (f-up: >36 mos)	Epidural Lead, Quadripolar 2-7mA, 30-85Hz, 210-300 µs, continuous/cycling, quadri/octopolar, parallel/perpendicular to CS
Lefaucheur et al (2009)	5 (4 incomplete, 1 complete)	Pain relief 2/4 (VAS −50-72%) Pain relief 1/1 (VAS −95%)	Epidural Lead, Quadripolar, perpendicular to CS, 2-3V; 60µs; 40-50Hz
Nguyen et al (2009) *(Creteil, Nguyen Group)* Includes: Nguyen et al (1997, 1999, 2000, 2004, 2008, 2009a) Drout et al (2002)	11	Pain relief 4/11 (VAS reduced at least 40%) (29-170 mo)	Epidural Lead, Quadripolar, perpendicular to CS, Neuronavigation, 1.0-3.5V; 60-150µs; 25-60Hz cyclical
Vesper (2010)	1	Pain relief (VAS −50%) (f-up: > 12 mos)	RTMS +
Fagundes-Pereyra et al (2010) Includes: Fagundes-Pereyra et al (2007)	11	Pain relief 6/11 > 50% VAS (23.4 mo)	Epidural Lead, Quadripolar, parallel to CS, 3D MRI reconstruction Robot assistance (in 6 patients) 2.2-5.1V; 100-500µs;45-60 Hz
André-Obadia et al (2014)	2	Pain relief 2/2 (6.1± 2.6 y) Improve QoL	Epidural Lead, Quadripolar (1 or 2) 3D MRI and neuronavigation, 1.5 – 4.5V; 60µs; 25-50Hz (whole mixed series)
TOTAL	63	34	-

9.1.3 Phantom and stump pain

Here, again, ICS can only be considered after failed attempts at spinal cord stimulation and intrathecal drug infusion. The efficacy (Table 9.3) appears to be equivalent to DBS.

Table 9.3: Post-amputation Phantom Limb (PLP) and Stump (SP) Pain.

Authors	Type of pain (number of patients)	Results (follow-up)	Notes/Parameters
Meyerson et al. (1993)	PLP (1)	0%	Epidural Lead, Quadripolar, parallel to CS 70-80% MT, 300μ, 50 Hz Intermittent
Sol et al (2001) Includes: Roux et al (2000)	PLP (2) PLP+BPA (1)	Pain relief 3/3 (drugs reduced) (activity/rest) 1 = 80/100% 1 = 40/70% 1 = 80% after repositioning (paddle on face M1 area: however for 4 mos, analgesia) (f-up: 24 - 29 mo)	Epidural Lead, Quadripolar, fMRI, neuronavigation, 3V;180-210μs; 40 Hz SCS ineffective in all iBS up to 12 mA: no motor response
Smith et al (2001) Includes: Carroll et al (2000)	PLP (2) PLP+SP (1)	Pain relief 2/3 (70 and 75%) (27-30 mo) SP: no relief	Epidural Lead, Quadripolar, parallel to CS 2.5-7V; 450μs; 25-75Hz, cycling mode, Electrodes repositioned in 2 pts. Two-stage procedure (craniotomy + electrode implantation)
Katayama et al (2001)	PLP (5: 2 with BPA)	Pain relief: 2 (both with BPA) A: >80% (>24 mos) B: <50% (> 24 mo)	Lead epidural, Quadripolar, parallel 2-8V; 100-500s; 25-50Hz SCS ineffective in all Vc DBS less effective in A, more in B
Canavero e Bonicalzi (2002)	PLP+SP (1)	Pain relief 1/1 (months)	Epidural Lead, Quadripolar, parallel to CS

continued Table 9.3: Post-amputation Phantom Limb (PLP) and Stump (SP) Pain.

Authors	Type of pain (number of patients)	Results (follow-up)	Notes/Parameters
Nandi et al (2004)	PLP+SP (1)	Pain Relief VAS from 8.9 to 1.9 (48 mos)	Epidural Lead, Quadripolar, parallel to CS, Parameters ns After 4 years no more pain relief and submitted to DBS
Pirotte et al (2005)	PLP (2)	Pain relief 1/2 (<75%) (22 mos)	
Nuti et al (2005) Includes: García-Larrea et al (1997) García-Larrea et al (1999) Mertens et al (1999) Sindou et al. (1999) Montes et al (2002)	PLP (2)	Pain relief 1/2 80% VAS <20% VAS (2 – 6 mos)	Subdural Lead (Interhemispheric), Quadripolar, parallel to CS, 1.3-4V; 25-55 Hz cycling
Koppelstaetter et al (2007)	PLP (1)	Pain relief VAS −70% (6 mos)	SCS ineffective
Hosomi et al. (2008) Includes: Saitoh et al (2000) Saitoh et al (2001) Saitoh et al (2003) Saitoh et al (2006)	PLP (3) PLP+SP (1)	Pain relief 1/4 90% VAS (54mos)	Subdural lead (Interhemispheric), 1 or 2 electrodes grids. Pharmacological tests 0.9-5V; 200μs, 25-50 Hz removal in 2 patients after 6 mos
Finet & Raftopoulos (2009)	PLP+SP (1)	Pain relief (excellent)	Subdural lead (8 contact)
Fagundes-Pereyra et al (2010) Includes: Fagundes-Pereyra et al (2007)	PLP (3)	Pain relief 2/3 (21-36 mos)	Epidural Lead, Quadripolar, parallel to CS, 3D MRI reconstruction Robot assistance (in 2 patients) 2-3.3V; 100-500μs;45-60 Hz
Sakas et al (2010)	PLP (1)	Pain relief 1/1 (90% relief with M1+S1 ICS; M1/S1>S1>M1) (9 mos)	Interdural Lead, 2 octopolar, perpendicular to CS, 3D MRI reconstruction Neuronavigation 3.5mA; 250μs;180 Hz
TOTAL	28	17	-

9.1.4 Postherpetic Neuralgia

Data is not yet sufficient to make a strong statement, but ICS appears to carry benefit for these patients (Table 9.4).

Table 9.4: Postherpetic Neuralgia (PHN)

Authors	**Posthepetic Neuralgia (Number of patients)**	**Results (follow-up)**	**Notes/Parameters**
Henderson et al (2004)	1	Pain Relief 1/1 (FU ns)	Epidural Lead, parallel to CS 1.7-9.5mA; 240-390µs; 50-110Hz
Brown and Pilitisis (2005)	2	Pain relief 2/2 Drug intake reduction (3 – 24 mos)	Epidural Lead, parallel to CS 2.0-8.0mA; 90-240µs;40Hz
Cioni and Meglio (2007)	2	0%	Epidural Lead Multipolar grid Several combinations
Velasco et al. (2008)	3	Pain relief 3/3 (56%, 75% and 80% on VAS) Improvement on MQP scores (12 mos)	Epidural Lead Quadripolar, parallel to CS 2.0-7.0V; 90µs; 40 Hz, cycling Prospective, randomized, double blind-trial
Nguyen et al (2009) Includes: Nguyen et al (1997, 1999, 2000, 2004, 2008, 2009a) Drout et al (2002)	2	Pain relief 1/2 40% VAS = 1 (29-170 mos)	Epidural Lead Quadripolar, perpendicular to CS Neuronavigation 1.0-3.5V; 60-150µs; 25-60Hz cycling
Lefaucheur et al (2009)	1	0%	Epidural Lead, Quadripolar, perpendicular to CS 2-3V; 60µs; 40-50Hz
Esfahani et al (2011)	1	Pain relief 1/1 VAS from 9-10 to 0 (FU ns)	Subdural Lead, Quadripolar, parallel to CS, Neuronavigation 3-T fMRI 1.6V; 93µs; 43Hz
TOTAL	12	8	-

9.1.5 Complex Regional Pain Syndromes

Neuromodulation plays a role in the treatment of these conditions, but ICS must be considered -at present- investigational (Table 9.5).

Table 9.5: CRPS I & II

Authors	**CRPS (Number of patients)**	**Results (follow-up)**	**Notes/Parameters**
Son et al (2003)	CRPS II (1)	Pain relief 1/1 (VAS9.5 to 1) Improvement in hyperalgia and allodynia (12 mos) hemisoma pain (burning and evoked pain) relieved (10-20% leg-90% arm)	Epidural Lead, Quadripolar, parallel to CS, neuronavigation 2.5V;450μs; 50 Hz cycling (50'ON, 10'OFF), 0-3+ motor deficit regressed
Velasco et al. 2009 Includes: Velasco et al (2008)	CRPS I/II due to: BPA (3) Parkes-Weber (hemangiectasia) Syndrome (1) Scleroderma (1)	Pt 1 (BPA): VAS9 to 1-4 (relapse due to fibrosis, excision, VAS 1-3, back to work; f-up: 84 mos) Pt 2 (PWS): VAS10 to 0, drugs OFF (60 mos), relapse due to migration, repositioning,VAS0 at long term, drugs OFF Pt 3(BPA): 0% Pt 4 (BPA): VAS10 to 2,breakage due to head trauma, DREZ Pt 5 (SD): VAS10 to 2 (36 mos) Sympathetic signs disappeared shortly after starting ICS Both spontaneous and evoked pains allayed	Epidural Lead, Quadripolar, parallel or perpendicular to CS, cycling (1h ON, 4h OFF), 2.0-3.5V (median 2.8V); 90μs; 40 Hz (up to 7V, 450μs,130Hz during test in unresponsive pt; up to 10.5V, 450μs, 6-10Hz in 2 reoperated pts with impedance>2000Ω) 20 contact-grid-contact during test period Analgesia only if motricity preserved at least partially and no area of anesthesia inside the painful territory *Relief always with contacts separated by 1-2 cm* Prospective, double blind-trial
Fonoff et al (2011) Includes: Fonoff et al (2007)	(2)	Pain relief 2/2 VAS 9 to 3 and 10 to 4 Improvement in allodynia (27-36 mo)	Epidural Lead, quadripolar, parallel to CS, 3-3.6V; 210μs; 10 Hz

9.1.6 Miscellaneous PNPs

Again, ICS appears to have effects (Table 9.6), but the case-load is still too limited to draw overarching conclusions.

Table 9.6: Miscellaneous PNPs

Authors	Type of pain (number of patients)	Results (follow-up)	Notes/Parameters
Meyerson et al. (1993)	- Peripheral nerve injury (shoulder) (1)	Pain relief > 50%	Epidural Lead Quadripolar, parallel to CS, 70-80% MT, 300μs, 50 Hz Intermittent
Rainov et al (1997)	- Glossopharyngeal neuralgia (after cervical lymph-node biopsy) (1)	Pain relief 1/1 VAS from 8 to 2 (18 mos)	Lead epidural 5-6V, 400μs, 100Hz Intermittent use (6-7h/daily) Seizure episode
Smith et al (2001) Includes: Carroll et al (2000)	- Brachialgia post-neurofibromatosis and previous cervical laminectomy (1)	0%	Epidural Lead, Quadripolar, parallel to CS, 2.0-7.0V; 450 μs; 15-75Hz
Hosomi et al. (2008) Includes: Saitoh et al (2000) Saitoh et al (2001) Saitoh et al (2003) Saitoh et al (2006)	- Peripheral nerve injury (1)	Pain relief 1/1 60% VAS (17 mos)	Subdural Lead (Interhemispheric), Quadripolar 0.9-5V; 200μs, 25-50 Hz
Delavallée et al (2008)	- Posttraumatic cubital neuropathy (1)	Pain relief <40%	Subdural Lead, Octopolar, neuronavigation oblique, intermittent 3V, 210 μs, 60Hz
Nguyen et al (2009) *(Creteil, Nguyen Group)* Includes: Nguyen et al (1997, 1999, 2000, 2004, 2008, 2009a) Drout et al (2002)	- Peripheral nerve injuries (12)	Pain relief 7/12, (58.3%) (29-170 mos)	Epidural Lead, Quadripolar, perpendicular to CS, Neuronavigation 1.0-3.5V; 60-150 μs; 25-60Hz cycling

continued Table 9.6: Miscellaneous PNPs

Authors	Type of pain (number of patients)	Results (follow-up)	Notes/Parameters
Lefaucheur et al (2009)	- Neurofibromatosis 1 (3) - Peripheral limb nerve trauma (1)	Pain relief 3/4 91% and 93% (neurofibromatosis) 31% (peripheral nerve trauma) (ns)	Epidural Lead, Quadripolar, perpendicular to CS, 2-3V; 60 µs; 40-50Hz
Fagundes-Pereyra et al (2010) Includes: Fagundes-Pereyra et al (2007)	- Peripheral nerve trauma (1)	Pain relief 1/1 90% VAS (24 mos)	Epidural Lead, Quadripolar, parallel to CS, 3D MRI reconstruction Robot assistance 3-4.5V; 100-500 µs;45-60 Hz
Louppe et al (2013)	- Pudendal entrapment syndrome (perineal pain) (2)	Pt 1 : VAS −45% (40 mos), analgesics -70% Pt 2 : VAS −40-50% (19 mos), analgesics unchanged	Pt 1 : rTMS + (20' 20x10s trains,10Hz,80%MT,50sITI, 2000 stimuli), SCS ineffective, Pt 2: rTMS + (twice, 3 weeks and 2 days) Epidural Lead, perpendicular to CS, 2-2.5V, 60µs, 40Hz, cathode on M1
André-Obadia et al (2014)	- peripheral nerve (ulnar) (1)	Pain relief 1/1 (6.1)	Epidural Lead, Quadripolar (1 or 2) 3D MRI and neuronavigation 1.5 – 4.5V; 60µs; 25-50Hz (whole series)
TOTAL	23	16	-

QoL= quality of life; y=years; mo=month; fMRi=functional magnetic ressonance imaging; MEG magnetoencephalography; VAS=visual analog scale; MT= motor threshold; NS=not specified; ADL= activities of daily life; PG= pulse generator; FU= follow-up; DBS=deep brain stimulation; MQP= McGill pain questionnaire; NA=not available.

9.2 Conclusion

Since 1993, several groups have applied ICS to PNP conditions. M1 ICS can be proposed on the basis of pain severity and refractoriness to conventional therapies, in disabled patients with high ratings on pain scales, previously submitted to adequate conservative procedures. Efficacy of M1 ICS for PNP can be predicted –as already discussed in Chapter 8- by screening patients through rTMS. Although a positive response to rTMS strongly suggests subsequent analgesia with ICS, a negative trial should not rule out ICS either, especially for trunk and leg pains, which are less targetable with rTMS (Lefaucheur et al, 2009). André-Obadia et al (2014) observed that some patients with ineffective rTMS may have later good analgesia by ICS. The level of pain relief observed during the first month after ICS has been proposed as a strong predictor of long-term relief (Nuti et al 2005, Lefaucheur et al 2009), but there are exceptions: a gradual decrease in efficacy with long-term stimulation is not uncommon, generally within about 6 months, but sometimes even years. André-Obadia et al. (2014), in a long-term follow up study, observed a half of patients still retain a significant benefit after 2-9 years of continuous M1 ICS. On the other hand, Lefaucheur et al (2009) noticed a progressive improvement of analgesia at 1 year as compared to 6 months. Many patients benefit by reprogramming the parameters, either by increasing the amplitude of stimulation (though this entails the risk of inducing fits) or altering the dipole orientation or spacing without the need of an amplitude increase. In sum, about 50% of patients submitted to ICS evince about 50% pain relief and 50% of them will retain this result at long term. These rates are encouraging in this difficult group of chronic and refractory patients. In this context, it is important to consider that even 30–40% of pain relief may be a good result. It is also important to consider other aspects of ICS efficacy, such as functional recovery, quality of life and drug intake.

References

Anderson WS, Kiyofuji S, Conway JE, et al. Dysphagia and neuropathic facial pain treated with motor cortex stimulation: case report. Neurosurgery. 2009;65:E626

Andre-Obadia N, Mertens MP, Lelekov-Boissard T, et al. Is Life Better After Motor Cortex Stimulation for Pain Control? Results at Long-Term and their Prediction by Preoperative rTMS. Prospective Evaluation. Pain Physician 2014; 17:53-62

Brown JA, Pilitsis JG. Motor cortex stimulation for central and neuropathic facial pain: a prospective study of 10 patients and observations of enhanced sensory and motor function during stimulation. Neurosurgery 2005;56:290-7

Canavero S, Bonicalzi V. Therapeutic extradural cortical stimulation for central and neuropathic pain: a review Clin J Pain 2002; 18:48-55

Carroll D, Joint C, Maartens N, et al. Motor cortex stimulation for chronic neuropathic pain: a preliminary study of 10 cases. Pain 2000; 84:431-7

Cioni B, Meglio M. Motor cortex stimulation for chronic non-malignant pain: current state and future prospects. Acta Neurochir 2007; S97:45-9

Delavallée M, Abu-Serieh B, de Tourchaninoff M, et al. Subdural motor cortex stimulation for central and peripheral neuropathic pain: a long-term follow-up study in a series of eight patients. Neurosurgery. 2008;63:101-5

Delavallee M, Rooijakkers H, Koerts G, et al. Motor cortex stimulation in a three-year-old child with trigeminal neuropathic pain caused by a malignant glioma in the cerebellopontine angle: case report. Neurosurgery 2011; 69: E494-6

Drouot X, Nguyen JP, Peschanski M, et al. The antalgic efficacy of chronic motor cortex stimulation is related to sensory changes in the painful zone. Brain 2002; 125:1660-4
Ebel H, Rust D, Tronnier V, et al. Chronic precentral stimulation in trigeminal neuropathic pain. Acta Neurochir 1996; 138:1300-1306
Esfahani DR, Pisansky MT, Dafer RM, et al. Motor cortex stimulation : functional magnetic resonance imaging-localized treatment for three sources of intractable facial pain. J Neurosurg 2011; 114 :189-195
Fagundes-Pereyra WJ, Teixeira MJ, Reyns N, et al. The use of robotic system to pre-central cortex localization to the motor cortex stimulation for neuropathic pain treatment. Thesis to Doctorate Degree, presented to the Federal University of Sao Paulo, 2007.
Fagundes-Pereyra WJ, Teixeira MJ, Reyns N, et al. Motor cortex electric stimulation for the treatment of neuropathic pain. Arq. Neuro-Psiquiatr 2010; 68: 923-9
Fonoff ET, Teixeira MJ, Lin T, et al. Motor cortex stimulation for complex regional pain syndrome (CRPS type 1) results in pain relief and functional recovery. European Journal of Pain 2007; 11(S1):183
Fonoff ET, Hamani C, Andrade DC, et al. Pain Relief and Functional recovery in patients with complex regional pain syndrome after motor cortex stimulation. Stereotact Funct Neurosurg 2011; 89:167-72
Finet P, Raftopoulos C. Interhemispheric subdural motor cortex stimulation : 2 cases. Surg Neurol 2009; 72:522-3
Fontaine D, Bruneto JL, El Fakir H. Short-term restoration of facial sensory loss by motor cortex stimulation in peripheral post-traumatic neuropathic pain. J Headache Pain 2009; 10: 203-206
García-Larrea L, Peyron R, Mertens P, et al: Positron emission tomography during motor cortex stimulation for pain control. Stereotact Funct Neurosurg 1997; 68:141-8
García-Larrea L, Peyron R, Mertens P, et al: Eletrical stimulation of motor cortex for pain control: a combined PET-scan and electrophysiological study. Pain 1999; 83:259-273
Gharabaghi A, Hellwig D, Rosahl SK, et al. Volumetric image guidance for motor cortex stimulation: integration of 3D cortical anatomy and functional imaging. Neurosurgery. 2005: 57(1 Suppl):114-20
Gonzalez-Martínez J, Sharan A, Henderson J, et al. Epidural motor cortex stimulation for atypical facial pain. Neurosurgery 2002; 51:567 (abstr)
Herregodts P, Stadnik T, De Ridder F,et al. Cortical stimulation for central neuropathic pain: 3-D surface MRI for easy determination of the motor cortex. Acta Neurochir [Suppl] 1995; 64:132-135
Hosomi K, Saitoh Y, Kishima H, et al. Electrical stimulation of primary motor cortex within the central sulcus for intractable neuropathic pain. Clin Neurophysiol. 2008: 119(5):993-1001
Katayama Y, Yamamoto T, Kobayashi K, et al. Motor cortex stimulation for phantom limb pain: a comprehensive therapy with spinal cord and thalamic stimulation. Stereotact Funct Neurosurg 2001;77:159-161.
Koppelstaetter F, Siedentopf CM, Rhomberg P, et al. [Functional magnetic resonance imaging before motor cortex stimulation for phantom limb pain] Nervenarzt. 2007;78:1435-9.
Lefaucheur JP, Drouot X, Cunin P,et al. Motor cortex stimulation for treatment of refractory peripheral neuropathic pain. Brain 2009;132:1463-71
Louppe JM, Nguyen JP, Robert R, et al. Motor cortex stimulation in refractory pelvic and perineal pain: report of two successful cases. Neurourol Urodyn 2013;32:53-7.
Mandat T, Koziara H, Barszcz S, et al. Motor cortex stimulation in the treatment of neuropathic pain. Neurol Neurochir Pol 2012; 46:428-35
Mertens P, Nuti C, Sindou M, et al. Precentral cortex stimulation for the treatment of central neuropathic pain: results of a prospective study in a 20-patient series. Stereotact Funct Neurosurg. 1999; 73(1-4):122-5
Meyerson BA, Lindblom U, Linderoth B, et al. Motor cortex stimulation as treatment of trigeminal neuropathic pain. Acta Neurochir (Wien) 1993 Suppl 58: 150-153.

Mogilner AY, Rezai AR: Epidural motor cortex stimulation with functional imaging guidance. Neurosurg Focus 11: article 4, 2001
Nandi D, Yianni J, Humphreys J, et al. Phantom limb pain relieved with different modalities of central nervous system stimulation: a clinical and functional imaging case report of two patients. Neuromodulation.2004; 7(3):176-83
Nguyen JP, Keravel Y, Feve A,et al. Treatment of deafferentation pain by chronic stimulation of the motor cortex: report a series of 20 cases. Acta Neurochir suppl 1997;68:54-60.
Nguyen JP, Lefaucheur JP, Decq P, et al: Chronic motor cortex stimulation in the treatment of central and neuropathic pain. Correlation between clinical, eletrophysiological and anatomical data. Pain 1999; 82:245-251
Nguyen JP, Lefaucheur JP, Le Guerinel C, et al. Treatment of central and neuropathic facial pain by chronic stimulation of the motor cortex: value of neuronavigation guidance for the localization of the motor cortex. Neurochirurgie 2000; 46: 483-491.
Nguyen JP, Lefaucheur JP, et al. Motor cortex stimulation for the treatment of deafferentation pain. Neuromodulation.2004;7:146.
Nguyen JP, Velasco F, Brugières P, et al. treatment of chronic neuropathic pain by motor cortex stimulation: results of a bicentric controlled crossover trial. Brain Stimul 2008; 1:89-96
Nguyen JP, Lefaucheur JP, Raoul S, et al. Treatment of trigeminal neuropathic pain by motor cortex stimulation._Neurochirurgie. 2009; 55:226-30
Nuti C, Peyron R, Garcia-Larrea L, et al. Motor cortex stimulation for refractory neuropathic pain: four year outcome and predictors of efficacy. Pain 2005; 118: 43-52.
Osenbach RK. Motor cortex stimulation for intractable Pain. Neurosurg Focus 21: E7:1-12, 2006.
Pirotte B, Voordecker P, Neugroschl C, et al. Combination of functional magnetic resonance imaging-guided neuronavigation and intraoperative cortical brain mapping improves targeting of motor cortex stimulation in neuropathic pain. Neurosurgery 2005; 56: 344-359.
Pirotte B, Voordecker P, Brotchi J, et al. Anatomical and physiological basis, clinical and surgical considerations, mechanisms underlying efficacy and future prospects of cortical stimulation for pain. Acta Neurochir 2007; Suppl 97(2): 81-89.
Rainov NG, Fels C, Heidecke V, et al. Epidural eletrical stimulation of the motor cortex in patients with facial neuralgia. Clin Neurol Neurosurg 1997; 99:205-9
Rainov NG, Heidecke V. Motor cortex stimulation for neuropathic facial pain. Neurol Res 2003; 25: 157-161
Rasche D, Ruppolt M, Stippich C, et al. Motor cortex stimulation for long-term relief of chronic neuropathic pain: a ten year experience. Pain 2006; 121: 43-52.
Rasche D, Tronnier VM. Extradural cortical stimulation for peripehral (including trigeminal) neuropathic pain. In: Canavero S 8ed) Textbook of therapeutic cortical stimulation. New York: Nova Sci., 2009, 161-168
Raslan AM, Nasseri M, Bahgat D, et al. Motor cortex stimulation for trigeminal neuropathic or deafferentation pain: an institutional case series experience. Stereotact Funct Neurosurg. 2011;89:83-8.
Roux FE, Ibarrola D, Lazorthes Y, Berry I: Chronic motor cortex stimulation for phantom limb pain: a functional magnetic resonance imaging study: technical case report. Neurosurgery 2001; 48:681-8
Saitoh Y, Shibata M, Hirano SI, et al. Motor cortex stimulation for central peripheral deafferentation. J Neurosurg 2000; 92:150-5
Saitoh Y, Hirano SI, Kato A, et al: Motor cortex stimulation for deafferentation pain. Neurosurg Focus 11: article 1, 2001.
Saitoh Y, Kato A, Ninomiya H, et al. Primary motor cortex stimulation within the central sulcus for treating deafferentation pain. Acta Neurochir 2003; 87:149-52

Saitoh Y, Yoshimine T. Stimulation of primary motor cortex for intractable deafferentation pain. Acta Neurochir Suppl 2007 ; 97: 51-56.

Sakas DE, Flaskas TN, Panourias IG, et al. Bifocal cortical electrical stimulation for pain by interdural implantation of the electrodes. J Neurosurg 2011; 114:180-5

Smith H, Joint C, Schlugman D, et al. Motor cortex stimulation for neuropathic pain. Neurosurg Focus 11: article 2, 2001.

Sol JCH, Casaux J, Roux FE, et al. Chronic motor cortex stimulation for phantom limb pain: correlations between pain relief and functional imaging studies. Stereotact Funct Neurosurg 2001; 77:172–6

Son BC, Kim MC, Moon DE,et al. Motor cortex stimulation in a patient with intractable complex regional pain syndrome type II with hemi-body involvement. J Neurosurg. 2003;98:175-9.

Teixeira MJ, Fonoff E, Macri F, et al. Prediction of results of motor cortex stimulation in treatment of brachial plexus avulsion pain by trans-cranial magnetic stimulation. European Journal of Pain.2007;11 (S1) p.s192

Teixeira MJ, Fonoff ET, Macri F, et al. Prediction of results of motor cortex stimulation in treatment of brachial plexus avulsion pain by transcranial magnetic stimulation. Acta Neurochir (Wien) 2008; 150: 966, A01 (Duplicates)

Velasco M, Velasco F, Brito F, et al. Motor cortex stimulation in the treatment of deafferentation pain. Localization of the motor cortex. Stereotact Funct Neurosurg 2002; 79:146-167.

Velasco M, Velasco F, Arguelles C, et al. Efficacy of motor cortex stimulation in the treatment of neuropathic pain: randomized double-blind trial. J Neurosurg 2008;108:698-706

Velasco F, Carrillo-Ruiz JD, Castro G, et al. Motor cortex electrical stimulation applied to patients with complex regional pain syndrome. Pain. 2009;147: 91-8.

Vesper J. Chronic motor cortex stimulation and predictive value of rTMS. Eur J Pain 2010; S4 p135 A476

Angelo Lavano, Domenico Bosco, Marisa De Rose, Giusy Guzzi,
Giorgio Volpentesta, Sergio Canavero

10 Movement Disorders: Parkinson and Tremor

Parkinson's disease (PD) is a progressive neurological disorder that affects 1% of the population over the age of 65. In PD, two primary sources of dysfunction are identified: a reduction of DA projections from the midbrain to the basal ganglia and from the midbrain to the primary motor cortex (MI). After about 5 years (the "honeymoon period"), L-Dopa (introduced in 1967) and dopaminergic agonists, the mainstays of therapy, lead to dyskinesias or motor fluctuations that can be even worse than the disease itself.

In 1979, Woolsey et al wrote: "*Subthreshold electrical stimulation through implanted electrodes might be used to control marked tremor and strong rigidity in parkinsonian patients*". Twenty years later, Canavero performed the first such surgery in a PD woman (see history in Canavero 2009). Currently, extradural motor cortex stimulation (M1 ICS) represents an alternative neurosurgical treatment for PD with zero disabling morbidity-mortality. It is a valuable and safer option when DBS cannot be employed or patients are unresponsive or do not fulfill DBS inclusion criteria or simply refuse it.

10.1 Literature Review

About 130 patients have been submitted to Motor Cortex Stimulation (M1 ICS) for advanced PD. The published literature include case reports, single-center experiences and the Italian Multicenter Study (Table 10.1). Almost all studies are unblinded, with two exceptions. Inclusion criteria have been quite homogeneous in all studies: idiopathic PD (PDSBB criteria), at least 5 year-long disease history, advanced stage (UPDRS in off>/=40/180; Hoehn and Yahrs>/=3, motor complication fluctuations and disabling dyskinesia), positive response to L-Dopa, DBS not accepted by the patient or contraindicated, patient ability to give informed consent.

M1 ICS achieves a significant and sustained improvement in motor symptoms, with a remarkable effect on axial symptoms, L-dopa induced dyskinesias and quality of life. It must be stressed how the UPDRS III and Hoehn-Yahr scales appear inadequate in assessing the true clinical benefit of M1 ICS. In the only totally negative study, from Toronto (Moro et al 2011), an unsafe subdural approach was elected, with high-frequency, short pulse width stimulation, which is known to be ineffective or deleterious, as highlighted by Canavero et al (2002,2003).

Full clinical benefits observed with M1 ICS are always delayed. Although rigidity and, less so, tremor improve within several minutes of stimulation, the full effect on bradykinesia, gait and axial symptoms grows with time (days to weeks).

Table 10.1: Studies of M1 ICS for PD

Authors/date	Number of patients	Stimulation site	MCS operative technique	Parameters of stimulation	Configuration	Results
Canavero et al. 2000 Canavero et al. 2002 Canavero et al.2003	3	M1 (hand knob)	Unilateral (contralateral to worst clinical side) extradural	2-3,5 V 20-30 Hz 90-180 µs Continuous	Bipolar (3+/0-), OFF during sleep	Abolition of rigidity and tremor (bilateral); partial improvement of gait, bradykinesia, dysarthria and hypophonia; 50% decrease of UPDRS motor score; 40-80% decrease of LEDD
Verhagen et al. 2006	9	M1(hand knob)	Unilateral extradural (contralateral to worst clinical side)	20-127 Hz 250 µs (fixed)	-	24 week-long prospective multicenter study. The UPDRS III score OFF medication was 42.13 +/- 13.78 compared to 38.78 +/- 8.08 at baseline.
Benvenuti et al. 2006	1	M1 (knob)	Unilateral Extradural	-	Bipolar (?)	Improvement of 35% on the UPDRS scale: rigidity, dyskinesia and motor fluctuation were reduced significantly as well as standing, gait and motor performance.
Cioni, 2007	7	M1 (hand knob)	Unilateral (contralateral to worst clinical side) extradural in 3 pts; Bilateral extradural in 4 pts	3-4 V 80 Hz 120 µs continuous	Bipolar 0/3	Prospective study. Follow –up at 1, 3, 6 and 12 months. Five patients showed an improvement during MCS, while 2 patients resulted unresponsive. At 12 months follow-up UPDRS III in "off-med" decreased by 22%, as well as the dosage of l-dopa. Axial symptoms were ameliorated. Effect of unilateral MCS bilateral. After 1 year of unilateral stimulation, 2 patients underwent bilateral MCS that restored the clinical effect.
Cilia et al. 2007	5	M1 (left) (hand knob)	Unilateral extradural	3,0-4,0 V 40-60 Hz 180-210 µs	Multiple unipolar in 4/5; bipolar in 1/5	Follow-up performed at 6 months after surgery on and off medication, with stimulator ON, and 2 weeks later with stimulator OFF by the same neurologist in a blinded fashion. Improvement of motor fluctuations(daily OFF time reduction) and of axial symptoms (freezing gait, stooped posture and postural instability) as well as a reduction of dyskinesia in 3 patients. L-dopa dosage reduced (mean) by 16 % and dopamine agonist dosage by 49%. Subjective clinical benefit was reported after variable interval after surgery.

contiuned **Table 10.1:** Studies of M1 ICS for PD

Authors/date	Number of patients	Stimulation site	MCS operative technique	Parameters of stimulation	Configuration	Results
Arle et al. 2008	4	M1 (hand knob)	Unilateral extradural in 1 pt Bilateral extradural in 3 pts	3,2-3,5 V 100-130 Hz 210-240 µs	Multiple unipolar in 3/5 electrodes; bipolar in 2/5 electrodes (initially all contacts were checked in a monopolar setting at 130 Hz and 210 mcs, with voltage slowly increased to 4 V. Later patient 1 was stimulated at 3.2 A, 240 mcs, 130 Hz; patient 2 at 3.5 A, 210 mcs, 130 Hz; patient 3 at 3.4 A, 210 mcs, 100 Hz. Patient 4 was not detailed)	Prospective study. Benefits seen within the first 6 months in UPDRS III scores (decreased by 60%), tremor was only modestly managed most benefits seen initially lost by the end of 12 months. 1 infection 3 months post implant. Patient M1 (implanted on the left) developed a superficial infection of the extension wire site and required removal of the device. This patient had improvement of about 50% (>75% of day to less than 10% of day) over baseline in dyskinesias and a 30% improvement in the UPDRS III score but significantly regressed when the device was removed (he was the unilaterally implanted patient). After reimplantation of the device several months later, he again improved over pre-operative baseline in both dyskinesia reduction and UPDRS III improvement. Overall at 6 months the mean UPDRS III improvement was 46.8% (+/- 24.7%) (this includes the patient M1 at their 6 month time period after re-implant). At 1 year the mean improvement was -14.2% (+/- 66.8%) with one patient asking to have his stimulator kept in the "OFF" state due to no significant improvement. Two patients had a 20-30% (M2 and M3, both implanted bilaterally) reduction in medication requirements at three months, yet patient M3 has started to need more medication at the 6 and 12 month time points. One patient (M5, implanted on the right), however, had a 37% increased medication requirement. One patient had a return of dyskinesias after 3 months (M5); they had initially improved, but then the amplitude of stimulation was reduced and the benefit was lost. Once the patient's stimulation amplitude was increased again, dyskinesias were again better controlled.
Fasano e t al. 2008	1 (F/72)	M1 (hand knob)	Bilateral extradural	3-60-130 Hz (benefit at 130Hz only) 120 µs	Bipolar	Stimulation at 130 Hz improve axial akinesia and walking but benefits gradually disappeared In baseline med-off condition the patient was unable to rise from a chair and to stand without assistance. Consistent axial akinesia and walking amelioration. HMPAO SPECT: increase of rCBF in SMA during stimulation at 130 Hz. After five months, benefit gradually disappeared.

contiuned **Table 10.1:** Studies of M1 ICS for PD

Authors/date	Number of patients	Stimulation site	MCS operative technique	Parameters of stimulation	Configuration	Results
Pagni et al. 2005 *(Initial results of Italian Multicenter Study)*	16	M1 (hand knob)	Unilateral extradural (contralateral to worst clinical side)	2,5-6 V 25-40 Hz 150-180 μs	Bipolar	Patients evaluated only in the On-Med state from 4 months to 2,5 years. The improvement was bilateral: global UPDRS decreased by 42-62%, the UPDRS III score decreased by 32-83%, l-dopa dosage decreased by 11-33% in 3 patients and by 70-73% in 2 patients (Turin experience) Very advanced PD, aged 46-81, 15 of which were not eligible for DBS, evaluated at 3-30 months after implantation. Tremor and rigidity in all limbs and akinesia reduced, bilaterally. Standing, gait, motor performance, speech and swallowing improved. Also dyskinesias, motor fluctuations and other side effects of l-dopa administration were improved. Effect of stimulation persistent and not fading over time. Quality of life markedly improved.
Pagni et al. 2008	41	M1 (hand knob)	Unilateral extradural in 33 pts Bilateral extradural in 8 pts	2,5-6,0 V/3-4 V 25-40 Hz/60-80 Hz 150-180μs /90-120 μs	Bipolar/monopolar	Pts with good response to previous L-dopa treatment. There were 21 male and 20 female, aged 56-81. The study reported only the results of the unilateral stimulation. Follow-up at 1, 3, 6, 12 months and then at least every 6 months. There was no worsening of the total UPDRS score off medication/on stimulation at long term follow-up in each patient. A significant reduction in the off-medication UPDRS III score was observed after stimulation and persisted at long term; improvement was only very moderate in the on-medication state. Improvement in activities of daily living, posture, gait, rising from a chair, balance, bradykinesia. Marked attenuation of levodopa-induced dyskinesia and dystonia. Antiparkinsonian drugs expressed in terms of LEDD showed a trend to reduction when compared to doses used before surgery. Benefits on limbs tremor and rigidity bilateral, more evident in the limbs opposite to the stimulated side and in those patients presenting with lower UPDRS scores. Long term levodopa syndrome symptoms, dyskinesia and painful dystonia reduced in most patients and up to 90% in some of them.
Gutiérrez et al. 2009	6	MI (hand knob)	Unilateral (contralateral to worst clinical side) extradural	3,0-4,5 V 10-30 Hz 330-450 μs	All bipolar (3+/0-, except 1: 2+/1-)	Globally, mild daily life activities improvement with a slightly lower levodopa equivalent dose UPDRS part III scores: no significant modification.

contiuned **Table 10.1:** Studies of M1 ICS for PD

Authors/date	Number of patients	Stimulation site	MCS operative technique	Parameters of stimulation	Configuration	Results
Moro et al. 2011	5	Left M1 in 4 pts Right M1 in 1 pt	Unilateral subdural	3.5+/-0.9 V, 114+/-36 Hz, 78+/-27μs	Acutely tested mono and bipolar, chronically not specified	Evaluation 3 months after implantation with double-blinded assessment and after 1 year with an open assessment. No changes in the OFF medication/on stimulation motor scores compared with off stimulation. At 1 year no improvement. 1 cortical venous infarct., 3 self-limiting seizures with aggressive trials of stimulation in the period of parameters adjustment
De Rose et al. 2012	10	M1	Unilateral extradural	3,5-4,7 V 40-80 Hz 180 μs (continuous)	All bipolar (0-/3+)	Single-center prospective observational study. F-up: 36 months (8 pts), 2 died within 24 mos of unrelated causes. Improvement mainly of axial symptoms: UPDRS III items 27-31 off medication: mean percentage of decrease: 25% at 1 month, 30% at 3 months, 20% at 6 months, 22% at 12 months, 26% at 18 months, 24% at 24 months and 28% at 36 months; L-dopa-induced dyskinesia and dystonia: significant reduction of UPDRS IV score up to 18 months : mean percentage of decrease: 29.6% at 6 months, 40.9% at 12 months, 31.8% at 18 months, 15.9% at 24 months and 11.4% at 36 months, quality of life and global condition. Eight patients reported reduced OFF time in clinical fluctuations (UPDRS IV item 39 score from 3 to 1); evident reduction of L-dopa and dopamine agonist dosage: mean percentage of decrease: 39% at 6 months, 38% at 12 months, 33% at 18 months, 37% at 24 months and 29% at 36 months. The benefit on distal tremor, rigidity and bradykinesia bilateral but not significant, with a slight prevalence in the hemibody opposite to the stimulated side. No complications or adverse effects.

contiuned **Table 10.1:** Studies of M1 ICS for PD

Authors/date	Number of patients	Stimulation site	MCS operative technique	Parameters of stimulation	Configuration	Results
Di Giuda et al. 2012	6 (all under 70 years of age)	Right M1 in 5 pts Left M1 in 1 pt	Unilateral (contralateral to worst affected side) extradural	3,0-4,0 V 80 Hz 120 µs Continuous	All bipolar 0 (cathode) and 3 (anode)	^{123}I-FP-CIT SPECT preoperatively, 8 and 13 months after MCS. The effect of unilateral M1 ICS was bilateral and clinically evident after a 2-week stimulation. Pts evaluated 8 and 13 months under OFF-MED and ON-STIM conditions: significant improvement in total UPDRS scores (reduced by 22% at 8 months and by 16% at 13 months) and UPDRS part II (improved by 22% at 13 months). Dosage of antiparkinsonian drugs (LEDD) significantly reduced after 8 months, with a tendency towards preoperative values at 13 month evaluation. No significant differences in ^{123}I-FP-CIT uptake ratios between baseline and follow-up found, except for a progressive reduction in ^{123}I-FP-CIT uptake ratios in the striatum contralateral to the implant. No further decrease in ^{123}I-FP-CIT uptake ratios detected in the striatum ipsilateral to the implant. No correlations between changes in ^{123}I-FP-CIT uptake ratios with disease duration, changes in medication dosage and motor UPDRS scores.
Bentivoglio et al. 2012	9 (initially 11)	M1	Unilateral (contralateral wo worst clinical side) extradural	3,0-5,0 V 80 Hz 120 µs	All bipolar (distal contacts as cathode and anode)	Single-center prospective study. Assessment: after 1,3,6, and 12 months. In the MED-OFF condition, UPDRS motor score at baseline significantly reduced by 14,1%, 23.3%, 19.9% and 13.2% at 1,3,6 and 12 months, respectively. The improvement in motor score mostly related to a reduction of the contralateral and axial scores. Significant reduction of the limbs score by 19.3% at 6 months and by 10.0% at 12 months with beneficial effects on bradykinesia of the upper limbs at 3 and 6 months and of the lower limbs at 6 months. As to midline motor function, significant effect for UPDRS III item "arising from chair". Post-op LEDD reduced by 6.3%, 2.5%, 13.5%, 2.5% at 1,3,6 and 12 months, respectively. UPDRS II scores of the item "walking" at 3, 6 and 12 months and "FOG" at 6 and 12 months significantly reduced as compared to baseline. MCS also improved the global condition and quality of life. In the MED-ON condition, no significant effect found in any of the explored outcome measurements.

NB all authors implanted a quadripolar paddle electrode, except Verhagen et al in which only the 0 and 3 contacts were available. All electrodes parallel to central sulcus.

There is also a suggestion that M1 ICS may benefit Multiple System Atrophy-Associated Parkinsonism. Canavero et al (2003) improved for 9 months a single patient with extradural, bilateral M1 ICS (continuous stimulation, 2-2.5V, 90-180 µs, 25-40Hz), and Kleiner-Fisman et al (2003) reported subjective improvement in 3 out of 5 patients over 6 months.

In all published papers, the surgical technique involved the implantation of a four-contact strip electrode over the hand-knob of M1, extradurally, with one exception (Moro 2011: subdural). The implant was performed through a single burr-hole or two burr-holes drilled in front of the central sulcus under local or general anesthesia or, much less frequently, through a small craniotomy made on the central sulcus under general anesthesia. The subdural implant was performed under local anesthesia with conscious sedation (Moro 2011).In all cases the electrode was placed parallel to the motor strip over the hand knob or the upper limb area. In several cases, the correct position of the electrode was verified neurophysiologically using somatosensory evoked potentials (SSEPs) and/or motor evoked potentials (MEPs).

Surgery has always been performed contralaterally to the most affected side, with the exception of Cilia et al (2007)'s series, in which the dominant (left) hemisphere was elected. In a few patients, the implant was bilateral, but the stimulation was simultaneously on both sides only in two cases. It is known that in early PD one side is more affected, with higher M1 excitability: asymmetric motor involvement is also associated with excessive involuntary mirroring and defective interhemispheric inhibition, both unfavoring the more affected side (Spagnolo et al 2013).

The stimulation parameters differed in the studies. The frequency ranged from 10 to 130 Hz (most commonly 40-80Hz), the pulse duration from 60 to 450 µs (most commonly 120-240 µs) and the intensity from 2.5 to 6 V (always subthreshold for movements and sensory feelings). The stimulation was delivered continuously, in almost all cases with bipolar configuration, through the most distal contacts (0-/3+), or, in few cases, with multiple unipolar configurations.

Extradural M1 ICS has proved to be a very benign procedure, in stark contrast to the subdural approach (Moro et al 2011). Local stimulation-induced pain at the site of implantation has been reported.

10.2 DBS vs M1 ICS

Subthalamic (STN) DBS improves rigidity in 63% of patients and bradykinesia in 52% and, when dopaminergic treatment is added concomitantly, 73% and 69% respectively. Decrease in dyskinesia (70% - 90%), reduction of the required equivalent dose of levodopa (mean 55.9%, up to 63%) and reduction in 'off' periods (10%-90%) are reported. Yet, improvements are limited to the cardinal symptoms of PD, with balance (postural instability) and gait (freezing) or non-motor symptoms poorly controlled and limited benefit in activities of daily living. Neuropsychiatric effects (depression, apathy, anxiety, addictions, eating behavior alterations, dementia) have all been correlated to STN DBS (Castrioto et al 2014).

DBS cannot be offered to all PD patients: age over 70 years of age, a poor response to levodopa (less than 40-50% on the Levo-Dopa challenge test), or a score less than 30-40 in the Off-condition on UPDRS III, brain atrophy, dementia, psychiatric and medical co-morbidities represent contraindications to this procedure. Thus, roughly half of all Parkinsonian patients cannot benefit from DBS. DBS has a non-trivial mortality rate (0,4%, up to 1,8%): causes of death include intracranial hemorrhage, pneumonia, pulmonary embolism and suicide (Arle and Shils 2011) (see Box 10.1). Given the progressive nature of PD and the purely symptomatic effects of DBS, the long-term clinical evolution of these surgical patients currently seems to be associated with a new PD phenotype, mainly characterized by axial motor problems and cognitive impairment (Rodriguez-Oroz et al 2012). In a series (Rizzone et al 2014), at 11 years, DBS was still improving the motor symptoms by only 35.8%, as compared to the preoperative off-state, with an 84.6% improvement of dyskinesias and a 65.8% improvement of motor fluctuations; on the other hand, the UPDRSII-on score worsened by 88.5%, mainly due to advancing poorly levodopa-responsive symptoms.

Intraoperative:

---Hypertension (59%)/ Hypotension (7,9%), Tachycardia (6,2%)/ Bradycardia (18%)

---Venous infarction (caused by the transection or coagulation of large draining veins at the site of the burr hole): 0,9%

---Deep infarcts: case reports but incidence unknown (probably because they remain asymptomatic or are difficult to recognize on the post-operative scans)

---Seizures:2.4% (0-14%) (intra-or post-operative, usually instigated by cortical irritation at the lead entry site or ischemic\hemorrhagic damage)

---Subdural hemorrhage: <1%

---Intracerebral bleeding: 0,7% - 3,3% per lead, with a permanent morbidity of 0,6-0,8% (increased risk of hemorrhage due to the use of the microelectrode recording, especially with multiple micro-electrodes passes)

---Venous air embolism (DBS is usually performed in a semi-seated position that requires continuos anesthesiological monitoring, since it can occur just after the burr hole placement and can be istigated by accidentally coughing): rare

---Pulmonary embolism: rare

Postoperative:

---Infections: 4-12,2% incidence per patient or 1,5-9,7% risk per lead. Usually Staphylococcus Aureus and superficial. Overall 2,8% infection rate, with 1,4% of superficial skin infection. Need for removal: 4,6%. Combined deep infection and erosion rates: 1,5-15,2%.

---Lead fracture: 2-9,9% per patient or about 1,8% per lead implanted. DBS lead migration: 1,5%-6,3% of patients or approximately 4,4% of leads implanted. Migration from 6 months to 3 years after the initial surgery.

---Hardware complications (misplaced lead, loss of effect, lack of efficacy, lead fracture, lead migration and infection): 7,8%.32,9% of patients or 8% per lead-year.

---STN DBS: impairments in executive functions, verbal fluency and Stroop naming time, dysarthria, paresthesia, blepharospasm; Gpi DBS: visual disturbance, paresthesia, gait and speech difficulties, confusion an depression

---Increased suicide rate

---Post-operative confusion, speech difficulties and mental status/cognitive changes

---

Box 10.1: Complications of DBS

The clinical effect of DBS cannot be compared with that of M1 ICS due to different inclusion criteria. DBS is usually contraindicated in those submitted to M1 ICS, because of age or MRI anatomical abnormalities (e.g. cerebral atrophy and vascular lesions). M1 ICS appears to have some advantages over STN DBS: it is more suitable in elderly patients due to minimal surgery-related side effects and lower complications and adverse event rates; verbal fluency is not impaired, axial symptoms and gait disturbances that are poorly responsive to DBS are allayed. Unilateral M1 ICS induces clinical effects bilaterally and it is more cost-effective because it does not require stereotactic equipment.

10.3 rTMS vs M1 ICS

Non-invasive brain stimulation (e.g. repetitive transcranial magnetic stimulation - rTMS, transcranial direct current stimulation - tDCS) can be effective in improving motor symptoms in patients with PD. The analysis of TMS studies has shown that this result is consistent across controlled and uncontrolled trials, but the effect is modest, with a 20% reduction of motor scores at frequencies of 5-25Hz and greater effects with multiple sessions over a longer duration of time (Khedr 2009). Compared to rTMS, M1 ICS guarantees precise stimulation of the target, provides continuous stimulation without interfering with daily activities and reduces the need of repeated treatments as for rTMS. However, rTMS could help select responders for ICS (Canavero and Bonicalzi 2007).

10.4 Mechanism of Action

Several mechanisms of action can be envisioned (Canavero and Bonicalzi 2007, Canavero 2009, Cerasa and Quattrone 2014) (see chapter 18 and Box 10.2). What is important to remember, though, is that even STN DBS works by alleviating the PD-associated pathological M1 state (Li et al 2014).

In PD, both increased L-Dopa-responsive cortical facilitation (hyperactivity) and concomitant impaired non-L-Dopa-responsive GABA-A inhibition coexist (Ni et al 2013). M1 ICS can up-regulate this defective GABA tone (Canavero 2009). Interestingly, L-Dopa exerts different and opposite effects on cortical excitability within M1 compared to S1, with subtle changes in sensory and motor behavior (Nelson et al 2012). On the other hand, M1 ICS can modulate both M1 and S1 by way of U-fibers.

Several studies posit that synchronized oscillations at multiple frequencies within spatially segregated regions of the M1-basal ganglia circuit relate to distinct components of clinical impairment in PD: the relationship hitherto reported between β activity and bradykinesia-rigidity might be tightly locked with (phase amplitude coupling) or even secondary to effects at both lower and higher γ frequencies (cross-frequency interactions), with an exaggerated coupling of β phase in the STN and M1 and broad band γ amplitude in M1 specific to PD (Oswal et al 2013). Cortical stimulation may engage these oscillatory patterns (Canavero 2009, Thut and Miniussi 2009).

In M1 ICS the clinical changes are delayed for several days after switching the stimulator ON or OFF or after modifying the parameters of stimulation, whereas they are durable after stopping long-term stimulation (After-Effects). This points to plastic rearrangements induced by M1 ICS (which makes the parameters search stage more labor-intensive than DBS). Transcallosal pathways – and to a minor extent interhemispheric connections at brainstem, thalamic and basal ganglia levels, including a pathway connecting the subthalamic nuclei (Canavero 2009, Groppa et al 2013)- account for the bilateral effects of unilateral stimulation; particularly strong interhemispheric conduction pathways exist between the hand representations of M1s, which explains why the hand area should be targeted for M1 ICS in PD (Canavero 2009, 2011).

Another reason for targeting the hand area is that stimulation involving electrodes overlying the anatomic hand knob has a lower stimulation threshold when compared with stimulations of electrodes overlying M1 outside the hand knob area (2.1m vs 2.8mA) (Kovac et al 2011).

Importantly, Di Giuda et al. (2012) demonstrated that no further DAT (dopamine) level reduction occurred in the striatum ipsilateral to the implant during chronic M1 ICS, suggesting a "neuroprotective" effect.

---

modulation of the hyperdirect pathway from MI to STN (see also Baudrexel et al 2011)
restoration of deficient inhibition (GABAergic interneurons) in M1, abolition of M1 hyperactivity and reduction of hyperglutamatergic tone
reversal of dysfunctional MI plasticity
functional restoration of motor maps in M1 and SMA
interhemispheric compensation
desynchronization of β (antikinetic) frequency and increase of γ (prokinetic) synchrony between M1 and striatum

---

Box 10.2: Possible Mechanisms of Action

10.5 Conclusions

Extradural M1 ICS can relieve all three major symptoms of PD (akinesia, rigidity, tremor) on both sides simultaneously, with zero disabling morbidity-mortality, unlike DBS, although results vary widely. It has a particular and significant effectiveness on axial symptoms, freezing and dyskinesias, whereas DBS appears to have stronger effects on distal symptoms. However the clinical effects of MCS cannot be compared with those of DBS, due to the different inclusion criteria (age, older in M1 ICS series, MRI anatomical abnormalities,...).

Canavero (2009) suggests that that left MI ECS might be preferable. A fMR study found that in patients with right-sided – but not left-sided- dominant symptoms the brain tries to compensate by employing alternative ipsilateral pathways (Kalmar et al 2011). Also, in right-handers the depth of the CS is greater in the left hemisphere than in the right and the motor hand knob is larger and metabolically more active in the left hemisphere (Caulo et al 2007).

In early stages, maladaptive/compensatory changes take places in M1 and plasticity deteriorates as the symptoms progress (Kojovic et al 2012). Also, older patients –constituting the great majority of patients submitted to MCS- exhibit less distinctive cortical representations and decreased basal interhemispheric inhibition (Bernard and Seidler 2012). These two factors may, in undetermined ways, interfere with M1 ICS and lead to suboptimal results.

PD patients, who very often do not fulfill the inclusion criteria for DBS, may be eligible for M1 ICS. M1 ICS can be performed without the need of general anesthesia, does not require stereotactic frames or microelectrode recording, and virtually eliminates the possibility of intracranial hemorrhage. As opposed to rTMS and its need for repeated treatments, minimally invasive M1 ICS guarantees precise stimulation of the target, along with the possibility of a continuous stimulation. *Subdural MCS is strongly discouraged.* Parameters search should follow the TANG recommendations (Box 10.3): different parameters differentially modulate intracortical and/or interhemispheric processing in M1 and these must be explored as thoroughly as possible.

What emerges clearly is that M1 ICS results cannot be assessed with the same criteria of DBS, given the discrepancy between the UPDRS III and Hoehn-Yahr scales and subjective reports from the patients. M1 ICS effects, unlike DBS, are almost never immediate. Assessment after a change of parameters must be undertaken after about 2-4 weeks due to long after-effects setting in as a result of neuroplastic changes. Moreover, effects, particularly on akinesia, grow over time. After 1-3 months of stimulation, UPDRS scores can be evaluated, after changing parameters, only at -at least- 1 month intervals; at least initially, effects of M1 ICS on motor scores should not be evaluated off medication (Canavero 2009).

Failures of M1 ICS could be put down to individual variations in the organization of MI, i.e. mosaicism, inverted disposition of MI functional areas, wide somatotopic variability of individual distal arm representations, not only between individuals, but also between hemispheres in the same individual (Canavero 2009). Also, state-dependency in brain stimulation (Kundu et al 2014) is even more important in PD where the cognitive state of the patient impacts the course of the illness. Interestingly, in rTMS studies, the shape of the hand knob in M1 determines the physiologic response to coil orientation: the inverted Ω shape responds preferentially to a 45° coil angle, the ε shape to a 90° coil angle (Opitz et al 2013): it remains to be seen how the hand knob shape bears on M1 ICS. Also, the presence of bridging veins may divert part of the electric charge injected.

According to Canavero (2009), new targets are possible, for instance the premotor cortex or the somatosensory cortex SI could be assessed for clinical effects.

According to the model suggested by Zwartjes et al (2012), activation of either the basket cell or pyramidal tract (PT) type axons is involved in the clinical effect of M1 ICS. To selectively target the basket cell axons, either cathodal or bipolar stimulation with the electrode strip placed perpendicular rather than parallel to the gyrus and the cathode overlying M1 seems indicated; selectivity can be increased by using multiple cathodes either adjacent or with an inactive contact in between. PT type axons (hyperdirect pathway) can be selectively targeted with anodal stimulation using electrodes with large contact sizes. Selective stimulation of the PT type axons is reduced when using subdural stimulation and bipolar stimulation with the strip oriented parallel as well as perpendicular to the gyrus: thus, subdural stimulation is discouraged.

Ultimately, the recent proposal of closed-loop cortical stimulation in PD opens new perspectives in this field: modulation, but not suppression, of pathological rhythms (10Hz μ range) might be beneficial, although the causal relationship between M1 activity and PD tremor still remains to be demonstrated (Beuter et al 2014; Chapter 17).

-Paddle implanted contralateral to side of initial symptoms; also evaluate implant contralateral to less affected side in nonresponders
-Bipolar stimulation: electrode setting: 0+/3-
-BLOCK A (4 days)
60μs
0.5V 10,20,30,40,50, 80, 130 Hz; 1V 10,20,30,40,50, 80, 130 Hz; 2V 10,20,30,40,50, 80, 130 Hz; 3V 10,20,30,40,50, 80, 130 Hz
each setting kept 1hour
-BLOCK B (4 days)
180 μs
0.5V 10,20,30,40,50, 80, 130 Hz; 1V 10,20,30,40,50, 80, 130 Hz; 2V 10,20,30,40,50, 80, 130 Hz; 3V 10,20,30,40,50, 80, 130 Hz
each setting kept 1 hour
-BLOCK C (4 days)
450 μs
0.5V 10,20,30,40,50, 80, 130 Hz; 1V 10,20,30,40,50, 80, 130 Hz; 2V 10,20,30,40,50, 80, 130 Hz; 3V 10,20,30,40,50, 80, 130 Hz
each setting kept 1 hour
-12 day block repeated with the reverse setting, 0-/3+ (total: 24 days) and then for other settings (1-/2+ and 2+/1-...)
-For definitive stimulation: either continuous or cyclical stimulation (1h On, 1h OFF or the like), with switch-off at night

---

Box 10.3: M1 ICS for PD: Tang Guidelines (Canavero 2009)

References

Arle JE, Apetauerova D, Zani J, et al. Motor cortex stimulation for Parkinson disease: 12 months follow up in 4 patients. J Neurosurg 2008; 109: 133-139

Arle JE, Shils J. Motor Cortex stimulation for pain and movement disorders. Neurotherapeutics 2008; 5:37-49

Arle JE, Shils J (eds). Essential neuromodulation. San Diego: Academic Press, 2011

Baudrexel S, Witte T, Seifried C, et al. Resting state fMRI reveals increased subthalamic nucleus-motor cortex connectivity in Parkinson's disease. Neuroimage 2011;55:1728-38

Bentivoglio AR, Fasano A, Piano C, et al. Unilateral extradural motor cortex stimulation is safe and improves Parkinson's disease at 1 year. Neurosurgery 2012;71:815-25.

Benvenuti E, Cecchi F, Colombini A, et al. Extradural motor cortex stimulation as a method to treat advanced Parkinson's disease: new perspectives in geriatric medicine. Aging Clin Exp Res 2006; 18:347-348

Bernard JA, Seidler RD. Evidence for motor cortex dedifferentiation in older adults. Neurobiol Aging. 2012;33:1890-9

Beuter A, Lefaucheur JP, Modolo J. Closed-loop cortical neuromodulation in Parkinson's disease: An alternative to deep brain stimulation? Clin Neurophysiol 2014; 125:874-885

Canavero S, Paolotti R. Extradural motor cortex stimulation for advanced Parkinson'sdisease. Mov Disord 2000; 152169-171

Canavero S, Paolotti R, Bonicalzi V, et al. Extradural motor cortex stimulation for advancedParkinson's disease: report of two cases. J Neurosurg 2002; 97 21208-121 1

Canavero S, Bonicalzi V, Paolotti R, et al. Therapeutic extradural cortical stimulation formovement disorders: a review. Neurol Res 2003; 25: 118-122

Canavero S, Bonicalzi V. Cortical stimulation for parkinsonism. Arch Neurol 2004; 61: 606

Canavero S, Bonicalzi V. Extradural cortical stimulation for movement disorders. In: D Sakas, B Simpson, E Krames, Eds. Operative Neuromodulation. II Neural Networks Surgery. Wien: Springer-Verlag, 2007, 223-232

Canavero S. Invasive cortical stimulation for Parkinson's disease (PD): why, where and how. In: Canavero S (ed) Textbook of therapeutic cortical stimulation. New York: Nova Science, 2009, 217-227

Canavero S Cerebral-Surface. In J Arle and J Shils Eds. Essential Neuromodulation, Elsevier, 2011, 19-42.

Castrioto A, Lhommée E, Moro E, et al. Mood and behavioural effects of subthalamic stimulation in Parkinson's disease. Lancet Neurol. 2014;13:287-305.

Caulo M, Briganti C, Mattei PA, et al. New morphologic variants of the hand motor cortex as seen with MR imaging in a large study population. AJNR 2007; 28: 1480-1485

Cerasa A, Quattrone A. May Hyperdirect Pathway Be a Plausible Neural Substrate for understanding the rTMS-related Effects on PD Patients With Levodopa-induced Dyskinesias? Brain Stimul 2014; 7: 488-9

Cilia R, Landi A, Vergari F, et al. Extradural motor cortexstimulation in Parkinson's disease. Mov Disord 2007; 22:1 1 1-114

Cilia R, Marotta G, Landi A, et al. Cerebral activity modulation by extradural motor cortex stimulation in Parkinson's disease: a perfusion SPECT study. Eur J Neurol 2008; 15: 22-28

Cioni B. Motor cortex stimulation for Parkinson's disease. In: D Sakas, B Simpson, EKrames, eds. Operative Neuromodulation. II Neural Networks Surgery. Wien: Springer-Verlag, 2007, 233-238

De Rose M, Guzzi G, Bosco D, et al. Motor cortex stimulation in Parkinson's disease Neurology research International 2012;12:502096

Di Giuda D, Calcagni ML, Totaro M, et al. Chronic motor cortex stimulation in patients with advanced Parkinson's disease and effects on striatal dopaminergic transmission as assessed by ^{123}I-FP-CIT SPECT: a preliminary report Nuclear Medicine Communications 2012, 33:933-940

Fasano A, Piano C, De Simone C, et al. High frequency extradural motor cortex stimulation dramatically improves axial symptoms in a patient with Parkinson's disease. Mov Disord 2008; 23:1916-9

Groppa S, Muthuraman M, Otto B, et al. Subcortical substrates of TMS induced modulation of the cortico-cortical connectivity. Brain Stimul. 2013;6:138-46.

Gutierrez JC, Seijo FJ, Alvarez Vega M, et al. Therapeutic extradural cortical stimulation for Parkinson's disease: report of six cases and review of the literature. Clinical Neurology and Neurosurgery 111 (2009) 703-707

Kalmar Z, Kovacs N, Perlaki G, et al. Reorganization of motor system in Parkinson's disease. Eur Neurol 2011; 66: 220-226

Khedr EM. Noninvasive stimulation for treatment of movement disorders. In: Canavero S (ed) Textbook of therapeutic cortical stimulation. New York: Nova Science, 2009, 183-200

Kleiner-Fisman G, Fisman DN, Kahn FI, et al. Motor cortical stimulation for parkinsonism in multiple system atrophy. Arch Neurol 2003;60:1554-8.

Kojovic M, Bologna M, Kassavetis P, et al. Functional reorganization of sensorimotor cortex in early Parkinson disease. Neurology 2012;78:1441-8.

Kovac S, Scott CA, Maglajlija V, et al. Extraoperative electrical cortical stimulation: characteristics of motor responses and correlation with precentral gyrus. J Clin Neurophysiol 2011;28:618-24

Kundu B, Johnson JS, Postle BR. Trait-like Differences in Underlying Oscillatory State Predict Individual Differences in the TMS-evoked Response. Brain Stimul 2014 (in press)

Li Q, Qian ZM, Arbuthnott GW, Ke Y, Yung WH. Cortical effects of deep brain stimulation: implications for pathogenesis and treatment of Parkinson disease. JAMA Neurol. 2014;71:100-3

Moro E, Schwalb JM, Piboolnurak P, et al. Unilateral subdural motor cortex stimulation improves essential tremor but not Parkinson's disease Brain 2011; 134(Pt 7):2096-105

Munno D, Caporale S, Zullo G, et al. Neuropsychological assessment of patients withadvanced Parkinson Disease submitted to extradural motor cortex stimulation. Cog Behav Neurol 2007; 20: 1-6

Nelson AJ, Premji A, Rai N, et al. Dopamine alters tactile perception in Parkinson's disease. Can J Neurol Sci 2012; 39: 52-57

Nguyen JP, Pollin B, Fève A, et al. Improvement of action tremor by chronic cortical stimulation. Mov Disord 1998; 13:84-88

Ni Z, Bahl N, Gunraj CA, et al. Increased motor cortical facilitation and decreased inhibition in Parkinson disease. Neurology. 2013;80:1746-53

Opitz A, Legon W, Rowlands A, et al. Physiological observations validate finite element models for estimating subject-specific electric field distributions induced by transcranial magnetic stimulation of the human motor cortex. Neuroimage 2013;81:253-64.

Oswal A, Brown P, Litvak V. Synchronized neural oscillations and the pathophysiology of Parkinson's disease. Curr Opin Neurol. 2013;26:662-70.

Pagni CA, Zeme S, Zenga F, et al. Extradural motor cortex stimulation in advancedParkinson's disease: the Turin experience. Neurosurg 2005; 57 (ONS Suppl 3): ONS-402 (includes Canavero's cases)

Pagni CA, Altibrandi MG, Bentivoglio A, et al. Extradural motor cortex stimulation (M1 ICS) for Parkinson's disease. History and first results by the study group of the Italian neurosurgical society. Acta Neurochir 2005 93:113-119 (includes Canavero's cases)

Pagni CA, Albanese A, Bentivoglio A, et al. Results bymotor cortex stimulation in treatment of focal dystonia, Parkinson's disease and post-ictalspasticity. The experience of the Italian Study Group of the Italian NeurosurgicalSociety. Acta Neurochír Suppl. 2008; 101:13-21

Rizzone MG, Fasano A, Daniele A, et al. Long-term outcome of subthalamic nucleus DBS in Parkinson's disease: From the advanced phase towards the late stage of the disease? Parkinsonism Relat Disord 2014 (in press)

Rodriguez-Oroz MC, Moro E, Krack P. Long-term outcomes of surgical therapies for Parkinson's disease. Mov Disord 2012;27:1718-28.

Spagnolo F, Coppi E, Chieffo R, et al. Interhemispheric balance in Parkinson's disease: a transcranial magnetic stimulation study. Brain Stimul 2013;6:892-7.

Thut G, Miniussi C. New insights into rhythmic brain activity from TMS-EEG studies. TICS 2009; 13: 182-189

Verhagen Metman L, Pahwa R, Lyons K, et al. Motor cortex stimulation in Parkinson's disease: a pilot study. Neurology 2006 (suppl 2) 66: A47

Woolsey CN, Erickson TC, Gilson WE. Localization in somatic sensory and motor areas of human cerebral cortex as determined by direct recording of evoked potentials and electrical stimulation.J Neurosurg. 1979;51:476-506.

Zwartjes DG, Heida T, Feirabend HK, et al. Motor cortex stimulation for Parkinson's disease: a modelling study. J Neural Eng. 2012;9:056005

Giuseppe Messina, Michele Rizzi, Miryam Carecchio,
Roberto Cordella, Angelo Franzini

11 Movement Disorders: Dystonia

Different forms of dystonia, including primary focal and generalized dystonia and secondary dystonia due to ischemic or traumatic brain injuries generally respond poorly to medical and conservative treatments. Mobile forms of dystonia, characterized by twisting, repetitive movements which result in abnormal, often painful postures, are classified according to the anatomical distribution of abnormal movements (focal, segmentary, generalized), presence or absence of a clear etiology (idiopathic or secondary), and age at onset (early or late forms). Medical therapies include the use of triexylphenidyl, tetrabenazine, benzodiazepines and baclofen. Focal dystonias, such as writer's cramp, may also benefit from local botulinum toxin injections, but generalized forms cannot and often do not respond satisfactorily to medical treatment.

A great heterogeneity exists with regard to the etiology of abnormal fixed postures of several body segments: they may develop following different focal brain lesions involving the basal ganglia, be psychogenic, or occur in the context of the so-called fixed dystonia (FD) syndrome. The prominent clinical feature seen in FD is the permanent abnormal posture of the affected body segments that never revert to normal positions. Accordingly, it is important to differentiate it from segmentary spasticity, which shows a typical pattern of muscular involvement, and from primary forms of dystonia that tend to be mobile and lack, by definition, structural abnormalities on brain imaging. FD is clinically and often etiologically different from mobile dystonia because it is more frequently focal and less frequently segmentary. It often causes a significant level of functional impairment, also due to poor response to medical treatment (Schrag et al 2004). FD can be idiopathic or be part of other conditions including corticobasal degeneration, advanced-stage primary dystonia and causalgia-dystonia syndrome. FD can also be accompanied by severe psychiatric disorders, thus being frequently misdiagnosed as somatization disorder or psychogenic dystonia. Prognosis is poor. In a series, only 6% of patients reached remission, 25% improved and 33% continued worsening (Ibrahim et al 2009).

The main surgical options that can be offered to these patients are Deep Brain Stimulation (DBS) and Implantable Cortical Stimulation (ICS). DBS of the posteroventrolateral (somato-sensory) portion of both GPs is considered a well-established and effective surgical procedure for the treatment of primary and secondary generalized dystonia, as well as of primary cervical dystonia. In this chapter, we address the results of extradural ICS.

11.1 Overview

Fixed dystonia (FD), which is poorly responsive to DBS (Romito et al 2007, Lalli et al 2012), has been observed to improve in patients with thalamic hand syndrome and in post-stroke fixed postures (Franzini et al 2000). Good control of involuntary movements has been reported by one Japanese group (Katayama et al 2002, Yamamoto et al 2011): in 2 of 3 patients with hemichoreo-athetosis, 2 of 2 patients with distal resting or action tremor, and 1 of 3 patients with proximal postural tremor. Two patients with chronic pain had their dystonic posture improved (Nuti et al 2012). The acute effects of M1 ICS in a patient with spasmodic torticollis unresponsive to thalamotomy are on record (Canavero et al 2003). The theoretical basis of application of CS in dystonia relies on the modulatory role of the pre-motor or primary motor cortex on sensori-motor cortico-strio-pallido-thalamic circuits.

Two targets are possible for CS: the primary motor cortex (M1) or the premotor cortex (PMC). Both have been implicated in the genesis of dystonia by non-invasive CS studies (Khedr 2009; Murase et al 2005, Huang et al 2004).

We recommend localization of M1 by preoperative fMRI because of the frequent aberrant representation of the affected area resulting from abnormal intracortical plasticity underlying dystonia. The latter variable could thus affect the actual position and size of M1. We perform intra-operative EMG by delivering electrical current from various combinations of the epidural contacts, to ascertain which is capable, singly or in combination, to evoke motor potentials in the affected part of the body. Delivered current is gradually increased until motor potentials are recorded; partial or generalized seizures are not an uncommon occurrence, and they can be abolished either by local administration of cold saline or by IV diazepam. At the end of this procedure, the electrode can be secured to the burr-hole with a titanium miniplate. In case of a craniotomy, the electrode(s) can be directly sutured to the underlying dura mater. Surgery is then completed by subcutaneously tunneling the connection cable (in the lateral cervical region) to an infraclavicular pocket, where the IPG is positioned.

Our group has previously reported (Lalli et al 2012) an overall improvement in 7 patients affected by primary pure focal dystonia (6 with cervical dystonia (Table 11.1) and 1 with upper limb dystonia), who underwent extradural PMC ICS under general anesthesia.

Table 11.1:

	Patients number	BFMDRS improvement at 12 months	TWSTRS improvement at 12 months	QOLI improvement (SIP scale)
Neurostimulation group	6	17%	15%	50%

Cervical dystonia patients received a bilateral epidural cortical electrode implant of the PMC, the patient with limb symptoms a unilateral implant on the contralateral cortex. The target was set 2 cm anterior to the hand area in M1. The electrodes were all perpendicular to the precentral gyrus, after electrophysiological localization of the central sulcus (N20-P20 phase reversal). In cervical dystonia cases, monopolar stimulation was performed with 2 active contacts on the PMC (0-,1-, case +); in the upper limb dystonia patient, there were 3 active contacts (0-,1-,2-, case +). Stimulation was continuous for 24 hours. The improvement was rated by the Burke-Fahn-Mardsen scale (BMFS) and by the Toronto Western Spasmodic Torticollis Rating Scale (TWSTRS) and was observed after a 12-months' follow-up period. *No effect on dystonia was observed immediately upon start of stimulation.* There was an improvement on the BFMS at 6 months that remained unchanged at 12 months. ICS was substantially ineffective in the patients with a mainly fixed posture of the dystonic body segment. The patient with limb dystonia improved 51% at 1 year. Though non significant, *working visual memory, phonemic fluency, anxiety and depression showed an improvement.* We also found baseline (pre-operative) and bilaterally increased cortical metabolism in S1/M1 - as compared to controls- on ^{18}F-fluoro- deoxy-glucose positron emission tomography (FDG PET). This metabolic increase was found to be reduced during a 12 month post-surgery follow up, suggesting a modulatory or rebalancing role of epidural stimulation on hyperactive S1/M1.

We (Messina et al 2012) then submitted 10 patients affected by secondary fixed dystonia (FD) of the upper limb to M1 ICS. Here, we include a further patient affected by an ischemic thalamic stroke, for a total of 11 cases. The rationale for M1 ICS was based on the hypothesis that an abnormal cortical representation of the affected body segment could follow deep brain lesions (Opavsky et al 2006). Also, we reported on a patient affected by fixed hemidystonia who was unresponsive to Gpi DBS but not to M1 ICS (Romito et al 2007). All patients treated were refractory to conventional medical and non-invasive treatments (benzodiazepines, baclofen, motor rehabilitation, and botulinum toxin injections) and did not fulfil the Fahn and Williams's criteria for psychogenic dystonia. All were severely disabled: 5 patients had fixed dystonia secondary to cortical or subcortical ischemic stroke; in 1 patient to birth anoxia; in 2 patients to iatrogenic post-surgical syndromes; in 1 patient to postencephalitic syndrome; in 1 patient to long-term neuroleptic treatment (tardive dystonia); and in the last patient secondary to brain trauma. A movement disorder neurologist evaluated all patients both pre-operatively and post-operatively. These evaluations confirmed the phenotypic characteristics of unilateral upper limb fixed dystonia, involving, with various degrees of severity, shoulder, arm, forearm, and hand. Polygraphic EMG recordings showed tonic muscular co-contractions in the affected muscles at rest in all patients. Extensive psychiatric examination excluded the diagnosis of psychogenic dystonia, and complex regional pain syndrome (CRPS)-associated dystonia.

11.1.1 Surgical Procedure

In all patients, a unilateral quadripolar paddle electrode (Resume II, Medtronic, Minneapolis, Minnesota) was positioned on the dural surface corresponding to the "hand-knob" area of M1 of the side contralateral to the affected upper limb. Surgery was performed under general anesthesia in all patients without curarization, under neuronavigation guidance (Stealth Station System, Medtronic, Minneapolis, MA, USA) and through intraoperative electromyography (EMG) for localization of the hand-knob area. A 3-cm skin incision was made 4 cm behind the coronal suture and 3 cm lateral from the midline. A burr hole was performed to expose the dura mater overlying the postero-medial portion of the central gyrus. After dural dissection, from the internal cranial bone, the quadripolar electrode was placed parallel to the premotor cortex and along its main axis (as indicated by the navigation system); when a motor response was unelicitable, we changed the orientation of the paddle electrode until recording the appropriate upper limb's EMG responses (abductor pollicis brevis muscle). Muscular sites monitored intra-operatively with EMG were the orbicularis oris, brachioradialis, abductor pollicis brevis, rectus femori, tibialis anterior, and extensor digitorum brevis. After the electrode's initial positioning, a set of stimulation trials was delivered to evoke EMG responses in the affected muscles, specifically in the abductor pollicis brevis. In all cases, electric stimulation through the epidural quadripolar strip (60 Hz, 1 ms pulse width) evoked selective motor response and EMG activation of hand and upper limb muscles with 4 to 7 mA (Fig.11.1). Every procedure was completed with the subcutaneous implantation of a single-channel IPG and its connection cable to the epidural electrode. The day after surgery, the IPG was activated in all patients, and stimulation parameters adjusted to the threshold for the elicitation of side effects (such as paresthesias) and to the clinical effects during follow-up.

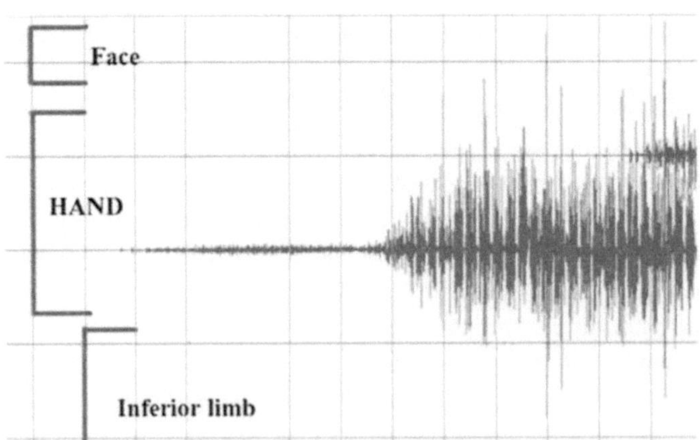

Fig. 11.1: Intraoperative EMG showing activation of hand muscles after stimulation with epidural paddle electrode.

11.1.2 Assessment and Outcome

Patients were evaluated using the Disability of Arm, Shoulder and Hand (DASH) scale and the Short Form-36 Physical Activity subscale. 7 out of 11 patients evinced a >30% improvement on the DASH scale and an overall 70% increase on the latter. A postoperative CT scan was merged with the preoperative 3D MR scan and the correct positioning of the epidural electrode was confirmed in all patients (Fig.11.2-11.3). The postoperative course was uneventful in all but 1 patient, who required surgical evacution for an acute epidural hematoma; after 6 months the whole system was re-implanted. No patient experienced seizures during parameters' search. The final stimulation parameters were set at the 6-month follow-up examination in all patients and the configuration was quadruple monopolar (Case as Anode, contacts 0,1,2, 3 as Cathodes). The follow-up ranged from 1 to 9 years. Periodic reassessment was carried out monthly in the first 6 months and then on a 6-month basis. The DASH Scale was employed, together with a self-report questionnaire to measure physical function and symptoms (SF-36). Higher DASH scale scores indicate greater disability. This scale focuses on the whole functionality of the affected segment of the body, better than more traditional scales employed for classical predominantly "mobile" dystonia. The overall degree of disability of patients was high due to total refractoriness to conservative treatment: an improvement of 30% of the DASH scores is thus significant and 7 patients reached this level of improvement at the latest follow-up (Table 11.2). The overall improvement on the SF-36 scale may indicate the high degree of interference resulting from this pathological condition on overall well-being. Although differences between pre- and postoperative DASH scores found in this series do not seem impressive if only numerical data are taken into account, nevertheless, even small changes in DASH score reflected a significant higher quality-of-life score (Table 11.2). Placebo effects cannot be discounted, but given refractoriness to conventional treatments this seems unlikely.

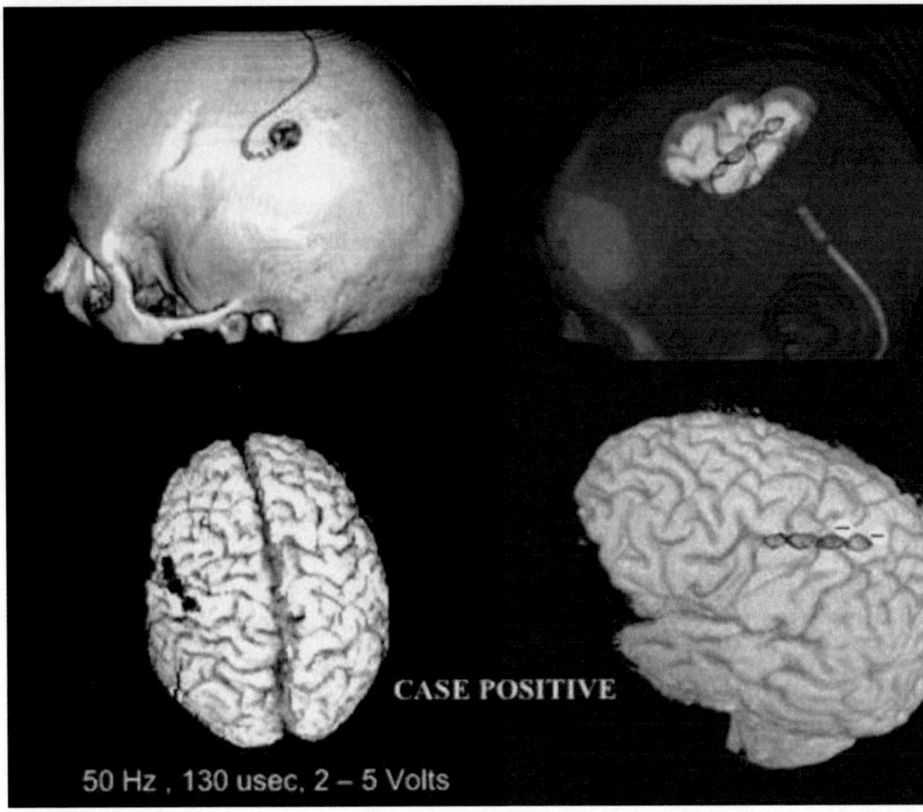

Fig. 11.2: 3-dimensional postoperative reconstruction showing the placement of the chronic leads over the motor cortex.

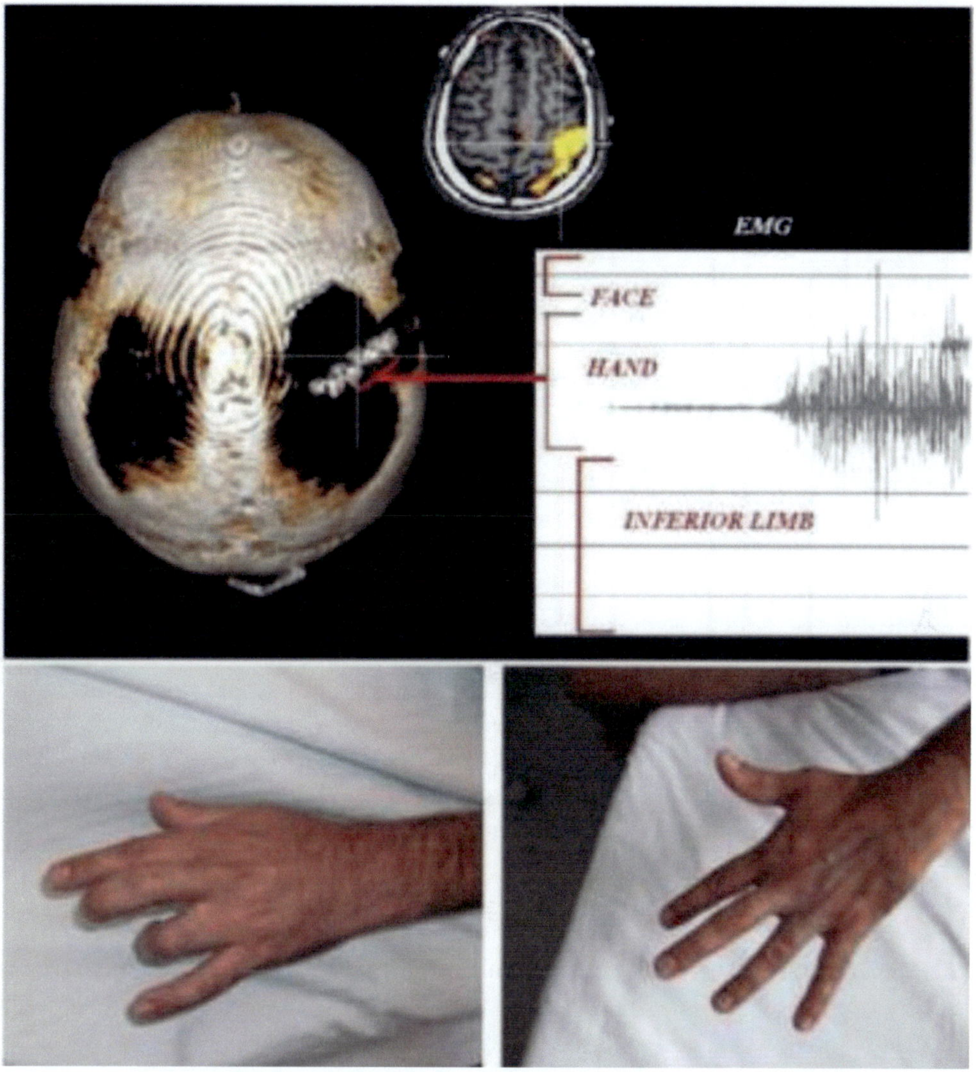

Fig. 11.3: *Top*: 3-dimensional reconstruction of the post-operative Computerized Tomography showing the contacts of the paddle electrode which allowed stimulation of contralateral hand muscle; above, an axial functional MRI image showing aberrant activation of hand motor cortex in the affected contralateral hand; *Bottom:* the affected hand of the patient before (left) and 4 months after MCS (right).

Rieu et al (2014) reported a double-blind, crossover, multicenter study involving 5 patients affected by dystonia secondary to focal post-ischemic basal ganglia (BG) lesions, who underwent extradural CS (Table 11.3). All the patients suffered from hemidystonia secondary to a basal ganglia vascular lesions. For every patient, two parallel quadripolar electrodes were positioned in the epidural space overlying both MI and PMC, parallel to the central sulcus, under neuronavigation guidance. The anode was positioned over the motor representation of the most affected limb on M1; PMC-wise, the electrodes were positioned over the superior and the middle frontal gyri. In all patients, post-operative CT confirmed optimal positioning of the electrodes. In this case series, the BFMS, the Ashworth scale for spasticity, Visual Analogue Scale (VAS) for Pain and SF-36 for quality of life were used for pre- and postoperative evaluations. After one month from implantation, patients were randomly assigned to two groups: stimulation-on and stimulation-off groups; such condition was maintained for three months; after a washout period of one month, a clinical evaluation was performed and the on-off condition was reversed; again, this was maintained for other three months and, then, a second follow-up was carried out. The above-mentioned scales scores were not significantly modified at any evaluation time, thus no patient benefited from the procedure. Given the study design and the negative results obtained, the Authors concluded that Class I evidence exists that epidural CS failed to improve dystonia secondary to BG lesions. This is untenable, since these patients presented with mobile rather than fixed dystonia, the sample size was limited (5 patients) and the follow-up period relatively short (3 months). Also in light of the slow build-up of effect, the 1-month intervals may have been too short

11.2 Conclusion

How CS achieves its results remains unknown, but similar arguments to Parkinson disease can be made (see Chapter 10). Increased M1 excitability has been demonstrated in patients with dystonia secondary to focal lesions of the basal ganglia and thalamus (Trompetto et al 2012). An involvement of cerebellar pathways should also be considered.

The generator of FD could be an increased thalamocortical drive resulting in hyperexcitability of the sensorimotor cortex; the overactivation of glutamatergic input to the cortex could be caused by an unbalance between the so-called direct and indirect corticonuclear pathways, although why in some patients this may result in fixed postures rather than typical mobile dystonic movements remains unexplained. In fact, according to the direct-indirect pathways theory, lesions localized in the motor portion of the thalamus (such as those found in 3 of our patients) would more likely suppress movements instead of increasing the thalamocortical drive. Moreover, not all patients affected by acquired basal ganglia lesions present with FD, and spasticity, tremor, myoclonus, and athetosis can develop as well. Complex interactions between

Table 11.2:

Pt nr.	Origin	Stimulation Parameters	DASH pre	DASH post	Improvement %	SF-36 Physical Activity Subscale pre	SF-36 Physical Activity Subscale post	SF-36 Mental Scale Subscale pre	SF-36 Mental Scale Subscale post	Follow-up
1	Striatal stroke	120 µs, 30Hz, 2.5V	86	57	34	0	85	64	88	36
2	Parieto-temporal stroke	90 µs , 50Hz, 3.5V	90.5	77.6	15.1	0	40	24	72	48
3	Temporo-occipital and thalamic stroke	120 µs, 50Hz, 3V	92	49.1	47	30	85	28	48	24
4	Viral meningo-encephalitis	120 µs, 30Hz, 3.1V	72.4	64.2	12.4	10	75	36	60	24
5	Bulbopontine cavernoma	90 µs, 30Hz, 3V	32.5	18.1	44.4	20	65	36	44	24
6	Perinatal hypoxia	120 µs, 50Hz, 3V	48.3	30.8	36	75	100	40	52	24
7	Neuroleptic-induced dystonia	90 µs, 50Hz, 3.3V	87.1	28.4	67	0	95	4	100	24
8	Thalamic oligoastrocytoma	120 µs, 50Hz, 3.5V	66.4	44.8	32	20	75	28	60	24
9	Thalamic stroke	120 µs, 30Hz, 2.8V	75	28.4	62	60	80	44	76	24
10	Post-Traumatic putaminal stroke (bilat.)	150 µs, 30Hz, 4V	84	66	22.3	40	40	56	60	120
11	Thalamic stroke	150 µs, 40Hz, 4V	80	74	7.5	40	40	50	64	4

the different subcircuits of the cortico-striato-pallido-thalamo-cortical loops are likely at work. Maladaptive cerebral plasticity may subtend secondary FD. In one of our patients, FD developed after surgery for a right bulbopontine cavernous hemangioma; the role of brainstem lesions in the pathophysiology of dystonia has not been elucidated, but several reports point to a role of dysfunction of ascending and descending pontomesencephalic pathways such as the central tegmental tract and the dentatothalamic fascicle, as well as the pedunculopontine nucleus and the nucleus interstitialis of Cajal (Loher and Krauss 2009). The problem of CS-refractory patients can be explained by maladaptive plasticity extending beyond the targeted areas, perhaps even bilaterally, and this must be explored in future studies.
In sum, surgical CS is a new alternative for the management of FD.

Table 11.3:

Pt nr.	Origin	Stimulation Parameters	BFM (global) at baseline	BFM at 3 months (Stim OFF)	BFM at 3 months (Stim ON)	VAS at baseline	VAS at 3 months (Stim OFF)	VAS at 3 months (Stim ON)
1	Right subthalamic and cerebral peduncle stroke	60 µs, 40Hz, 3.8V	22	20	17	8.2	3.72	6.38
2	Right globus pallidus stroke	60 µs, 40Hz, 3.8V	14	18.5	20	6.2	7.98	0
3	Right striatum stroke	60 µs, 40Hz, 3.8V	20	20	24	6.1	5.67	7.55
4	Right striatum and frontotemporoparietal cortex stroke	60 µs, 40Hz, 3.8V	22	15	15	7.1	3.62	4.15
5	Right striatum and right parietal cortex stroke	60 µs, 40Hz, 3.8V	28	24	32.5	7.1	4.95	9.25

References

Canavero S, Bonicalzi V, Paolotti R, et al. Therapeutic extradural cortical stimulation for movement disorders: a review. Neurol Res 2003;25:118-22.

Franzini A, Ferroli P, Servello D, et al. Reversal of thalamic hand syndrome by long-term motor cortex stimulation. J Neurosurg. 2000;93:873-875

Franzini A, Ferroli P, Dones I, et al. Chronic motor cortex stimulation for movement disorders: a promising perspective. Neurol Res. 2003;25:123-126.

Franzini A, Messina G, Marras C, et al. Poststroke fixed dystonia of the foot relieved by chronic stimulation of the posterior limb of the internal capsule. J Neurosurg. 2009;111:1216-1219.

Huang YZ, Edwards MJ, Bhatia KP, et al. One-Hz repetitive transcranial magnetic stimulation of the premotor cortex alters reciprocal inhibition in DYT1 dystonia. Mov Disord. 2004 ;19:54-9

Ibrahim NM, Martino D, van de Warrenburg BP, et al. The prognosis of fixed dystonia: a follow-up study. Parkinsonism Relat Disord. 2009;15:592-7

Katayama Y, Oshima H, Fukaya C, et al. Control of post-stroke movement disorders using chronic motor cortex stimulation. Acta Neurochir Suppl. 2002;79:89-92.

Khedr EM. Noninvasive stimulation for treatment of movement disorders. In: Canavero S (ed) Textbook of therapeutic cortical stimulation. New York: Nova Science, 2009, pp 183-200

Lalli S, Piacentini S, Franzini A, et al. Epidural premotor cortical stimulation in primary focal dystonia: clinical and 18F-fluoro deoxyglucose positron eMIssion tomography open study. Mov Disord. 2012;27:533-8

Loher TJ, Krauss JK. Dystonia associated with pontomesencephalic lesions. Mov Disord. 2009;24:157-67

Messina G, Cordella R, Dones I, et al. Improvement of secondary fixed dystonia of the upper limb after chronic extradural motor cortex stimulation in 10 patients: first reported series. Neurosurgery. 2012;70:1169-75

Murase N, Rothwell JC, Kaji R, et al. Subthreshold low-frequency repetitive transcranial magnetic stimulation over the premotor cortex modulates writer's cramp. Brain. 2005 ;128(Pt 1):104-15.

Nuti C, Vassal F, Mertens P, et al. Improved dexterity after chronic electrical stimulation of the motor cortex for central pain: a special relevance for thalamic syndrome. Stereotact Funct Neurosurg 2012;90:370-8.

Opavsky R, Hlustik P, Kanovsky P. Cortical plasticity and its implications for focal hand dystonia. Biomed Pap Med Fac Univ Palacky Olomouc Czech Repub. 2006;150:223-226

Rieu I, Aya Kombo M, Thobois S, et al. Motor cortex stimulation does not improve dystonia secondary to a focal basal ganglia lesion. Neurology. 2014 ; 82:156-62

Romito LM, Franzini A, Perani D, et al. Fixed dystonia unresponsive to pallidal stimulation improved by motor cortex stimulation. Neurology. 2007;68: 875-876.

Schrag A, Trimble M, Quinn N, et al. The syndrome of fixed dystonia: an evaluation of 103 patients. Brain. 2004;127(Pt 10):2360-72.

Trompetto C, Avanzino L, Marinelli L, et al. Corticospinal excitability in patients with secondary distonia due to focal lesions of the basal ganglia and thalamus. Clin Neurophysiol. 2012;123:808-14

Yamamoto T, Katayama Y, Watanabe M, et al. Changes in motor function induced by chronic motor cortex stimulation in post-stroke pain patients. Stereotact Funct Neurosurg. 2011;89:381-9.

Sergio Canavero, Hyoung-Ihl Kim

12 Post-Stroke Recovery

More than half of all stroke survivors have remaining disabilities and roughly one third of stroke survivors suffer from aphasia. Rehabilitation gives modest improvement in leg function, but no clear benefit on arm function, and actual recovery slowly subsides after the first post-stroke month; no major spontaneous recovery can be expected beyond the 6-month mark. On the other hand, aphasia can improve further even several years after the initial stroke (i.e. longer window for recovery). The degree of recovery is idiosyncratic, despite similar rehabilitation protocols. This may depend on, among other factors, inter-individual variability in vascularization (e.g. a different extent of collaterals or different blood supply from adjacent arteries) or intrinsic reorganizational capability.

12.1 Premises

In a series of duplicate papers since 1993, a Japanese group (Katayama et al 2002, Yamamoto et al 2011) reported subjective improvements in motor performance in a subset (19%) of central post-stroke patients who had mild motor weakness submitted to extradural M1 ICS (<50 Hz). In particular, they examined the correlation between the duration of daily M1 ICS applied over 6 months and motor function assessed on the basis of the Fugl-Meyer Assessment (FMA) score of the patients. In the 6 patients with motor weakness, the FMA score of the upper extremity increased in 4 patients who underwent daily stimulation for less than 4 hours. On the other hand, two patients who were overstimulated to control their complicating post-stroke pain showed decreased FMA scores and worsened motor function due to increased rigidity and/or spasticity: both recovered their motor function after stimulation was restricted to less than 4 hours. Nuti et al (2012) – among others – reported that 10 out of 38 (26%) patients prospectively submitted to M1 ICS for chronic pain declared a benefit in their motor function. Eight presented objective evidence of recovered dexterity for rapid alternating movements, due to relief of spasticity. They found a significant correlation between thalamic lesions and benefits in motor performance. Thus, ICS per se may partially contribute to overall improvement.

Over the past decade or so, noninvasive cortical stimulation (rTMS, tDCS) has been employed in order to enhance recovery from stroke, especially subcortical stroke. However, a review of published controlled studies found no consistent beneficial effects of rTMS (8-30% transient benefit), a trend only for improvement in activities of daily living and only limited evidence for a beneficial effect of rTMS on aphasia and neglect (Raffin and Siebner 2014). Anodal tDCS has been found to benefit arm motor function in chronic stroke paretics, but the small sample size and the very low to low quality of the studies (n=15; 455 patients) mitigate this conclusion (Raffin and Siebner 2014, Elsner et al 2014). In addition, there is also substantial intersubject variability in their effects. Regardless, experience with noninvasive CS suggests that:

1. *targeting may depend on the stage of stroke,*
2. *multisite stimulation should be an option, e.g. stimulating simultaneously or consecutively M1 or premotor, parietal and cerebellar cortex in the ipsi or contralesional hemisphere,*
3. *repeated daily sessions* might be better - with prolongation of the aftereffects and *cumulative effects*- but nonetheless suboptimal,
4. *a night of sleep* might be indicated to resensitize the brain to stimulation (Night stim-OFF),
5. *CS and rehabilitation can be additive, with the choice of activity critical for the success of the therapy (constraint-induced therapy not additive)*
6. while stimulation applied after 12 months of stroke incurs no risk of interfering with spontaneous neuroplastic changes, there is some sparse evidence that benefit might accrue from subacute stimulation (within 2 weeks), although at this point negative consequences cannot be ruled out. Direct stimulation around lesioned MI might increase metabolism and trigger excitotoxicity in the penumbra.
7. right Pars Triangularis (BA 45), a site in the inferior frontal gyrus, is the most effective target for aphasics.

12.2 Clinical Studies of Extradural Cortical Stimulaton

Direct stimulation of the cortex via implanted extradural electrodes (ICS) has been simultaneously and independently attempted for the first time in 2002 by Canavero (Canavero et al 2006) and, under the aegis of NorthStar Neuroscience, a now defunct US neurostimulation company, Brown, as an adjunct to standard rehabilitation. This line of research has been then pursued by Kim and a few other groups (Table 12.1).

The conclusion is that, while simple stimulation may be beneficial, combined protocols of temporary cortical stimulation and physiotherapy produce the best results. Rehabilitation with stimulation may cement these improvements by causing persistent anatomical changes, also explaining persistence of functional improvement after withdrawal of ICS. Importantly, improvement after ICS is observed long after further recovery is thought to be no longer possible (Fig.12.1-4).

Table 12.1: Studies of Epidural Cortical Stimulation for post-stroke rehabilitation

Authors Year	N	Infarct Location	Aim of CS Device	Target structures	Duration of CS	Parameters Of CS	-Effect of CS -Complications
Brown et al (2003)	1	SCI (implanted 2002)	-Upper arm motor recovery -Grid + EPG	Ipsi MI (fMR hotspot)	3 weeks	4,5mA, 50Hz, 100 μs stimulation during rehabilitative training	-UEFM improved by 10 points, Hand dexterity ↑ -none -able to grasp a pen and to write letters. This improvement persisted for at least four weeks after conclusion of rehab.
Canavero et al (2006)	1	CI (implanted 2002)	-Motor and language -Double Strip + IPG	Bilateral M1/PMC	6 months	Continuous, 3-3,7 V, 50 or 130 Hz, 210μsec	-Modest improvement of motor arm impairment & aphasia -none
Brown et al. (2006)	8 (+8 ctrls: rehabilitation only) Time since CVA: 9-33 mos	SCI or CI	-Upper arm motor recovery -Paddle + IPG	Perirolandic fMRI-activated area	3 weeks	Bipolar stimulation during rehabilitative training Half-threshold or 6.5 mA, 50Hz, 250μsec	-UEFM from 35.3±7.8 to 45.5 ± 10,8 -1 infection, 1 breakage -prospective, randomized, multicenter study. Improvements persisted throughout the 12-week follow-up assessment (study week 16). In comparison, lesser improvements in control patients occurred within the first two weeks and then seemed to decrease over time.

continued **Table 12.1:** Studies of Epidural Cortical Stimulation for post-stroke rehabilitation

Authors Year	N	Infarct Location	Aim of CS Device	Target structures	Duration of CS	Parameters Of CS	-Effect of CS -Complications
Levy et al (2008) Huang et al. (2008)	12 (+12 ctrls) Time since CVA: 4 mos-8 yrs	SCI or CI	-Motor recovery -Paddle + IPG	Perirolandic fMRI-activated area	6 weeks	Bipolar stimulation + rehabilitative training (2.5 hours daily); Half-threshold or 6.5 mA, 50 or 101 Hz, 250µsec. 3 anodes + 3 cathodes (1.8 cm2 stimulation area)	-prospective, randomized, multicenter study. AMAT (a measure of activities of daily living focusing on upper extremity paresis): improved by 0.4 (+/-0.6) points vs 0.2 points in controls (p=0.2) = 67% of pts had UEFM improvement (=/> 3.5- point increase) vs 25% of ctrls. 50% of patients had clinical improvement in both UEFM and AMAT scores (including 0.21 point improvement on AMAT) vs 8% of controls. Patients in the treatment arm began at a baseline UEFM of 35 points. This indicates moderate to severe impairment. These patients improved by 5.5 points (range 0-17). A two-point improvement is equal to an improvement from no activity to full activity. This implies that even a small improvement in UEFM score can be significant functionally. Control patients improved from a baseline of 32.4 to 34.3 points, (p=0.03).. Patients with left-side stroke who were stimulated showed more language improvement than controls, as measured by the Wechsler Abbreviated Scale of Intelligence vocabulary t-score (1.3 versus control score -3.8, p=0.05). 1 seizure

continued **Table 12.1:** Studies of Epidural Cortical Stimulation for post-stroke rehabilitation

Authors Year	**N**	**Infarct Location**	**Aim of CS Device**	**Target structures**	**Duration of CS**	**Parameters Of CS**	**-Effect of CS -Complications**
Northstar's Everest Pivotal Study (press release, 2008) Harvey et al (2009) Nouri and Cramer (2011)	91 (+55 ctrls) Single-Blind 21 US centers 2004-2008	SCI or CI (moderate-severe: UEFM 20-50 points) at least 4 months after stroke	-Motor recovery -Paddle + IPG	Perirolandic fMRI-activated area (pts without perirolandic hotspot excluded)	6 weeks (5 days/week in weeks 1-4 and 3 days/week for weeks 5-6)	Bipolar stimulation + task-oriented rehabilitative training (2.5 hours daily); Half-threshold or 6.5 mA, 50 Hz, 250μsec. 3 anodes + 3 cathodes (1.8 cm2 stimulation area)	At the 4-week follow-up, 30.8% of active group obtained =/>4.5 points improvement (UEFM) and =/>0.21 points (AMAT) versus 29.1% of controls (Δ= 1.7, P 0.41= NS; preset primary end point: 20% absolute difference). Responders had a smaller fraction of the CST injured vs non-responders (44% vs 72%, p<0.04) and rarely had severe tract injury. Responders had more often preserved motor responses on intraoperative stimulation (67% vs 27%, p<0.05); responders with elicitable motor responses also had lower rate of MI injury vs those without motor responses (0% vs 33%, p<0.05) and higher gray matter volume in areas including MI.
Kim et al (2008)	2	SCI & CI	-Motor & language -Paddle + IPG	Ipsi MI+PMC & Broca's area	6 months	Unipolar & Continuous 5V, 50Hz, 200μsec	-UEFM from 8 to 27 in one; 35 to 42 in the other Marked language improvement -none

continued **Table 12.1:** Studies of Epidural Cortical Stimulation for post-stroke rehabilitation

Authors Year	N	Infarct Location	Aim of CS Device	Target structures	Duration of CS	Parameters Of CS	-Effect of CS -Complications
Kim et al (2010)	2	SCI & CI (infarct was too large to be improved with single perirolandic stimulation)	Pt 1: severe hemiplegia associated with large cortical infarct in the right frontoparietal area. The patient could neither stand independently or walk; Pt 2: hemiplegia and aphasia due to cortical infarct in the left middle cerebral artery territory.	Two paddle electrodes covering frontal and parietal area were implanted, followed by dual cortical stimulation with concurrent rehabilitative training in patient 1. Two paddle electrodes were implanted to cover pre-motor and motor cortex in patient 2.	6 months	NA	Both patients had intensive rehabilitative training for more than 6 months with no beneficial results. Pt 1: after 6 months of stimulation, the patient could walk with a good posture. Pt 2: After similar treatment, the motor function was markedly improved.
Cherney et al (2010)	4 pts (vs 4 ctrls) time since CVA (left carotid artery): =/>12 mos			FMR hot spot intersecting activations during tasks overlying BA6 ventral. Craniotomy flap. 2x3 grid (2.6x2.7com in total area).	Rehab: 3h/die, 5 days a week, 6 weeks	50 Hz, 6.5 mA (4.75 mA in 1).	Single-blind. Randomised, controlled safety study. Non-fluent aphasia, slow agrammatic output & apraxia of speech. NorthStar Neuroscience study. Mean WAB-AQ change from baseline: 8 points (6 week f-up) and 12.3 points (12 week f-up). Underpowered! In matched patint pairs, none with mild-moderate aphasia achieved a 5 point change on WAB/AQ, but study pts had greater changes at all time points. Pts with moderate and moderate/severe aphasia reached a 5 point change on WAB/AQ. Ctrls had larger lesions (although nonsignificant). Most marked benefit in more severe aphasia. *Benefit associated with decrease in total brain activation during language tasks on fMR*

continued **Table 12.1:** Studies of Epidural Cortical Stimulation for post-stroke rehabilitation

Authors Year	N	Infarct Location	Aim of CS Device	Target structures	Duration of CS	Parameters Of CS	-Effect of CS -Complications
Balossier et al (2012, 2013)	1 pt	Left external capsular CVA	Control of pain	craniotomy, fMR aided neuronavigation. RESUME straddling MI and SI behind Broca's area		Continuous stimulation, 50 Hz, 60-120 μs, 3-3.65V	Pt developed central post-stroke pain, right periorbital region and cheek. Paroxysms triggered by cold and reading; allodynia. VAS 8-10. 5 years later: VAS 2-3. double-blind evaluation. Mild Broca's aphasia + severe speech apraxia. Aphasia regressed (verbal fluency, text reading) during stim ON At 5 years, semantic and phonemic improvement during stim ON less than initially seen After 6 years, sudden pain and aphasia relapse due to battery depletion. Benefit recaptured, with significant improvement in phonemic verbal fluency and text reading.

*SCI: subcortical infarct, CI: cortical infarct, Ipsi MI: ipsilesional motor cortex, Cont MI: contralesional MI, PMC: premotor cortex, IPG: internal pulse generator, EPG: external pulse generator, PD: pulse duration, UEFM: upper extremity Fugl Meyer, N: number of patients, CST: corticospinal tract, WAB-AQ: western aphasia battery/ aphasia quotient.

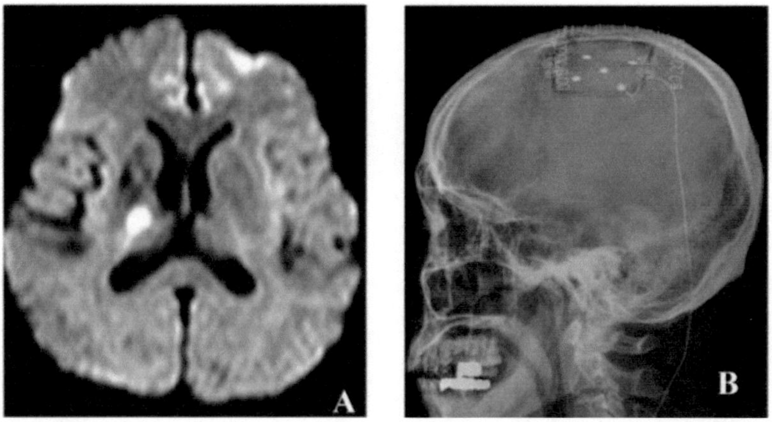

Fig. 12.1: Chronic subcortical infarct in the right internal capsule. This 51- year-old man with a chronic subcortical infarct 8 months before and moderately spastic arm and clumsy hand underwent ICS of the premotor and primary motor cortex. Diffusion imaging of MRI demonstrates the lesion in the right internal capsular area (A). fMRI images on a wrist flexion –extension task of the paretic arm failed to show activation of MI in both hemispheres. Six months' stimulation with rehabilitative training improved the mobility and spasticity of his hands, thus enabling him to drive a car again. In addition, his Functional Independence Measure (FIM) score improved in self-care, mobility, and locomotion. This patient had left hemiparesis with spastic upper extremity. A paddle electrode was implanted to cover premotor and hand/arm MI (B). After 6 months' stimulation and rehabilitative training, the patient can drive a car with improved FIM scores.

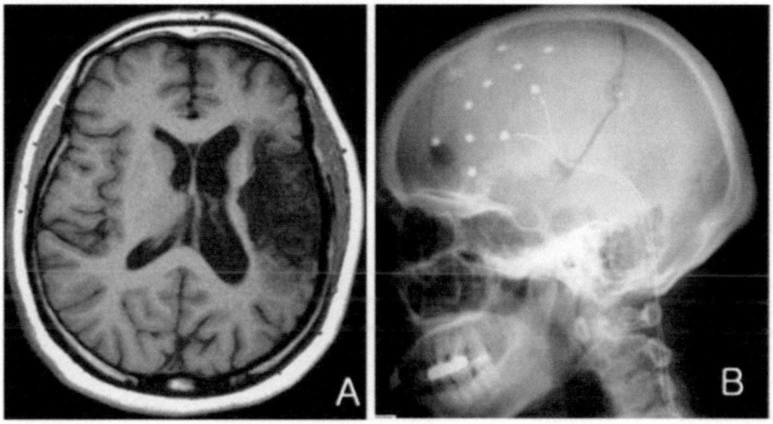

Fig. 12.2: Chronic cortical infarct in the left middle cerebral artery territory. T1-wighted image shows the cortical infarct in the left middle cerebral artery territory (A). This 39-year old patient with a cortical infarct 18 months earlier presented severe dysphagia and hemiparesis. Two 4x4 cm paddle electrodes were implanted to cover Broca's area plus premotor and MI cortices (B). After 6 months of stimulation (1 to 5Vover 1 month, 200 μs, 50 Hz) and rehabilitation (two hours every day), the patient regained communication ability and improved motor function of the right limbs.

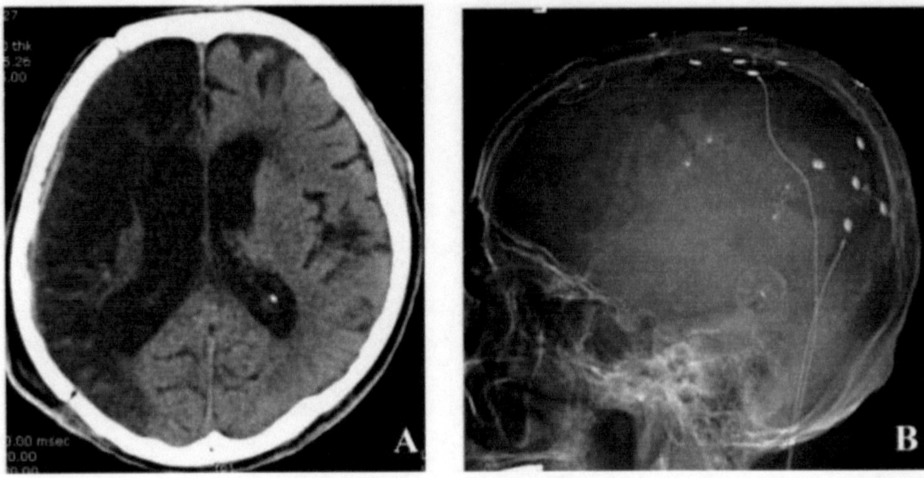

Fig. 12.3: Massive cortical infarct in the right hemisphere. T1-weighted image shows a diffuse fronto-parietal cortical infarct (A). This 67 year old patient could only stand with maximal assistance, otherwise he was bed-ridden, despite long-term intensive rehabilitation. fMRI on flexion-extension of the knee showed diffuse activation in posterior parietal areas. Two paddle electrodes were implanted to cover the frontal (near supplementary motor cortex) and posterior parietal area (network stimulation) in order to achieve maximal coverage (B). After stimulation and rehabilitative training for 6 months, he began to stand independently and walk 200 m.

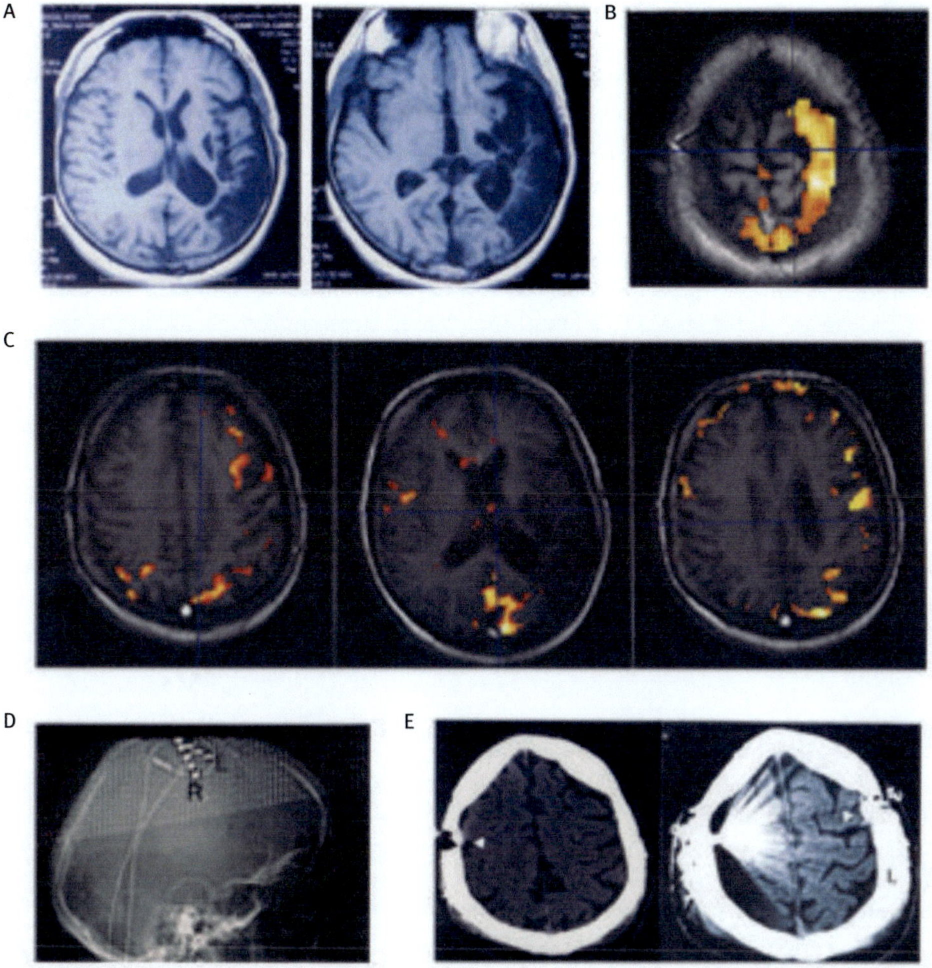

Fig. 12.4: Massive corticosubcortical infarct in a young adult (A). fMR scans showing a widespread hotspot on moving the paretic shoulder (rest of the arm plagic) (B,C). Bihemispheric stimulation covering frontal motor areas (D,E)

12.3 Mechanisms Subserving Recovery

The mechanisms subserving recovery are not well understood and it appears that several mechanisms may be at work simultaneously. ICS is known to modulate GABA and reactivate lesional and perilesional plasticity (Canavero et al 2006); the role of plasticity is also evinced by the long (months) after-effects of ICS. Long-Term Potentiation (LTP) and a cause-effect link between excitability changes and motor behavior have not been proven directly in man. Strengthening of latent neural pathways is another possibility. ICS, like other stimulation techniques, can also act via stochastic resonance, i.e. a small increase in noise improves signal processing in nonlinear systems that work in a context of low signal-to-noise ratio; this biases endogenous and cortical and corticosubcortical neural oscillations.

Intraoperative stimulation may immediately induce observable finger contractions that were not voluntarily possible prior to stimulation, implicating marginally effective circuits. In cases where no contractions are elicited, benefits may nonetheless be obtained by inducing new cortico-cortical connections to form new local networks by incorporating perilesional areas. Likewise, improvement would not occur only as an indirect result of electrical inhibition of confounding regions of hyperactivity.

12.4 Surgical Technique

12.4.1 Preoperative Evaluation

Candidates for ICS are chronic stroke patients who do not show further clinical improvements six months following a stroke. Although most patients reported in the literature underwent ICS no later than 3 years post-stroke, at least one received surgery 8 years later. Perhaps, there is no upper limit to duration of chronic stroke for ICS. Patients should be cognitively competent and motivated to adhere to long-term rehabilitation. Exclusion criteria are medical comorbidities that contraindicate rehabilitation or general anesthesia, epilepsy, other neurological diseases and compound strokes. Candidates should be evaluated with MR Tractography (DTI) and single-pulse TMS to assess the pyramidal tract. Motor activation fMR is indicated, but the task should correspond with the parts of the body targeted by rehabilitation. Noninvasive stimulation may have prognostic value as of subsequent ICS and help select the best parameters by highlighting facilitatory or inhibitory effects: this has yet to be explored in this context.

12.4.2 Targets

Targets employed in the published literature include the premotor cortex (PMC), MI (when spared) and SI, posterior parietal cortex, singly or combined (bifocal or network stimulation), uni- or bi-hemispherically. Yet, the ideal way to improve on blinded application of CS is provided by optimal site-finding protocols, either rTMS- or neuroimaging-driven, as these account for individual variability (Cramer et al 2003) in clinical factors such as lesion size and volume that could differentially influence the mechanisms of neuroplasticity in each patient. For example, one site that may be optimal in a patient with a small lesion may not be appropriate for another patient with more extensive damage. The extent of transcallosal disinhibition, or propensity of involvement of the perilesional and potentially beneficial contralateral homologs, differs among patients, and therefore, site-finding protocols help to meet individual treatment needs. The choice of the appropriate site for stimulation is key, as the electrode paddles usually employed are not large enough to cover extensive target areas singly. Both stimulating large or focal areas may have theoretical advantages and disadvantages. One should also be reminded that scars (and CSF) may shunt the induced current with mislocalization of stimulation.

Spontaneous improvement is mediated either by reintegration or increased connectivity within perilesional areas. Yet, both published evidence and our experience prove that *the perirolandic cortex does not qualify as a universal target for all patients*, despite similar presentation of imaging and clinical findings. Peri-infarct activation is not directly correlated with the magnitude of motor recovery (Cramer et al 2006) and lack of motor-task activations on fMRI cannot be relied upon for selection of patients: one of Kim's patients showed no activation on fMRI, yet was markedly improved, whereas in many patients, intraoperative stimulation elicited no motor response (Levy et al 2008), despite fMR hot spots. Data suggest that patients presenting near normal MI/SI activation on fMR would not be good candidates, as maximal usage implies no further reserve (Loubinoux 2007). In this sense, a low baseline cortical activity may represent underuse of surviving cortical resources (but also damage with little available resource to activate or enhance). A simple increase in corticospinal excitability might facilitate volitional recruitment of corticomotor output neurons, but effects of stimulation are not mediated by simply changing motor cortex excitability. *Presence or absence of fMR activation is not directly related to surgical outcome* and *selection of target based on the results of fMR may be confusing*, as areas of fMRI activation may really be a specific reorganization of motor representation or just a by-process unrelated to actual recovery. In other words, *while functional neuroimaging data can demonstrate the process of functional reorganization –generally over multiple, bilateral areas, they cannot be used to make a definitive surgical decision*. Likewise, results of ICS in chronic stroke patients with cortical infarcts may show variable results: perirolandic cortex stimulation produces variable results in patients with apparently similar neurologic conditions. *Modulating ipsilesional M1 is unlikely to benefit all patients.*

PMC has a direct connection with spinal motor neurons, although of lesser magnitude than the primary motor pathways: unmasking of this latent pathway may form a new motor pathway (Leuthardt et al 2009: ipsilesional PMC). Also, it is heavily connected with both MI and SMA (engaged in the temporal organization of movements) and a restitution of ipsilesional effective connectivity between SMA and M1 underlies improved motor performance after stroke (Grefkes et al 2010). Yet, ICS centered on the premotor cortex does not guarantee clinical improvement, even for small subcortical infarcts. Interestingly, the coupling between SMA and M1 is inhibitory and the SMA may act as an interface between motor and limbic systems for processing emotionally rich cue for motor acts: therefore, emotionally rich visual cues could be more effective than neutral ones in motor rehabilitation (Oliveri et al 2003).

Enhancement of somatosensory input leads to improvement of motor performance in stroke patients. M1 and S1 display a striking capacity to reorganize and are anatomically and functionally highly interconnected. Direct electrical stimulation of the somatosensory cortex (S1) may be used as an amplifier to substitute for peripheral electrical stimulation in terms of strengthening the sensory input, leading to improved recovery. As for the posterior parietal lobe, this is connected with PMC, while the inferior parietal lobe with SMA.

The unaffected hemisphere is also known to be associated with post-stroke motor recovery. It is said that an abnormal increase in interhemispheric inhibition from the contralesional to the ipsilesional hemisphere contributes to motor impairment, including aphasia and neglect (*interhemispheric dysbalance model*). Thus suppressing cortical overexcitability in the contralesional hemisphere or boosting cortical excitability in the ipsilesional hemisphere will release the ipsilesional cortex from excessive interhemispheric inhibition and improve neural processing in the lesioned hemisphere. However, this simplistic theory is negated by studies reporting negative results and transcallosal mediated excitability changes do not occur in all patients. Moreover, suppressing activity in contralesional M1 may be contraindicated in more severe stroke patients –a fact contrary to the commonly held view that the contralesional hemisphere takes over in large strokes, since this might reduce the excitability of ipsilateral descending pathways that may be important in some patients (Bradnam et al 2013). In the only case of bihemispheric ICS (Canavero et al 2006), ICS with facilitatory parameters in the unaffected hemisphere produced mixed effects, both positive and negative, pointing to a complex role of the unaffected hemisphere in motor recovery.

The recovery of language follows similar lines. Targets of course differ depending on the type of aphasia (expressive vs receptive) and the extent of the infarct. In aphasia cases, 6 different sites in the right inferior frontal gyrus should be stimulated with rTMS (600 pulses, 1 Hz). Sites include the mouth area in the motor cortex, pars opercularis (POp; BA 44), three separate sites on pars triangularis (PTrdorsal posterior, ventral posterior and anterior PTr), and the pars orbitalis (BA 47). The same can be carried out contralesionally. In those with fluent aphasia, either the right or left superior temporal gyrus (STG) should be stimulated. Studies show that the perilesional area adjacent to Broca's area is the single most important area for the recovery of expressive aphasia and is the primary target for ICS (Kim et al. 2008). Intriguingly, there is growing evidence suggesting a functional connectivity between language areas (including Broca's and Wernicke's) and regions mediating hand motor function. It remains to be clarified whether stimulation of the perilesional area adjacent to Broca's area may enhance cortical hand function or vice versa (Kim et al, unpublished observations), although it is known that stimulation outside the language areas can improve aphasia (Canavero et al 2006). The right hemisphere may take up language all by itself, if areas of the left hemisphere responsible for language are extensively damaged. Yet, the right arcuate fasciculus is rudimentary (Schlaug et al 2011).

12.4.3 Single Vs Multi-Site Stimulation

Single-site stimulation of the perilesional area has been the major option in ICS. This strategy may work if the cortical infarct is not extensive or limited to the subcortical area. If the infarct area is large or involves cortical and subcortical areas simultaneously, with widespread disruption of corticocortical connections, premotor cortex or MI/SI stimulation often is ineffective. ICS of a larger area, or even network stimulation, is required. Combined stimulation including PMC + SI + PPC may be beneficial for improving the motor outcome. As the electrode cannot cover the entire brain, the number and placement of electrodes should be modified depending on the goal of treatment. For instance, a patient with complete hemiplegia may wish to regain locomotor ability rather than fine hand motricity. In this situation, the electrode(s) may be placed more superiorly to cover leg representation areas in MI or peri-infarct areas adjacent to leg function. Dual-site, ipsi- or bihemispherical, CS (Canavero et al 2006, Shin et al 2010) has the ability to recruit more corticospinal/bulbar fibers and simultaneous stimulation of functionally related areas might prove better.

12.4.4 Parameters of Stimulation

Since it takes several weeks to months to observe clinical recovery, the choice of parameters cannot be based on acute clinical effects. Also, inter-individual variability makes it difficult to determine uniformly optimal parameters. One important caveat is that brain atrophy is often observed among stroke patients and this must be taken into account when setting amplitude.

Stimulation should always be subthreshold, and parameters must be decided empirically (6.5 mA in Brown et al 2006 and Levy et al 2008). Kim generally employs continuous-mode stimulation at 5V, 50Hz, and 200μs of pulse duration. Canavero et al (2006) tried both low and high frequency stimulation and found mixed effects. Kim uses anodal and unipolar stimulation, in order to reach deeper regions, in particular deeper "leg representation areas" in the inter-hemispheric fissure. Finally, "inhibitory" CS does not always induce local inhibition, but may be facilitative in some patients.

12.4.5 Duration of Stimulation

We make a strong case for longer periods of stimulation, i.e. 4-6 months (Canavero et al 2006, Kim et al 2008) versus 4-6 weeks reported in other series (Brown et al 2006, Levy et al 2008). Three-to-four weeks of stimulation are, in our experience, of limited value. Some patients began to show improvement after four months of stimulation, with recovery continuing even after removal of the stimulation devices. ICS is usually provided during the rehabilitative training, as it is believed to support brain plasticity and facilitate the learning process. Thus, about three hours of stimulation with concurrent rehabilitative training has been reported (Brown et al 2006, Levy et al 2008). Alternatively, continuous stimulation has been employed and found beneficial, despite possible neuronal fatigue (Canavero et al 2006, Kim et al 2008). Data indicate that two hours of stimulation every twelve hours may achieve the same effects of continuous stimulation (unpublished data). We think that the duration of stimulation must be individualized, depending on the extent and location of the stroke. For larger infarcts, longer durations of stimulation may be required.

12.4.6 Technique of Implantation

12.4.6.1 Types of Electrodes

The strip electrode as usually employed for ICS is adequate to recruit cortical areas involved in functional reorganization. However, approximation of two or more strip electrodes may be indicated.

12.4.6.2 Preoperative Mapping

Identification of the intraparietal sulcus is important when planning fronto-parietal network stimulation. Similar to the junction between the precentral sulcus and superior and inferior frontal sulci in the frontal lobe, the post central sulcus is joined by the horizontally-running intraparietal sulcus. This sulcus divides the parietal lobe into the superior and inferior parietal lobes. However, it is not easy to identify the sulci without the aid of neuronavigation and curvilinear plus multiplanar imaging. In the end, the neurosurgeon's judgment is required to convert neuroimages to "real-life" surgery. If pairs of electrodes are elected, simple anatomical landmarks (using MRI combined with fMRI) can be employed to determine the target, without the use of neuronavigation.

12.4.6.3 Craniotomy and Electrode Implantation

Implantation of the electrode can be performed under either local or general anesthesia. General anesthesia may be risky in older patients with associated comorbidities. In such cases, neuro-leptoanalgesia is an option, particularly with non-flap techniques. Subdural placement would be indicated in severely atrophic brains, but is unsafe. One or two burr holes are enough when inserting the strip electrode extradurally. A burr hole is made based on the length of the strip electrode and the direction of placement over the cortex. Strip electrodes are usually positioned to cover the premotor and motor cortex, integrating imaging data. A burr hole is fashioned immediately anterior to M1. Alternatively, a small (3-5 cm) flap craniotomy may be fashioned. Intraoperative stimulation of M1 may not always evoke muscle twitches, depending on damage to the corticospinal tract. If two paddles are placed epidurally to cover the premotor and part of motor cortex areas, the anterior electrode can be placed just behind the coronal suture, and the upper and lower one can be adjusted, depending on the activation pattern on fMRI. If the electrode is positioned on the inferior frontal (Broca's) or other cortical areas, a similar procedure is employed. In case of a flap, electrodes need to be tightly anchored to increase the contact, to keep blood out of the space between electrode and dura, and to prevent the migration of the electrode. Seepage of blood into the space between the dura and the electrode may hinder delivery of the electrical stimulation and therefore decrease the efficacy of treatment. The electrode is connected with a lead, which is subcutaneously tunneled and connected to the neural stimulator, which is usually implanted subclavicularly in the anterior chest or axillary area.

12.4.6.4 Postoperative Management

Antibiotics are administered according to local policies and regulations. Two or three days following the procedure, the patient may be discharged, but is rescheduled for a parameters-setting session. Initially, the threshold for eliciting a motor response in the contralateral extremity is determined by trains of stimulation (3 seconds of a train at 50 Hz, 100-250μs, starting from 0.5 V). Amplitude is gradually increased until movement is observed or up to 10V. If the patient showed a positive response to movement during intraoperative testing, movement of the contralateral extremity can be expected; otherwise, even high voltages are likely to be ineffectual. Rehabilitation is usually started two weeks after the placement of electrode. The current is gradually increased up to half threshold for four weeks (up to 4-5V), while searching for side effects of stimulation. Stimulation for aphasia does not elicit motor responses and thus is ramped up to 5V only, to avoid possible side effects. The dose of stimulation can be modified depending on the severity of the neurological deficit. If the patient has a mild neurological deficit, two hours of stimulation every twelve hours may suffice. Continuous stimulation is indicated in severely compromised brains. It is important to administer rehabilitation while the stimulator is on, for synergy to occur. Noninvasive CS has been applied before physiotherapy to prime the cortex or during or after to consolidate. No noticeable stimulation–related complications such as seizures, abnormal behavior, or decline of neurological functions have been reported up to now, with the exclusion of one seizure in the trial of Levy et al (2008). Rehabilitation is usually performed using peripheral parts of the body. Given the limited scientific evidence, no indication can be offered as to which rehabilitative technique is best associated to ICS, except to underscore the need of individualization of the rehabilitative process to the patient's physical and cognitive disabilities. A few caveats apply: *1) behaviors can compete and training in one behavior can have negative consequences for another; 2) a plastic nervous system can respond positively, but also negatively, to suboptimal rehabilitation strategies; 3) the best rehabilitation should be general, not task-specific; 4) the effect of sleep for consolidation should be taken into account.* It has been suggested that, since plasticity saturates when neuronal circuits adapt to long-term stimulation, intensive rehabilitation during the all-important first three months after CVA, should be interrupted after 6 weeks by a week of no therapy (relaxation phase) (Butz et al 2009).

12.5 Outcome and Outcome Predictors

In general, after a stroke, initial mild leg paresis is four times as likely to recover compared with severe leg paresis and better outcomes may be expected in subcortical infarcts compared with cortical infarcts, whereas there is no significant difference between motor recovery in hemispheric and brain stem infarcts. Preservation of both parts of the corticospinal tract and thalamic circuitry is a major determinant of the quality of hand-motor recovery following acute brain ischemia in adults. Recovery of function after a stroke is also better for proximal arm function than distal. Sensory deficit is a poor prognostic sign. Currently, the only favorable prognostic sign is the ability to elicit intraoperative motor responses. It may be that more stimulation with more complex tasks is required needed in extensive strokes. ICS plus rehabilitation is said to promote recovery at a level above what is observed after CIMT (Levy et al 2008) and results of CS persist in time. It led to 5- 40% improvement of the original neurological deficit and activities of daily living in successful cases, with benefit persisting > 6 months in almost all cases. New predictive markers, perhaps based on

MR spectroscopy (GABA levels), resting state MR (connectivity analysis), DTI or EEG patterns are needed.

12.6 Conclusion

Although investigational, ICS may be indicated for chronic stroke patients whose neurological deficit has not improved after initial rehabilitative training. Unlike tDCS and rTMS, ICS can provide longer – even continuous- stimulation, because the stimulator is fully implanted. The failure of the EVEREST trial (Table 1) should not put off surgeons wishing to embark on this technique. The failure of this trial was likely due to too temporally short rehabilitation and faulty inclusion criteria, based on a one-size-fits-them-all approach.

Patients were only implanted on the affected MI/SI and a fixed frequency was set for all patients. EVEREST used the fMR hotspot for hand/wrist/finger movement, with rehabilitation targeting shoulder, elbow and distal joints during reach/grasp and self-care. As shown by available data, in several patients other cortical areas must be included (see above). Dual or triple stimulation of functionally-related areas may "salvage" patients that might not benefit from single stimulation. A TMS study found that bilateral rTMS exceeded the algebraic sum of the separate stimulation of each MI (Strens et al 2003). Also, in EVEREST, only 16% of patients showed evoked intraoperative movements as compared with 100% and 42% of patients in phase I and II trials respectively: those who did showed greater improvement than controls.

Future studies should explore concurrent drug administration (an, in the near future, stem cells) and even stimulation of neurogenesis. Reducing the excitability of the lesioned M1 before training (rather than enhance it) in order to increase the range of plastic changes triggered by physiotherapy is an option (Hummel et al 2008). Another interesting possibility lies in coupling Brain-Machine Interfaces with cortical stimulation for brain-state dependent stimulation (Gharabaghi et al 2014).

In conclusion, cortical stimulation to enhance recovery after ischemic stroke represents a new treatment paradigm that may extend our ability to reverse the devastating effects of cerebrovascular disease. Long-term stimulation is required to observe the effect of functional reorganization. Once the stimulation effect plateaus, further stimulation is unnecessary. Such stimulation may be effective long after recovery from the acute phase has ceased. A variety of disabilities follow stroke attacks, including cognitive impairment and depression: simple correction of motor or language deficits may fail to improve quality of life, but multi-target ICS might.

On the other hand, ICS does not hold promise for ALS: for instance, in one case, no effect was evinced (M1 ICS, hand knob, parallel, bipolar 0-3, 1 hour bid, 5-8V, 3Hz or 30Hz at 8V) (Di Lazzaro et al 2010).

References

Balossier A, Etard O, Descat C, et al.. Epidural electrical stimulationto improve chronic poststroke aplasia: a 5-year follow-up. Brain Stimul. 2012;5:364-8.

Balossier A, Etard O, Descat C, et al. Epidural electrical stimulation for the treatment of chronic poststroke aplasia: still compulsory 6 years later! Br J Neurosurg. 2013;27:246-8.

Bradnam LV, Stinear CM, Byblow WD. Ipsilateral motor pathways after stroke: implications for non-invasive brain stimulation. Front Hum Neurosci; 2013; 7 : art 184

Brown JA, Lutsep H, Cramer SC, Weinand M. Motor cortex stimulation for enhancement of recovery after stroke: case report. Neurol Res 2003;25:815-818.

Brown JA, Lutsep HL, Weinand M, et al. Motor cortex stimulation for the enhancement of recovery from stroke: a prospective, multicenter safety study. Neurosurgery 2006;58:464-473

Butz M, van Ooyen A, Wörgötter F. A model for cortical rewiring following deafferentation and focal stroke. Front Comput Neurosci. 2009 Aug 4;3:10. doi: 10.3389/neuro.10.010.2009. eCollection 2009.

Canavero S, Bonicalzi V, Intonti S, et al. Effects of bilateral extradural cortical stimulation for plegic stroke rehabilitation. Neuromodulation 2006; 9:28-33

Cramer SC, Benson RR, Burra VC, et al. Mapping individual brains to guide restorative therapy after stroke: rationale and pilot studies. Neurol Res 2003; 25: 811-814

Cramer SC, Benson RR, Himes DM, et al. Use of functional MRI to guide decisions in a clinical stroke trial. Stroke 2005;36:e50-52.

Cramer SC, Shah R, Juranek J, Crafton KR, Le V. Activity in the peri-infarct rim in relation to recovery from stroke. Stroke 2006;37:111-115

Di Lazzaro V, Di Leone M, Pilato F, et al. Long-term motor cortex stimulation for amyotrophic lateral sclerosis. Brain Stimul. 2010;3:22-7

Elsner B, Kugler J, Pohl M, Mehtholz J. Transcranial direct current stimulation for activities after stroke. What is the evidence? Stroke 2014; 45: e36-37

Gharabaghi A, Kraus D, Leao MT, et al. Coupling brain-machine interfaces with cortical stimulation for brain-state dependent stimulation: enhancing motor cortex excitability for neurorehabilitation. Front Hum Neurosci 2014; 8:122

Grefkes C, Nowak DA, Wang LE, et al. Modulating cortical connectivity in stroke patients by rTMS assessed with fMRI and dynamic causal modeling. Neuroimage. 2010;50:233-42

Harvey RL, Winstein CJ; Everest Trial Group. Design for the EVEREST randomized trial of cortical stimulation and rehabilitation for arm function following stroke. Neurorehabil Neural Repair. 2009;23:32-44

Huang M, Harvey RL, Stoykov ME, et al. Cortical Stimulation for Upper Limb Recovery Following Ischemic Stroke: A Small Phase II Pilot Study of a Fully Implanted Stimulator. Top Stroke Rehabil 2008;15:160-172

Hummel FC, Celnik P, Pascual-Leone A, et al. Controversy : noninvasive and invasive cortical stimulation show efficacy in treating stroke patients. Brain Stim 2008; 1: 370-382

Katayama Y, Oshima H, Fukaya C, et al. Control of post-stroke movement disorders using chronic motor cortex stimulation. Acta Neurochir Suppl. 2002;79:89-92.

Kim HI, Shin YI, Moon SK, et al. Unipolar and continuous cortical stimulation to enhance motor and language deficit in patients with chronic stroke: report of 2 cases. Surg Neurol 2008; 69:77-80.

Leuthardt E, Schalk G, Roland J, et al. Evolution of brain-computer interfaces: going beyond classic motor physiology. Neurosurg Focus 27(1): E4

Levy R, Ruland S, Weinand M, et al. Cortical stimulation for the rehabilitation of patients with hemiparetic stroke: a multicenter feasibility study of safety and efficacy. J Neurosurg 2008;108:707-714.

Loubinoux I. Can fMRI measures of brain motor activation add significantly to other variables in the prediction of treatment response? Stroke 2007; 38: 2032

Nouri S, Cramer SC. Anatomy and physiology predict response to motor cortex stimulation after stroke. Neurology 2011;77: 1076-1083

Nuti C, Vassal F, Mertens P, et al. Improved dexterity after chronic electrical stimulation of the motor cortex for central pain: a special relevance for thalamic syndrome. Stereotact Funct Neurosurg 2012;90:370-8

Oliveri M, Babiloni C, Filippi MM, et al. Influence of the supplementary motor area on primari motor cortex excitability during movements triggered by neutral or emotionally unpleasant visual cues. Exp Brain Res. 2003;149:214-21.

Raffin E, Siebner HR. Transcranial brain stimulation to promote functional recocery after stroke Curr Op Neurol 2014 27: 54-60

Schlaug G, Marchina S, Wan CY. The use of non-invasive brain stimulation techniques to facilitate recovery from post-stroke aphasia. Neuropsychol Rev 2011;21:288-301

Shin YI, Kim H, Moon SK, et al. Dual extradural cortical stimulation in chronic stroke patients with large infacts: technical case report. Neurol Res. 2010;32:556-60.

Strens LH, Fogelson N, Shanahan P, et al. The ipsilateral human motor cortex can functionally compensate for acute contralateral motor cortex dysfunction. Curr Biol 2003 15;13:1201-5.

Yamamoto T, Katayama Y, Watanabe M, et al. Changes in motor function induced by chronic motor cortex stimulation in post-stroke pain patients. Stereotact Funct Neurosurg. 2011;89:381-9.

Aurore Thibaut, Olivier Bodart, Steven Laureys, Sergio Canavero

13 Chronic Disorders of Consciousness

In Section 1 of this chapter, we will examine the use of nonimplantable brain stimulation (ie, transcranial magnetic stimulation - TMS and transcranial direct current stimulation - tDCS) to improve the recovery of patients with Disorders of Consciousness (DOC) (see Box 13.1-2). For details on this technology, the reader is referred to a comprehensive review (Canavero 2009). Whereas TMS is more focal and may reach up to 3 cm depth, tDCS stimulates a wider area more superficially. TDCS is simpler and appears safer in this context; it is also possible to conduct double-blind and sham-controlled trials, since both subjects and operators can be easily blinded. In section 2, we will examine the use of invasive CS. This allows for more continuous, multi-site stimulation and a much wider choice of stimulating parameters.

13.1 Non-Implantable Cortical Stimulation

13.1.1 Repetitive Transcranial Magnetic Stimulation (rTMS)

Pape et al (2009) delivered rTMS over 30 sessions (F8,300 trains per session, 100 ms interpulse interval, 5-second intertrain interval, 110% of motor threshold, 5 days per week for 6 weeks) onto the right dorsolateral prefrontal (DLPF) cortex in a 26 year old patient, who was initially in post-traumatic PVS/UWS (287 days after a TBI, SSEPs absent bilaterally). He improved to MCS after 15 sessions (+8 DOC points), with further improvements up to the 25th session. However, between the 25th rTMS session and the follow-up, there was a decline of functioning of 10 points. No side effects were reported. The same authors (Pape et al 2014) assessed the safety of rTMS in 2 other PVS/UWS patients (6 months and 9 years) targeting the right and left DLPFC respectively (110% MT, 30 sessions, 300 paired pulse trains per session, the rest as above). As a result, patient 1 showed purposeful vocalizations and obeyed simple commands, patient 2 turned the head towards speakers.

Piccione et al (2011) submitted a patient in a MCS for 5 years to an ABA design alternating between rTMS and peripheral nerve stimulation. rTMS (condition A) involved the delivery of 10 trains of 100 stimuli at 20 Hz using a stimulator with a 70-mm fig.-of-eight coil to elicit a contraction of the abductor pollicis brevis. Condition B used median nerve electrical stimulation. After peripheral stimulation, the patient did not exhibit clinical, behavioral, or electroencephalographic (EEG) changes. The frequency of specific and meaningful behaviors increased after rTMS, along with the absolute and relative power of the EEG δ, β, and α bands. These same authors (Manganotti et al 2013) studied 3 PVS and 3 MCS patients >12 months post-

S Canavero

The *vegetative state* (VS; other recent terms: *Unresponsive Wakefulness Syndrome* (UWS), and, for patients with clear imaging signs of responsiveness, *Non-Behavioral* or *Functional Minimally Conscious State* (NBMCS/ FMCS) or *Functional Locked-In Syndrome* (FLIS)), an artifact of intensive care units introduced in the 1960's, was described by Jennett and Plum in 1972. The VS is diagnosed when, after some days to weeks of brain injury, comatose patients open their eyes, but there is no apparent intentional interaction with the environment. VS may be permanent or a transition to the minimally conscious state (MCS), a conscious disabled state or full recovery. Traumatic VS has an incidence of 1-10/100000, with a prevalence lying between 56 and 140 per million: in the USA, at least 4200 new cases of VS and 29000 MCS cases are diagnosed yearly (Giacino et al 2014). Anoxic VS is always more severe than post-traumatic or post-hemorrhagic cases. The widely held notion that preserved consciousness does not occur in patients who have survived for many years after TBI is incorrect (Fernandez-Espejo and Owen 2013). Emergence from the VS later than 1 year is possible - although no better than a severely disabled fully dependent state of living (about 10 cases reviewed by Wijdicks and Cranford 2005), sometimes even 5 years after brain injury (Dyer 1997). Actually, many VS patients evolve to the MCS. A patient emerged from traumatic VS 20 months after the event: beginning from the sixth month, event related potentials (ERPs) to complex sensory and verbal stimulation started to improve, although the clinical examinations remained unchanged (Faran et al 2006). Sarà et al (2007) reported on a 44 year-old man with recovery of consciousness and severe diability 19 months after a nontraumatic brain trauma. Sancisi et al (2009) reported on a 22 year old male who recovered consciousness 19 months after brain injury, with further improvement over 7 years, attaining a condition of independent living. In Estraneo et al (2010)'s series, out of 50 pts, 6 patients in VS improved to MCS (though in a severely disabled state) beyond the 12-month mark. In 1 anoxic VS case, this happened 22 months later. Age younger than 39 years and post-traumatic VS were positive prognostic factors. In Luautè et al (2010)'s series, over 5 years, no VS patient improved, whereas one third of those in MCS improved after 12 months. Yet, it must be recognized that recovery mechanisms from VS and MCS remain poorly understood. Several experimental therapies, both pharmacological (LevoDopa. amantadine, zolpidem, baclofen), and stimulative (deep brain stimulation, DBS; spinal cord and peripheral nerve stimulation), have been attempted over the decades, occasionally successfully, but never with consistent, across-the-board results (Georgiopoulos et al 2010, Lemaire et al 2014), and without a real understanding of the mechanisms underlying their efficacy. Failures in large series have been reported (e.g. Thonnard et al 2014: zolpidem 10 mg ineffective in 28 VS and 32 MCS cases). Yet, the need to restore stable awareness to these patients has become vital, with the advent of virtual reality (VR) and brain-computer interfacing (BCI) and the possibility to eventually control exoskeletons and robotic motor actuators (Naci et al 2012, Rao 2013). BCI can only be applied in the presence of non-fluctuating, stable levels of arousal, awareness and cognition, and these vary dramatically between patients.

Box 13.1: Overview of Docs

S Canavero

Assessing the presence of intentionality and thus consciousness in the single patient is a daunting task. Consciousness may be present in more patients than previously thought, with qualitatively different levels thereof, although the existence of low level consciousness cannot be proven. Conscious and unconscious processing of verbal material employs largely overlapping brain structures, with conscious processing probably involving more cell assemblies of the same type simultaneously: the continuum is fluid, *no exact borders can be drawn* (Kotchoubey B, et al. News Physiol Sci 2002;17:38-42). Thus, clinical differentiation between VS and MCS is very difficult. Estimation of the presence of consciousness requires expert clinical interpretation of "motor responsiveness": VS patients can move extensively and differentiating reflex or automatic from voluntary or willed movements is thus hard. According to Laureys (Trends Cogn Sci 2005; 9:556-9), up to 40% of patients in apparent VS have some signs of consciousness. MCS is now classified as *MCS+ (obeys simple commands)* or *MCS- (visual pursuit, orientation to pain, smiling to family but not strangers),* recognizing that smiling and crying, in certain contexts, might be the only means of communication available to patients (i.e. volitional) (Owen AM and Coleman MR. Nature Rev Neurosci 2008; 9: 235-243) and that previous criteria to diagnose MCS (correct responses to 6 of 6 orientation questions on 2 consecutive examinations) were too stringent (Nakase-Richardson R et al. Neurology 2009; 73:1120-1126). Blinking to threat, when present, predicts recovery in 30% of the cases. Up to 43% of PVS patients (and 10% of MCS cases) are reclassified as MCS by specialized operators, using such scales as the CRS-R (Schnakers C et al. BMC Neurol 2009; 9:35; see also: Andrews K et al. BMJ 1996; 313: 13-16; Childs NL and Merger WN. BMJ 1996; 334: 13-16), yet even in the best hands some patients will likely remain erroneously diagnosed. The need to know the level of awareness of the subject is key, since emotional harm may come from bedside discussions of condition and prognosis and such knowledge would help customize treatment. fMR and EEG studies (Fernandez-Espejo and Owen 2013) have revealed a subset of VS patients who are aware (command following), but entirely physically unresponsive *(at least 17-19%),* even in the long-term, and some even communicated via these means. Activity in higher level associative cortices provides important positive prognostic information. Up to now, a*ll (but one) the reported patients shown to be covertly aware are post-traumatic.* Performing fMR in PVS patients remains exceptionally challenging and many patients may not be detected (negative studies) by these techniques, because of subclinical seizure activity, aphasia, motor deficit, pain, fatigue, lack of motivation or will, sensory or perceptual impairment, fluctuating arousal with sleep bouts, lack of the cognitive resources (sustained attention, language comprehension, response selection, working memory) required to understand and execute the study tasks. Moreover, patients are generally on several medications and this can alter neurovascular coupling. Also, a patient may not show a response in one modality, but can to another type. More simply, neuroimaging may be insensitive to small changes in brain activity in some patients. *No conclusions or claims about the preservation or loss of residual awareness in patients can be drawn on the basis of a negative finding. False negatives in functional neuroimaging are common even in healthy volunteers and MCS+.* Stender et al (Lancet, 2014, 384: 514-522) reported that ^{18}F-FDG PET has high sensitivity for identification of patients in MCS and high congruence with behavioral CRS–R scores, unlike fMRI. ^{18}F-FDG PET correctly predicted outcome in 74% of the cases and fMRI in 56%. 32% of the behaviorally unresponsive patients (ie, diagnosed as unresponsive with CRS–R) showed brain activity compatible with (minimal) consciousness on at least one neuroimaging test; 69% of these patients subsequently recovered consciousness. Event related potentials (ERPs), such as MMN, P300 and others, are another means to assess VS patients: it is important to remember, though, that these too are biased to underestimate patients'cognitive abilities. *ERP test data should be treated as the lowest limit of the patients' capabilities*. This means that one to two thirds of VS patients are capable of cortical differentiation of physical stimulus features and *at least 20%* of these patients can differentiate semantic stimuli (i.e. understood language) (Kotchoubey et al 2002). Similar figures (*25%* have nP300, *ca 20%* evince a MMN) have been reported by others (Fischer C et al. Clin Neurophysiol 2010; 121: 1032-1042). Within the first year, many patients show an intact P300 and several also an N400, indicating considerable residual information processing: at follow-up, about 25% recover (Steppacher I et al. Ann Neurol 2013; 73: 594-602). One of 8 VS and both MCS patients showed an increased hand EMG signal specifically linked to a verbal command (Bekinschtein TA et al. JNNP 2008; 79: 826-828).

Box 13.2: Assessing Consciousness Pre- and Post-treatment

A Perturbational Complexity Index (PCI) has been developed to classify the level of consciousness of patients or healthy subjects, by combining TMS and high-density EEG (Casali AG et al. Sci Transl Med 2013;5:198ra05, Gosseries O et al. Ann Rev Neurosci 2014; 37: 457-478). The PCI estimates brain complexity, including both the information content and the integration (long-range cortical effective connectivity) of brain activations, through algorithmic compressibility, with good spatio-temporal resolution. For example, the PCI is invariably above 0.31 in healthy awake subjects, in patients in MCS or patients in locked-in syndrome, as well as in healthy subjects in REM sleep. In contrast, the PCI is always below a 0.31 threshold during deep sleep, in both UWS patients and in those under general anesthesia using midazolam, propofol or xenon (Fig.5). Unfortunately, TMS-compatible EEG sets are not commonly found and hundreds of TMS pulses needed to compute a single PCI value, which can be a problem where consciousness fluctuates.

Several caveats are in order, that question recent efforts to characterize "markers" of conscious awareness. In too many studies, comparison has been made with healthy subjects, whereas the appropriate control should have been brain damaged patients with intact consciousness. Also, the choice of the resting condition (eyes closed vs eyes open) must be considered carefully, e.g. when comparing PVS with control subjects, because it fundamentally differs in network recruitment (exteroceptive vs interoceptive) on fMRI (Xu P et al. Neuroimage 2014; 90C:246-255). The sense of self is not the same as self-awareness and a state of consciousness that has no content is conceivable (e.g. certain kinds of epileptic states or meditative states). Nonconscious stimuli can evoke emotional states. In a study (Yu T et al. Neurology 2013; 80: 1-8), 5 of 44 VS patients showed consistent fMR responses to cognitive imagery instructions and 24 showed pain matrix activation by pain cries (sensory in 34% and affective in 30%). Thus, affective consciousness can remain in VS cases, even in the absence of cognition. There is much recent discussion about the importance of the default mode network and of binding synchrony of frontoparietal connectivity as markers of conscious awareness. Actually, while this is rather fashionable, there is ample evidence that casts a pall on any overenthusiastic acceptance of these imaging-driven constructs. In human studies, neither gamma power per se, nor synchrony per se correlated with consciousness (Pockett S, Holmes MD. Consciousness and Cognition 2009;18:1049-55) and there are no compelling reasons to assign functional cognitive roles to oscillatory synchrony in the gamma range beyond its generic functions at the level of infrastructural (activation) neural control (Merker B. Neurosci Biobehav Rev 2013;37:401-17). Reemergence from anesthesia (propofol) is not accompanied by large changes in neocortical function (i.e. comes before full recovery of neocortical processing) and what seems to count most is the midline thalamus, the hypothalamus and the brainstem (locus coeruleus / parabrachial area) (Langsjo JW, et al. J Neurosci 2012; 34: 4935-4943; see also Castaigne P et al. Ann Neurol 1981; 10: 127-148). This is in line with cases of hydranencephalia -where the thalamus and brainstem are intact-who appear conscious, although with deficits in rich contents (Merker B. Behav Brain Sci 2007; 30: 63-81). It has been shown how the insular cortex, anterior cingulate and medial prefrontal cortex are not required for most aspects of self-awareness; the thalamus and brainstem are relevant (along with the post cingulate / precuneus / retrosplenial cortex: Philippi CL, et al. PloS One 2012; 7: e38413; see also Silva S et al. Neurology 2010; 74: 313-320 and Fernandez-Espejo D et al Ann Neurol 2012 ; 72 : 335-343). A patient submitted to direct intraoperative stimulation of the posterior parietal cortex showed behavioral unresponsiveness with loss of external connectedness; upon reawakening the patient described himself as in dream, outside the operating room (Herbet et al. Neuropsychologia 2014; 56: 239–244). It should also be borne in mind that -arousal-wise – extrathalamic input from the brainstem can compensate for damaged thalamocortical transmission.

Finally, to further compound the problem, many (including this author) believe that consciousness is not generated by the brain, but merely filtered through it, a position variously expressed by Penfield, Eccles and many others.

continued **Box 13.2:** Assessing Consciousness Pre- and Post-treatment injury. R-TMS (1 session of 1000 stimuli in 10 trains of 20 Hz at motor threshold; F8 coil, PosteroAnterior orientation; earplugs on) of the MI (left or right depending on presence of MEPs; C3/4 and P3/4) achieved no clinical benefit, except in one MCS (post-hemorrhagic) patient (JFK CRS-R: auditory: from 2 to 4, visual from 2 to 4, motor from 3 to 6, arousal from 2 to 3, verbal axis and communication unchanged).

Giovannelli et al (2013) conducted a randomized, double-blind, sham-controlled, cross-over study on 11 patients classified as PVS (9 post-anoxic, 2 post-traumatic). RTMS (20 Hz, left MI, for 5 consecutive days, 10 min stimulation or 1000 pulses at 60% of maximum stimulator output). Slight changes in JFK CRS-R did not significantly differ between real and sham conditions. Also, there was disagreement on Clinical Global Impression changes between clinicians and patients'relatives.
Globally, the risk of seizure is very low. There was an atypical seizure that required lower intensity of stimulation in one patient of Pape et al (2014).

13.1.2 Transcranial Direct Current Stimulation (tDCS)

Two studies tested tDCS over the motor and the prefrontal areas of patients in PVS/UWS and MCS. Angelakis et al (2014) tested 5 days of anodal tDCS (25 cm2 rectangular sponge saturated with saline; cathode: rectangular sponge 35 cm2 over right orbit) at 1-2 mA for 20 minutes per day, 5 days per week, for 3 weeks in 10 patients (7 UWS and 3 MCS-). The authors stimulated the left primary sensorimotor cortex (C3 on the 10/20 EEG international system) (n= 5) or the left dorsolateral prefrontal cortex (F3) (n= 5). Follow-up was 1 year. Sham stimulation achieved no effects in all patients. Results were assessed with the JFK CRS-R scale. No patient in PVS improved, although one went from 8 to 9 points. Two patients in MCS- (posttraumatic and postoperative brain damage) went from 10 to 22 (conscious) and from 9 to 19 (conscious), respectively: the latter was submitted to two cycles of stimulation at a 3 month interval and effects were additive. Both these two patients were stimulated on C3. These authors concluded that more cycles may lead to additional benefit. Thibaut et al (2014) explored the effect of a single session of anodal tDCS during 20 minutes over the left prefrontal dorsolateral cortex (F3 on 10/20 EEG international system) on 55 patients with DOC (30 MCS, 25 UWS, 25 post-TBI, 35 chronic – more than 3months post insult). Two stimulations were performed, one anodal and one sham, in a randomized order, preceded and followed by a behavioral assessment with the Coma Recovery Scale-Revised. 13 (43%) patients in MCS and 2 (8%) patients in UWS further showed post-anodal tDCS related signs of consciousness, which were neither observed during the pre-tDCS evaluation nor during the pre- or post-sham evaluation (i.e., tDCS responder). Out of the 13 MCS responders, 5 were included more than 12 months after injury. One patient in UWS became MCS- and the other one became MCS+ and 4 patients in MCS- became MCS+. Clinical improvement of the tDCS responders are reported in Table 13.1.

Table 13.1: Clinical improvement of tDCS responders (n=15)

CRS-R SUBSCALES	RECOVERY	NUMBER OF PATIENTS
Auditory	Systematic command following	1
	Reproducible command following	4
	Localization to sounds	1
	Auditory startle	0
Visual	Object recognition	2
	Object localization	1
	Visual pursuit	5
	Blinking to threat	0
Motor	Functional use of object	1
	Automatic motor reaction	2
	Object manipulation	3
	Localisation to noxious stimulation	0
	Flexion withdrawal	1
	Abnormal posturing	0
Oromotor/Verbal	Intelligible vocalisation	0
	Vocalisation	3
	Oral reflexive movement	0
Communication	Functional communication	2

13.2 Implantable Cortical Stimulation

Canavero et al (2009a, 2009b) performed extradural bifocal cortical stimulation in two VS patients 20 months following traumatic brain injury (for which decompressive hemicraniectomy was performed in the female case). The N20/P25 components of the SSEPs were absent bilaterally in both cases. The female (born 1988) was scored 25 on the Disability Rating Scale/DRS (Category 9) and the male (born 1985) 23 (category 8). The male patient had been on intrathecal baclofen for severe spasticity for several months. His defensive blink reflex was present and brisk, whereas it was completely absent in the female patient. While the male could be fed regularly, the female only with great difficulty. The parietal gyri P1 and P2 and the middle frontal sulcus (F2), including Brodmann's areas 8 and 46, were targeted for ICS in order to functionally reconnect a widespread network connected via the superior longitudinal fasciculus and exploit remaining corticothalamocortical reentrant loops. Stimulation of DLPFC, via its connections with the supplementary motor area (SMA), was also expected to influence swallowing and axial tone. The female was stimulated on the left side and the male on the right to confirm the role of laterality in possible consciousness recovery. After induction of general anesthesia, a double sigmoid incision of the skin overlying the target areas was performed. Specifically, the left superior parietal lobule and dorsolateral prefrontal cortex were targeted (Fig.13.1-2). Four burr holes were fashioned and two stimulating paddles were inserted extradurally (Lamitrode 4, MOD. 3240, ANS, Plano, Texas). The paddles were linked via a dual extension to a subclavearly pocketed pulse generator (Genesis, MOD. 3608, ANS, Plano, Texas). Stimulation was started at a low power and then gradually increased (8-12 mA). It consisted of daily stimulation with switching off at night. Parameters were determined empirically, on the basis of our previous experience with MCS for other disorders (Canavero 2009). Low frequency stimulation was elected (6-16 Hz) with pulse widths trials ranging between 52 and 455 μs in the female patient. In the male patient, assessed parameters were 6-100 Hz, 65-455 μs, 8-13 mA, 0+1-2-3+ /0+1-2-3+. Clinical progression was evaluated over the following 10 months on 9 occasions by means of the Coma Recovery Scale-Revised and the Levels of Cognitive Functioning Scale. Within 48 hours of switching the stimulator on, a few days after surgery, both showed increased arousal during follow-up. On changing parameters during follow-up, it was observed that arousal, spasticity and other vegetative parameters could dramatically change (improve or worsen) within 12 hours. High frequency (100 Hz) stimulation was not tolerated (spasticity increased) in the male patient. Best parameters were 50-60 Hz, 65-208 μs, 8-10 mA. In the female, best parameters were 8-10 Hz, 65 μs, 11 mA, ++--/--++. Intensity was higher than reported in DBS studies (2-3 mA versus 8-13 mA). Effects emerged immediately, but strengthened in time. The female showed increased vigilance with clear improvements of swallowing and self-management of oral secretions. Oral feeding with both solids and liquids became possible and episodes of aspiration were not reported; weight increased by 4 Kg. Axial tone too increased dramatically. Most importantly, occasionally after the first month and on a more repeatable basis at study end, she could lift her left arm and hand on command, a clear sign of consciousness. On several occasions, the physiotherapists had the clear impression of the patient being "conscious and cooperative". The male could respond to emotionally charged stimuli with appropriate facial expressions. Consistent interaction with family was the most important change cited by family members. Resting state fMR (Cauda et al 2009), explored as a potential "marker" of self-consciousness, showed a clear improvement, with a pattern towards normalization in both cases (Fig.13.3a,b,c,d). Diffusion tensor imaging (DTI) did not show signs of fiber regrowth (Table 13.2). In the male, Magnetic Resonance Spectroscopy (MRS) showed signs of altered neuronal metabolism (Table 13.3). Importantly, at the end of study, stimulators were deactivated: the benefits persisted, a sign of neuroplastic effects seen also in Parkinson Disease and Central Pain, so-called *after-effect* (Canavero 2009).

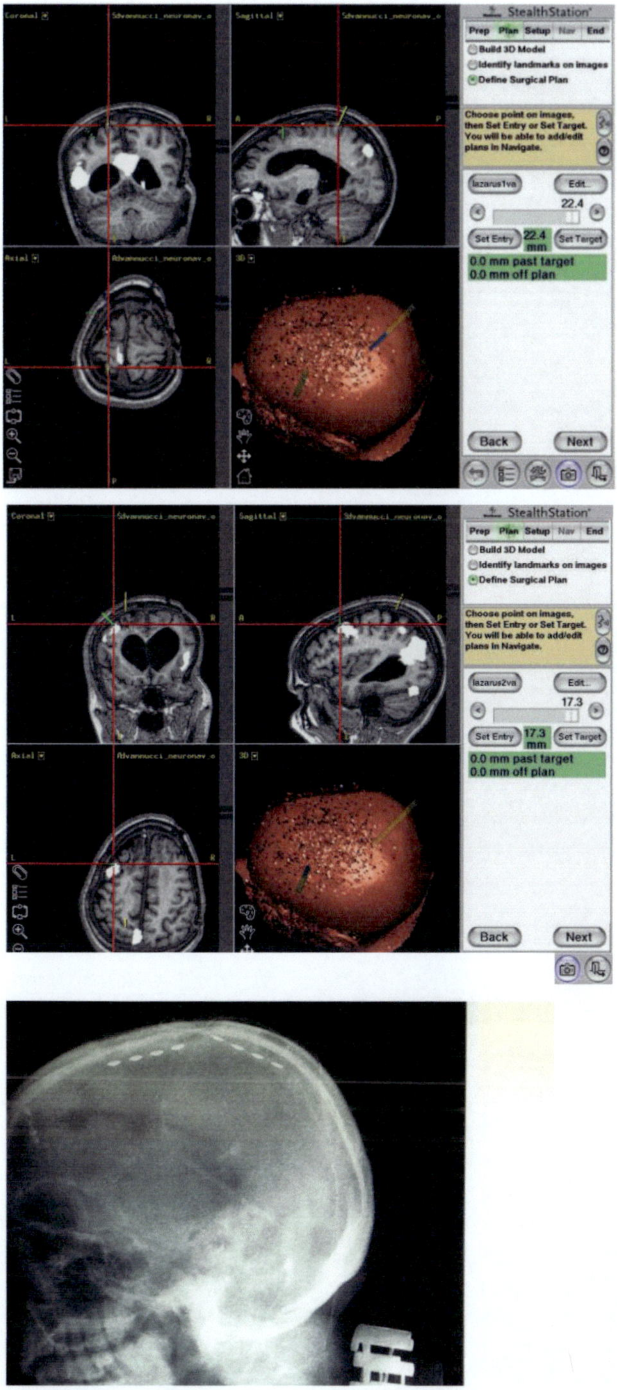

Fig. 13.1: case 1 (female). Neuronavigation images showing the parietal (a) and frontal (b) targets. Lateral skull x-rays showing the position of the two stimulating strips (c).

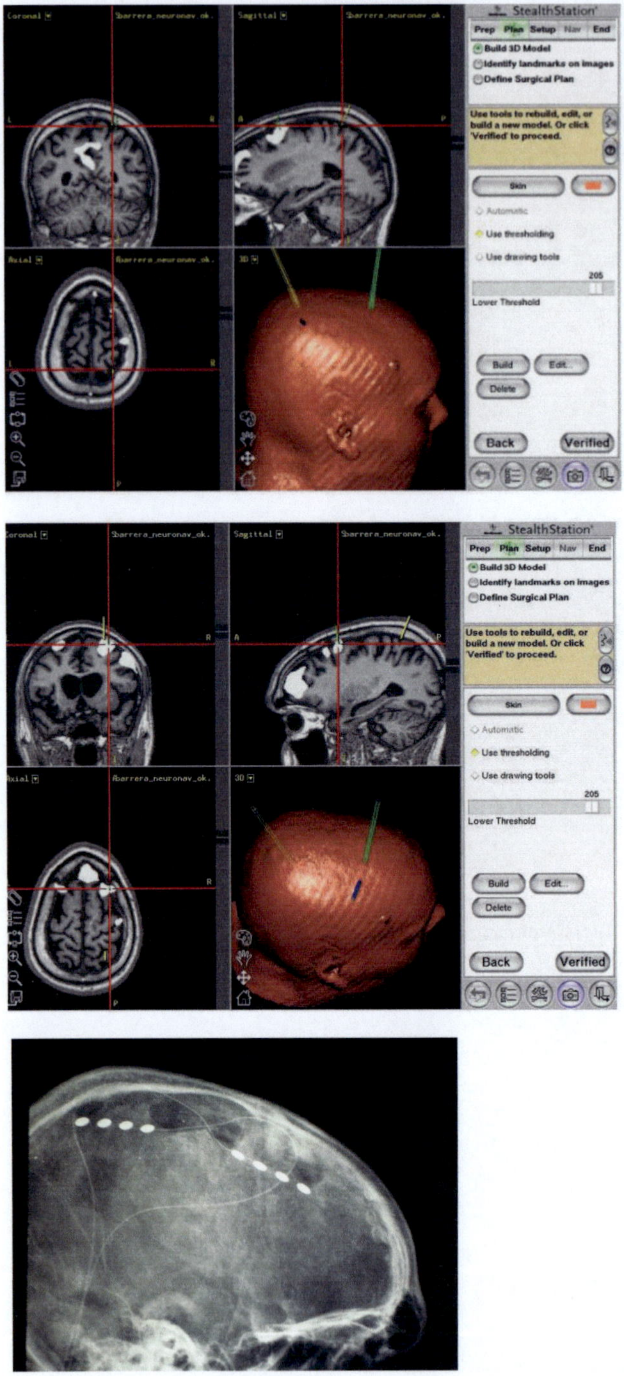

Fig. 13.2: case 2 (male). Neuronavigation images showing the parietal (a) and frontal (b) targets. Lateral skull x-rays showing the position of the two stimulating strips (c).

A

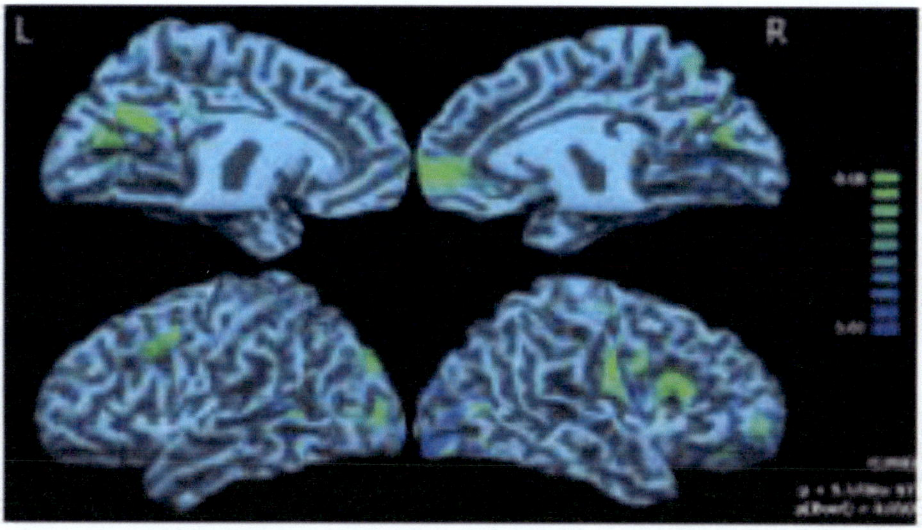

B

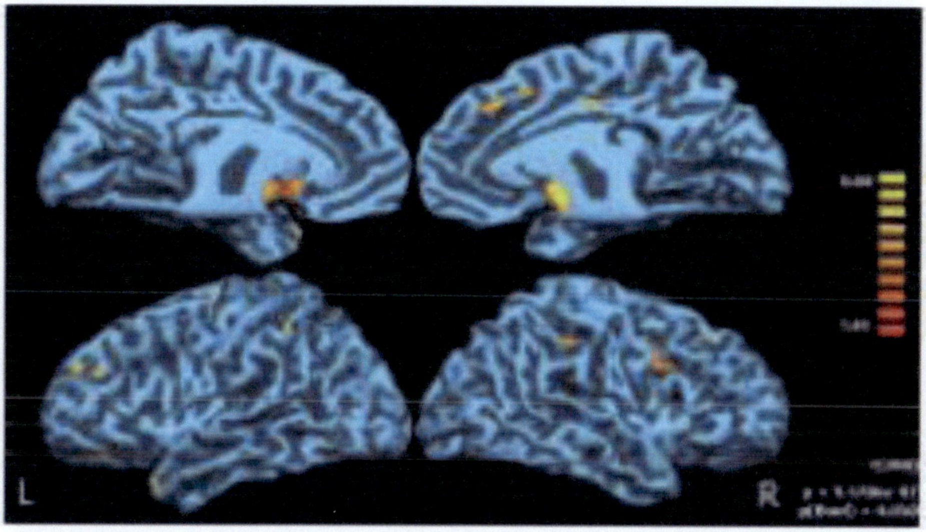

Fig. 13.3: Default Mode Network changes in the 2 patients. Female: increases (A) and decreases (B).

C

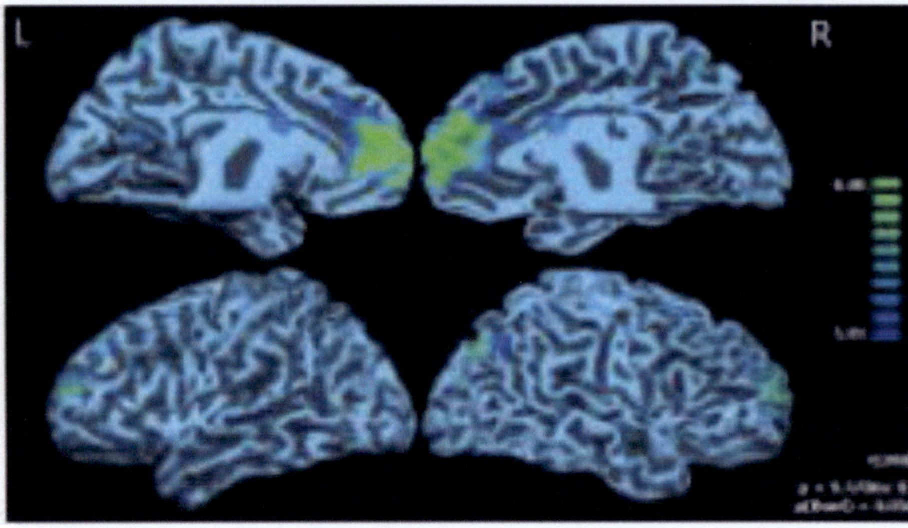

D

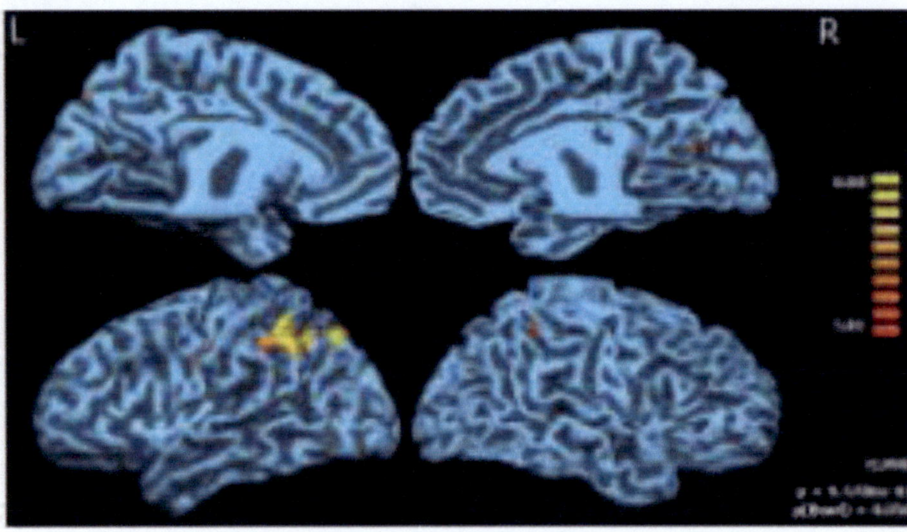

Fig. 13.3: Default Mode Network changes in the 2 patients. Male: increases (C) and decreases (D).

Chance recovery can be dismissed. Their level of functioning had been static for a significant amount of time before initiating therapy and there was a clear temporal relationship between the provision of stimulation and neurobehavioral gains. The girl died 4 years after implantation following antibiotic-resistant pneumonia.

Table 13.2A: Female patient. Bundle of interest statistics (mean and standard deviation): FA (Fractional Anisotropy), l (length), r (fibers density) for Cortico-Spinal Tract (CST), Corpus Callosum (CC) Superior Longitudinal Fasciculus (SLF) at pre and post treatment condition.

CST LEFT	**Pre mean**	**Pre SD**	**Post mean**	**Post SD**
FA	0.46	0.17	0.48	0.16
l [mm]	61	6	100	25
r [fibers/mm3]	0.010		0.008	
CST RIGHT	**Pre mean**	**Pre SD**	**Post mean**	**Post SD**
FA	0.44	0.17	0.44	0.18
l [mm]	63	17	60	14
r [fibers/mm3]	0.026		0.027	
CC	**Pre mean**	**Pre SD**	**Post mean**	**Post SD**
FA	0.37	0.26	0.40	0.16
l [mm]	28	18	40	27
r [fibers/mm3]	0.044		0.037	
SLF LEFT	**Pre mean**	**Pre SD**	**Post mean**	**Post SD**
FA	0.43	0.16	0.42	0.15
l [mm]	29	15	35	18
r [fibers/mm3]	0.033		0.040	
SLF RIGHT	**Pre mean**	**Pre SD**	**Post mean**	**Post SD**
FA	0.38	0.14	0.38	0.14
l [mm]	25	9	29	16
r [fibers/mm3]	0.038		0.032	

Table 13.2B: Male patient. Bundle of interest statistics (mean and standard deviation): FA (Fractional Anisotropy), l (length), r (fibers density) for Cortico-Spinal Tract (CST), Corpus Callosum (CC) Superior Longitudinal Fasciculus (SLF) at pre and post treatment condition.

CST LEFT	Pre mean	Pre SD	Post mean	Post SD
FA	0.47	0.17	0.49	0.17
l [mm]	105	15	110	12
r [fibers/mm3]	0.005		0.019	
CST RIGHT	**Pre mean**	**Pre SD**	**Post mean**	**Post SD**
FA	0.45	0.15	0.47	0.15
l [mm]	97	10	83	12
r [fibers/mm3]	0.006		0.011	
CC	**Pre mean**	**Pre SD**	**Post mean**	**Post SD**
FA	0.41	0.17	0.40	0.18
l [mm]	24	11	27	13
r [fibers/mm3]	0.044		0.053	
SLF LEFT	**Pre mean**	**Pre SD**	**Post mean**	**Post SD**
FA	0.39	0.15	0.40	0.15
l [mm]	28	13	28	17
r [fibers/mm3]	0.034		0.026	
SLF RIGHT	**Pre mean**	**Pre SD**	**Post mean**	**Post SD**
FA	0.44	0.15	0.43	0.15
l [mm]	40	21	49	23
r [fibers/mm3]	0.029		0.027	

Table 13.3: Magnetic Resonance Spectroscopy * data (male patient)

PREOPERATIVE MRS	POSTOPERATIVE MRS (6 weeks after surgery)
NAA/Cr 1.28	NAA/Cr 1.94
NAA/Cr(h) 1.32	NAA/Cr(h) 1.83
Cho/Cr 0.75	Cho/Cr 0.69
Cho/Cr(h) 0.69	Cho/Cr(h) 0.80
NAA/Cho 1.72	NAA/Cho 2.82
NAA/Cho(h) 1.92	NAA/Cho(h) 2.28
Cho/NAA 0.58	Cho/NAA 0.35
Cho/NAA(h) 0.52	Cho/NAA(h) 0.44

*posterior frontal white matter

13.3 Editor's Conclusion

The data reviewed in this chapter indicate that the severely injured brain has a capacity for recovery that exceeds current expectations and highlights the need for continuation of treatment efforts even years following injury.

CS might be combined with other stimulatory and pharmacologic therapies, and in the future, stem cells. CS can trigger neuroplastic changes (see Chapter 12). Despite a suggestion that fiber regrowth might be at work in the recovery of consciousness (Voss et al 2006), DTI data in two patients do not support this view. This is compatible with the "fast" improvement of level of consciousness in patients submitted to CS, both invasive and non. CS can force into resynchronization –"rebind"- (Slewa-Younan et al 2002) and rebalance activity across wide swaths of damaged hemispheres bilaterally (see Chapter 10), by altering thalamocortical transmission ipsilaterally and contralaterally via the corpus callosum and other deep structures. Cortico-cortical coherence between distant brain areas has been selectively enhanced by simultaneous bifocal 10Hz rTMS (Plewnia et al 2008). CS may also compensate for a loss of arousal regulation that is normally controlled by the frontal lobe in the intact brain.

The advantage of cortical stimulation over deep brain stimulation (DBS) is evident: DBS is more invasive and exposes the patient to more risks than CS (including death and further disability: Canavero 2010). CS can activate cortico-thalamo-cortical connectivity from the cortical side. Thalamic DBS is dependent on preserved metabolism in the thalamus, and thus is probably best reserved to MCS cases (Le Maire et al 2014).

As per the most appropriate targets of stimulation, three such targets have emerged: the prefrontal cortex (BA 9/46, possibly BA10), the posterior parietal cortex (BA 5/7) and M1, this latter being densely interconnected with both the prefrontal cortex and the thalamus, basal ganglia and brainstem. Areas BA 39/40 are another possible target, since they have been linked to the "will to move" (Desmurget and Sirigu 2012). Patients who survive a few months in PVS show gradual enlargement of the ventricular system: this may complicate targeting and affect electric conduction through the brain.

In sum, a VS patient may be submitted to tDCS/rTMS (also H-coil rTMS: Zangen et al 2005) of DLPFC, PPC and MI, on both sides, sequentially. If no benefit accrues or the benefit is limited, neurosurgical implantation of stimulating paddles centered on these same areas is possible (bifocal CS: M1 and PPC, MI and DLPFC, DLPFC and PPC), even on both sides (although this adds to overall cost). The search for effective parameters requires months and after-effects must be factored in. Finally, given recent speculation about the role of the claustrum in "binding" consciousness (Smythies et al 2014), this could become the focus of future neurostimulation studies.

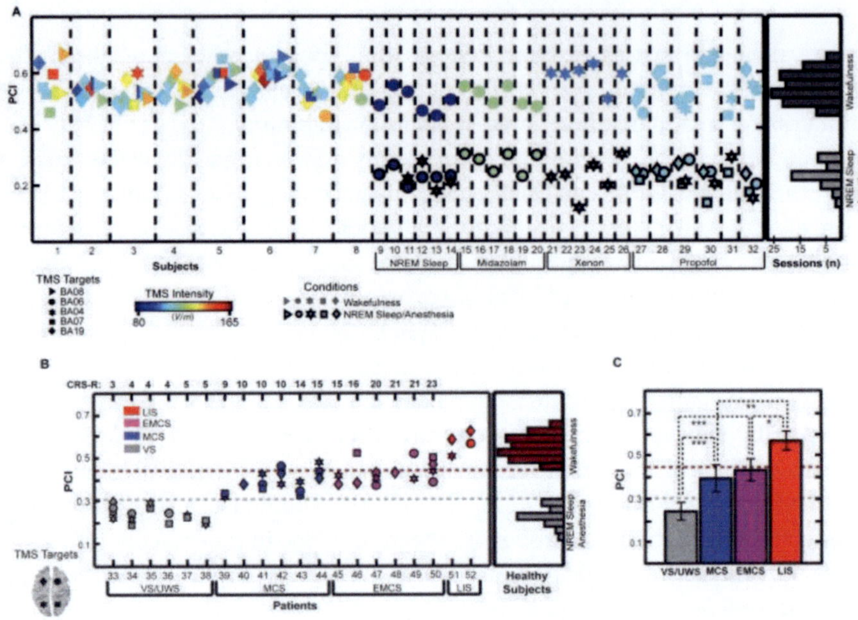

Fig. Box 13.1: PCI values in severely brain-injured patients. PCI progressively increases from VS/UWS to MCS and to recovery of functional communication (EMCS). PCI attains levels of healthy awake subjects in LIS patients (Coma Science Study Group, Liege, Belgium)

References

Angelakis E, Liouta E, Andreadis N, et al. Transcranial direct current stimulation effects in disorders of consciousness. Arch Phys Med Rehabil 2014; 95: 283-9

Canavero S. Textbook of therapeutic cortical stimulation. New York: Nova Science, 2009

Canavero S, Massa-Micon B, Cauda F, et al. Bifocal extradural cortical stimulation-induced recovery of consciousness in the permanent post-traumatic vegetative state. J Neurol 2009; 256: 834-6

Canavero S, Massa-Micon B, Cauda F, et al. Bifocal extradural cortical stimulation for the post-traumatic permanent vegetative state. In: Canavero S (ed). Textbook of therapeutic cortical stimulation. New York: Nova Science, 2009, 275-286

Canavero S (ed). Halfway technology for the vegetative state. Arch Neurol 2010; 67: 777

Cauda F, Massa-Micon B, Canavero S, et al. Disrupted intrinsic functional connectivity in the vegetative state. JNNP 2009; 80: 429-431

Desmurget M, Sirigu A. Conscious motor intention emerges in the inferior parietal lobule. Curr Op Neurobiol 2012; 22: 1004-1011

Dyer C. Hillsborough survivor emerges from permanent vegetative state. BMJ 1997; 314: 993

Estraneo A, Moretta P, Loreto V, et al. Late recovery after traumatic, anoxic, or hemorrahgic long-lasting vegetative state. Neurology 2010; 75: 239-45

Faran S, Vatine JJ, Lazary A, Ohry A, Birbaumer N, Kotchoubey B. Late recovery from permanent traumatic vegetative state heralded by event-related potentials. JNNP 2006;77:998-1000
Fernandez-Espejo D, Owen AM. Detecting awareness after severe brain injury. Nat Rev Neurosci 2013 14: 801-809
Georgiopoulos M, Katsakiori P, Kefalopoulou Z, et al. Vegetative state and minimally conscious state: a review of the therapeutic interventions. Stereotact Funct Neurosurg. 2010;88:199-207
Giacino JT, Fins JJ, Laureys S, Schiff ND. Disorders of consciousness after acquired brain injury : the state of the science. Nat Rev Neurol. 2014;10:99-114
Giovannelli F, Chiaramonti R, Bianco G, et al. Lack of behavioural effects of high-frequency rTMS in vegetative state: a randomised, double blind, sham-controlled, cross-over study. Clin Neurophysiol 2013; 124: p253, e185
Lemaire JJ, Sontheimer A, Nezzar H, et al. Electrical modulation of neuronal networks in brain-injured patients with disorders of consciousness: A systematic review. Ann Fr Anesth Reanim 2014; 33:88-97
Luautè J, Maucort-Boulch D, Tell L et al. Long-term outcomes of chronic minimally conscious and vegetative states Neurology 2010; 75: 246-252
Manganotti P, Formaggio E, Storti SF, et al. Effect of high-frequency repetitive transcranial magnetic stimulation on brain excitability in severely brain-injured patients in minimally conscious or vegetative state. Brain Stimul. 2013;6:913-21
Naci L, Monti MM, Cruse D, et al. Brain-computer interfaces for communication with nonresponsive patients. Ann Neurol 2012; 72: 312-323
Pape LBT, Rosenow J, Lewis G, et al. Repetitive transcranial magnetic stimulation-associated neurobehavioral gains during coma recovery. Brain Stimul. 2009;2:22-35.
Pape LBT, Rosenow JM, Patil V, et al. RTMS safety for two subjects with disordered consciousness after traumatic brain injury. Brain Stimul 2014; 7: 620-622
Piccione F, Cavinato M, Manganotti P, et al. Behavioral and neurophysiological effects of repetitive transcranial magnetic stimulation on the minimally conscious state: a case study. Neurorehab Neural Repair 2011; 25:98-102
Plewnia C, Rilk AJ, Soekadar SR, et al. Enhancement of long-range EEG coherence by synchronous bifocal transcranial magnetic stimulation. Eur J Neurosci 2008; 27: 1577-1583
Rao RPN. Brain-computing interfacing. An introduction. New York: Cambridge University Press, 2013
Sancisi E, Battistini A, Stefano CD, et al. Late recovery from post-traumatic vegetative state. Brain Injury 2009; 23:163- 6
Sarà M, Sacco S, Cipolla F, et al. An unexpected recovery from permanent vegetative state. Brain injury 2007;21:101-3
Smythies JR, Edelstein LR, Ramachandran VS (eds) The Claustrum. Amsterdam: Academic Press, 2014
Thibaut A, Bruno MA, Ledoux D, et al. tDCS in patients with disorders of consciousness: sham-controlled randomised double blind study. Neurology 2014; 82:1112-8
Thonnard M, Gosseries O, Demertzi A, et al. Effect of zolpidem in chronic disorders of consciousness: a prospective open-label study. Funct Neurol. 2013; 28:259-64
Voss HU, Uluc A, Dyke J, et al. Possible axonal regrowth in late recovery from the minimally conscious state. J Clin Invest 2006; 116: 2005-2011
Wijdicks EF, Cranford RE. Clinical diagnosis of prolonged states of impaired consciousness in adults. Mayo Clin Proc 2005; 80: 1037-1046
Zangen A, Roth Y, Voller B, Hallett M. Transcranial magnetic stimulation of deep brain regions: evidence for efficacy of the H-coil. Clin Neurophysiol 2005; 116: 775-9

Sharona Ben-Haim, Brian Harris Kopell

14 Psychiatric Disorders

Cortical targets represent important nodes within the neural networks that subserve psychiatric disorders. Although more invasive, surgical cortical stimulation allows for stimulation with increased spatial specificity. Current paradigms utilize electrodes implanted epidurally rather than subdurally, as the dura provides a barrier that increases the activation threshold of neural tissue, and reduces the risk of induced seizure (Bezard et al., 1999). Furthermore, the implantation of electrodes epidurally significantly decreases the risk of irritating or damaging underlying brain tissue, and eliminates the risk of subdural hematoma as well as cerebrospinal fluid leak. The mechanism of action of ICS is still poorly understood, particularly for psychiatric disorders in which neurophysiologic underpinnings are often ill defined.

14.1 Depression

14.1.1 Review of Studies

We conducted a prospective, longitudinal single-blinded analysis of the effect of epidural stimulation of the left DLPFC in patients with severe treatment-resistant depression (Kopell et al., 2011). The study included 12 patients, followed over the course of 104 weeks with the main outcome measure defined as at least a 40% decrease in the Hamilton-Depression Rating Scale - 28 (HDRS). As this was primarily designed to be a safety and feasibility study, only the subjects were blinded to the stimulation state during an 8-week sham-controlled phase. Patients selected were limited to those with the most severe, refractory depression and met a rigid series of inclusion and exclusion criteria (Table 14.1). Electrodes were implanted unilaterally through a small craniotomy, and consisted of a paddle with two platinum-iridium contacts 3.75 in diameter and spaced 15mm apart (Fig.14.1A). In addition to HDRS, the study also measured response in the Montgomery-Asberg Depression Rating Scale (MADRS), Global Assessment of Function (GAF), and Quality of Life Enjoyment and Satisfaction (QLES) questionnaire. Subjects were followed every two weeks from implantation to week 16, and subsequently every four weeks until week 104 with a variety of the above tests and, at pre-set intervals, the addition of a Mini-Mental Status Exam (MMSE) and repetition of the baseline neuropsychological battery. Moreover, PET scanning was performed at baseline, and in a treated state. Of note, one patient was excluded from the analysis because of a violation in study-protocol during the baseline period. After 8 weeks of active, *continuous stimulation* (week 8 for the study group, and week 16 for the sham-controlled stimulation group), the subjects entered an "adaptive protocol" and settings were adjusted based on subject response with attention to prolonging battery-life. All subjects were stimulated at 50Hz, with a pulse width varying from 150-250μs, and an amplitude setting of 5.5-6.5mA using either a bipolar or unipolar montage. In the evaluation of the 11 remaining patients over the 104-week period, 5 were randomized to the sham group and 6 were randomized into the active group. After week 8, all subjects received active stimulation. During the 8-week single-blinded sham controlled phase, a 20% mean improvement in HDRS scores was noted compared to a 3% improvement in the sham group, however this trend did not reach statistical significance ($p>0.1$). The fact that in this period of time outcomes were not significant may be a reflection of the small sample size, the variability in lead placement, and the short time course. In a post-hoc analysis of this data, it was determined that 20 weeks of stimulation are necessary to approach a 50% response probability (Pathak et al., 2013). During the first several months, it was noted that electrode placement was significantly correlated to response, and at week 52, patients with electrodes deemed to be sub-optimally located were offered revision surgery. Of the 6 patients identified, 3 underwent lead revision (see "Refining Techniques"). During the first 21 months of treatment, a significant improvement was noted in HDRS, MADRS, and GAF scores, however response rates in the QLES questionnaire remained unchanged. Overall, 6 patients (55%) achieved a greater than or equal to 40% improvement on the HDRS, the primary outcome measure, at some point during the trial and 5 patients (45%) achieved a greater than 50% improvement. Four subjects (36%) achieved remission at some point during the trial, defined as an HDRS score <10 (Table 14.2). Of the 3 patients that underwent revision surgery, there was an average of a 4-point improvement in the HDRS and a 0.1-point improvement in the MADRS; however, ultimately, none of these patients met the preset criteria for responsiveness. It is notable that despite the revision surgery, the electrode leads in these patients may still have been in a position posterior to the desired target cortex. Due to the dissolution of the parent company at the end of the trial (104 weeks), the study subjects were explanted per FDA mandate. During the active study phase, there were no reported surgical complications, however upon explantation, one patient developed a bone-flap infection necessitating further surgery for removal, antibiotic treatment, and eventual replacement with a synthetic prosthesis. One patient, who was initially excluded from the study secondary to violation of the protocol during the first 8 weeks (the patient was receiving concurrent TMS therapy), underwent a suicide attempt requiring hospitalization during the period of active stimulation, and completed suicide prior to explantation. This suicide attempt was thought to be caused by a myriad of extenuating personal circumstances, however the pending explantation of the ICS may have served as an additional constituent in her psychological decline.

Table 14.1: Inclusion Criteria

	Nahas, et al., 2010	Kopell, et al., 2011
Inclusion Criteria	HDRS score ≥ 20	HDRS score ≥ 20
	DSM IV diagnosis of MDD without psychotic features OR a major depressive episode as part of Bipolar Type I or II	DSM IV Diagnosis of MDD without psychotic features
	Failed response to ≥4 antidepressant treatments, with a minimum of 6 weeks of prior psychotherapy	Failed response to ≥4 antidepressant treatments*
	Current treatment regimen unchanged for at least 4 weeks prior to implantation	Current treatment regimen unchanged for at least 8 weeks prior to implantation
		At the time of the study, in a major depressive episode for >2 years, or >1 year with 4 or more lifetime episodes
		GAF <60
Exclusion Criteria		L- handed dominance**
		Pre-existing neurological disease (including epilepsy)
		Active comorbid Axis I psychiatric disorders
		Borderline or histrionic personality disorder
		MMSE < 24 or other evidence of cognitive disorder
		Active suicidal ideation
		ECT within 6 months of implantation
		Medical condition that may interfere with completion of the study

* Treatments include medications, ECT, VNS, or psychotherapy
** Defined as at least 75% dominance on the Edinburgh Handedness Inventory

Nahas et al (2010) submitted five patients with treatment resistant depression to open-label ICS. Notably different from the previous study, this study implanted two paddles with 4 electrode contacts each (Fig.14.1B), bilaterally, targeting the anterior and mid-lateral prefrontal cortices corresponding to Brodmann's areas 10 and 46 (Fig.14.2). All subjects underwent pre- and post-operative analysis using the HDRS and MADRS. Response was defined a priori as a greater than 50% reduction in mean HDRS and remission was defined as a score of 10 or lower. As in the prior study, a post operative CT scan was obtained and fused to the pre-operative MRI to evaluate electrode placement. No revision surgeries were deemed necessary, likely owing to the fact that there were 8 contact electrodes placed per side and more ability for programming across anatomical substrates. After an average of 2-3 weeks post-operatively, stimulation commenced and was tested for "optimal settings," guided by acute, subjective observations by the patients. The stimulation paradigm used differs from the previous study and more closely emulates rTMS protocols. Patients generally underwent chronic, intermittent bilateral stimulation of all four paddle leads at 60Hz, 2-4V, 30' ON 2.5 hours OFF from 8AM to 10PM. The group of five patients was followed for 7 months, after which patients showed a mean improvement in HDRS of 55±38% (p=0.009). Statistically significant improvements were also shown in the MADRS, Inventory of Depression Symptoms – Self Report (IDS-SR), and Clinical Global Impression (CGI). Interestingly, similarly to the previous study, no significant improvement was observed on the QLES. This may be a reflection of the lasting psychosocial effects in severe chronic depression, even after depressive symptoms have improved (Kopell et al., 2011). Of the 5 patients, 4 showed a greater than 40% improvement in HDRS scores at 7 month follow-up (80%), 3 showed a greater than 50% improvement and went on to achieve remission (60%) (Table 14.2). Increased time (28 weeks vs 16 weeks) was associated with improved HDRS scores and increase in likelihood to achieve remission (Table 14.3). Extensive neuropsychological testing was performed pre- and post-operatively and revealed no changes in cognitive functioning with the extensive pre-frontal stimulation. Two adverse events were noted. One was intraoperative and clinically insignificant, where the advancement of a paddle led to a small dural tear with no subsequent leakage of cerebrospinal fluid. The second event was a superficial purulent scalp infection 12 weeks post-operatively, which required debridement and explantation of the leads with no subsequent clinical consequence. Of note, this patient went on to achieve a 42% decrease in HDRS at 7 months follow-up despite explantation.

Fig. 14.1: Electrode design (A. Northstar Neuroscience Renova ® B. Medtronic Resume ®)

In both studies, ICS appears to have a potentially robust antidepressant effect in this patient population previously refractory to most forms of treatments. The combined 10/16 patients (62.5%) met criteria for a 40% decrease in HDRS score and 8/16 patients

(50%) met more rigid criteria for responsiveness with a greater than 50% decrease in score. Seven of 16 patients (43.8%) met criteria for remission. The relatively low surgical complications in both studies highlight the potential advantage of ICS over other surgical procedures, by its nature precluding the need to penetrate dura or brain parenchyma and thus decreasing the risk of hemorrhage and other potential complications. Both studies have proven to be prone to a dramatic variability in individual patient response, which may at least in part be attributed to the anatomical target chosen as well as individual anatomic variability, stimulation parameters as well as device limitations.

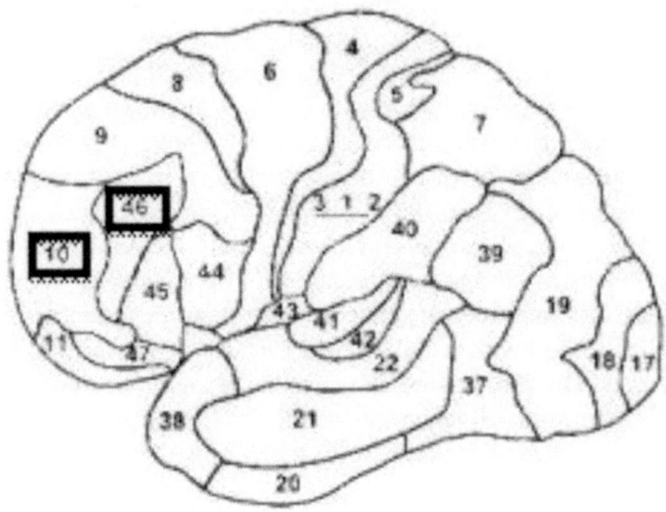

Fig. 14.2: Targeting the frontal pole and midlateral prefrontal cortex (BA 10 and 46)

Table 14.2: Clinical Outcomes

		Nahas, et al (n=5)	**Kopell et al (n=11)**
Partial Responders	>40% decrease in HDRS	4 (80%)	6 (55%)
Responders	>50% decrease in HDRS	3 (60%)	5 (45%)
Remitters	HDRS<10	3 (60%)	4 (36%)

Table 14.3: Average HDRS Scores Over Time

	Baseline (SD)	7 months (SD)	21 months (SD)	p-Value
Nahas et al	28.4 (4.8)	13 (11.4)	N/A	0.009
Kopell et al	34.25 (4.99)	N/A	15 (7)	<0.001

14.1.2 Surgical Technique

Good quality, pre-operative MR imaging is of paramount importance in the pre-surgical planning phase during which the target areas are localized. In the study conducted by Nahas et al (2010), the targets, which included the anterior frontal pole (BA10) and mid-lateral prefrontal cortex (BA46) were defined using an online atlas (MRIcro, http://mccauslandcenter.sc.edu/mricro) co-registered to the patients MRI (Fig.14.2). In the study performed by Kopell et al (2011), the target (L DLPFC – BA 9/46) which was localized to the mid-portion of the middle fontal gyrus, was identified using standard anatomic landmarks defined as 2cm anterior to the precentral sulcus, inferior to the sulcus frontalis superior, and superior to the sulcus frontalis inferior (Fig.14.3). Once the targets are identified, the patient is brought to the operating room and the MRI is co-registered with the patient's head using a stereotactic frameless system. The patient may be intubated and sedated, or minimally sedated if awake-intraoperative testing is deemed necessary. In the study conducted by Nahas et al, in which bilateral electrodes were placed, a coronal incision was made behind the hairline and slit-shaped craniotomies (3x0.5cm) were performed bilaterally to allow epidural insertion of the paddle leads. In the study conducted by Kopell et al, a 4-cm round craniotomy was performed centered directly over the predetermined area guided by stereotactic navigation. After insertion, the electrode leads are anchored by suture to the underlying dura. Subsequently, under general anesthesia a separate linear incision is made below the clavicle and a subcuteanous pocket is made for insertion of the pulse generator. Using standard procedures, the electrode extension leads are tunneled subcutaneously behind the ear and over the clavicle, and connected to the infraclavicular pulse generator. The system's impedance is then generally tested prior to the closing of the incision. The patients remain in the hospital for 24-48 hours post-operatively, and a post-operative CT scan without contrast is obtained and fused to the pre-operative MRI to ascertain the final lead placement and rule out intra-cranial hemorrhage.

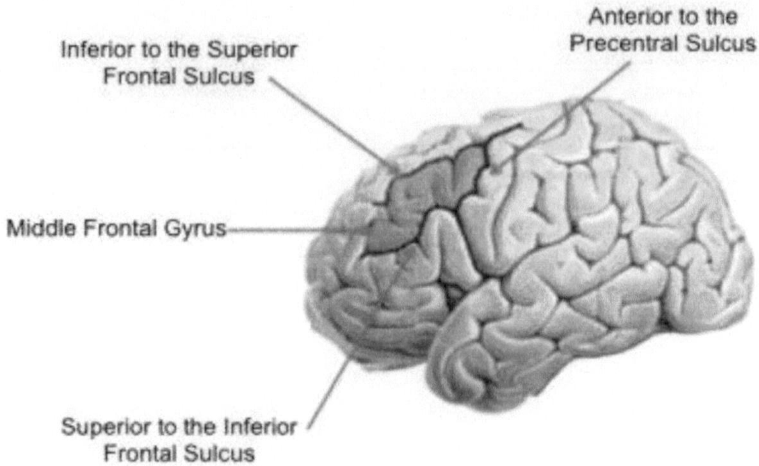

Fig. 14.3: Targeting the DLPFC (BA9/46)

14.1.3 Refining Techniques

Of the many sources of variability among studies and between patients, electrode location, stimulation settings and duration of stimulation are likely to play vital roles in the efficacy of this treatment modality.

The anatomical target of choice as well as the precise localization at that target has been postulated to be of utmost importance, possibly necessitating sub-centimeter accuracy to achieve optimal results (Herbsman et al., 2009; Kopell et al., 2011; Pathak et al., 2013). Given that the different targets chosen likely function within similar, if not interconnected, networks, *it is conceivable that differing anatomic locations will yield similar clinical outcomes*. Nonetheless, within a chosen anatomic location such as the DLPFC (see Box 14.1), targeting the lateral and anterior regions has correlated with better clinical outcomes (Herbsman et al., 2009; Pathak et al., 2013). In an analysis done at 16-weeks during the study conducted by Kopell et al, HDRS scores were significantly correlated with electrode distance from the pre-central sulcus with electrodes placed posterior to the initially defined target (2cm anterior to the pre-central sulcus) appearing to be less efficacious than those placed at or anterior to the target ($p = .03$) (Kopell et al., 2011). This distribution was so striking that it prompted the authors to offer revision surgery to the subjects in the cohort with electrodes deemed to be placed sub-optimally; however, those patients that underwent revision surgery did not ultimately yield the same distribution pattern of efficacy at the 104-week analysis. The use of functional imaging, specifically diffusion-tensor imaging (DTI), functional magnetic resonance imaging (fMRI) and magnetoencephalography

(MEG) may play a critical role in localizing cortical targets and accounting for inter-individual variability. The use of diffusor tensor imaging (DTI) may be of particular benefit in its capacity to delineate individual variability in circuitry (Fig.14.4). DTI has been investigated in the localization of sub-cortical targets in DBS for depression and successful placement with reference to tractographic findings has been shown to correlate with improved clinical outcome (Bhatia et al., 2012). DTI analysis with electromagnetic modeling has also been performed in TMS targeting of M1 (Nummenmaa et al., 2014).

In another source of variability, *stimulation sources and parameters varied significantly in between studies and* among patients. *In* the study conducted by Kopell et al, the stimulation was unilateral and sourced from two electrode contacts, was constant, and varied in montage with mixed polarity (anode/cathode) and full anodic modes found to be most effective (Kopell et al., 2011; Pathak et al., 2013). In contrast, the study by Nahas et al utilized stimulation delivered intermittently, bilaterally, and with a considerably more anterior target with 8 electrode contacts per side (Nahas et al., 2010). Nonetheless in both studies, stimulation was found to be effective.

Not secondarily, the devices themselves have significant limitations. The device used in one study (Fig.14.1A) incorporated only 2 contacts that were not independent in their capacity to stimulate (Kopell et al., 2011). These electrodes stimulated at a maximum of 6.5 mA and were not capable of providing a "burst" pattern of dosage. An improved electrode design would provide more avenues for personalized treatment protocols, and may obviate the need for revision surgery based on small discrepancies in anatomical targeting.

On average, effective stimulation parameters necessitated battery usage resulting in an average battery life of 9 months in one study (Kopell et al., 2011). However, rechargeable batteries may obviate this limitation.

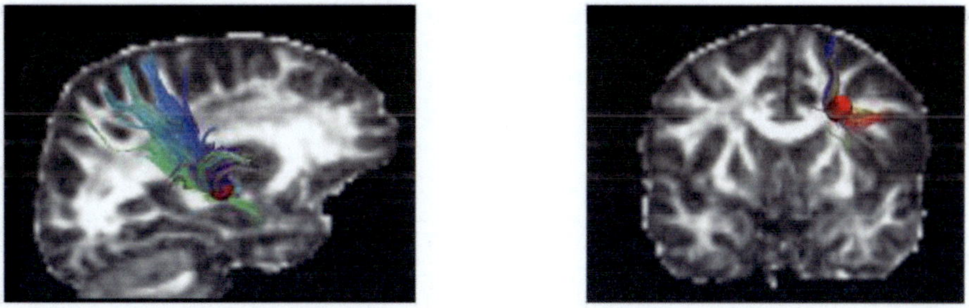

Fig. 14.4: Diffusion Tensor Imaging (DTI)

S Canavero
Current targets of stimulation for depression (DBS: subgenual cingulate cortex; CS: left DLPFC) have resulted from an emerging understanding of the neurophysiological basis of the disorder utilizing data from neuroimaging as well as neuropsychological studies to elucidate anatomical interconnectivity (Rogers et al. 2004). Several targets, postulated to be connected to centers of cognitive and emotional processing, have been implicated in the prefrontal cortex including: the frontopolar region (BA 10), midlateral prefrontal region (BA 46), and the dorsolateral pre-frontal cortex (DLPFC). The DLPFC lies at the junction of the lateral aspect of Brodmann's areas 9 and 46 (BA 9/46), makes up 10% of the surface of the frontal lobe and is functionally connected to the anterior cingulate cortex, the orbitofrontal cortex as well as having strong thalamic and other cortical connections (Fuster 2009). Imaging studies have revealed a consistent pattern between the right and left DLPFC, demonstrating hypometabolism of the left side and hypermetabolism of the right side in the resting state of patients suffering from MDD (Grimm et al., 2008). BA 10 has also shown a robust anatomic relationship to other limbic-related cortical and subcortical circuitry with connections to the anterior cingulate cortex, precuneus, posterior cingulate, orbitofrontal cortex and DLPFC (Fuster 2009). BA 46, which encompasses the DLPFC as well as ventral regions maintains connections to temporal areas, as well as to paralimbic circuitry (Fuster 2009). *Because it is thought to be an interconnected network, it is feasible that stimulation at a various number of anatomical points may yield similar effects.*Actually, resting state fMR studies have identified about 20 cortical networks in man: in depression, these are all dysfunctional. Thus, applying CS to any given node within these networks is expected to modulate the activity of other nodes via their shared anatomical connections: stimulating DLPFC also engages ACC, subgenual CC and basal ganglia, among others. The question whether CS restores cognitive control over limbic brain areas or enhances connectivity between them appears to have been answered.
Dysfunctional monoamine neurotransmitter systems are likely just downstream effects of another underlying disorder leading to the symptoms of depression and rTMS effects do not depend critically upon the central serotonergic tone.
Although the left DLPFC has been emphasized in imaging studies, actually both DLPFCs are dysfunctional and clinical studies evince no differences in depression after lesions to the right or left hemispheres. So either high-frequency (but also low frequency) left DLPFC or low-frequency right DLPFC (which is hyperactive) show antidepressant effects. Symmetrical DLPFC stimulation is thus an option, with an eye towards stimulating the brain broadly.
BA 10 has recently been affirmed to be the master-key in frontal lobe function, and this is an important new target for ICS.
Another potential target would be the rostral premotor cortex (rPMC:BA6/8). RPMC has fiber connections with both BA46 and caudalPMC/SMA, acting as a gateway between motor and cognitive networks (Hanakawa 2011).

Box 14.1: The DLPFC and Beyond

Closed-loop ICS will be available in the future for the treatment of psychiatric (and other) disorders. In order to make this possible, biomarkers are needed. It appears that increased interleukin 6 and decreased BDNF levels are among the most promising biomarkers of depression, decreased serum folate of treatment resistance, reduced ACC activity of treatment compliance and decreased total cholesterol of suicidal behavior. However, EEG based markers are required for closed loop systems to “kick in” when needed. CS effects can actually alter neuroplasticity, neurotransmission and CBF through an effect on cerebral oscillatory activity. Integration of brain activity across greater distances is coordinated by alpha or theta activity, while shorter-distance coordination is achieved by beta (12-20 Hz) and gamma (20-40Hz) oscillations. Synchronized alpha oscillations in particular play a key role in global top-down control of brain cognitive processes, probably via inhibition (8-10 Hz). Severity of depression correlates with degree of decrease of PFC rCBF and power of low frequency EEG. Yet, synchronization of rTMS to individual alpha frequency may be less effective than standard stimulation

References

Arns M, Spronk D, Fitzgerald PB. Potential differential effects of 9 Hz rTMS and 10 Hz rTMS in the treatment of depression.Brain Stimul. 2010;3:124-6.
Badre D, D’Esposito M Is the rostro-caudal axis of the frontal lobe hierarchical? Nat Rev Neurosci. 2009;10:659-69
Downar J, Daskalakis ZJ. New targets for rTMS in depression: a review of convergent evidence. Brain Stimul. 2013;6:231-40
Fuster J. The prefrontal cortex. San Diego:Academic Press, 2009
Grimm S, Beck J, Schuepbach D, et al. Imbalance between left and right dorsolateral prefrontal cortex in major depression is linked to negative emotional judgment: An fMRI study in severe major depressive disorder. Biol Psych 2008;63:369-376.
Hanakawa T. Rostral premotor cortex as a gateway between motor and cognitive networks. Neurosci Res 2011; 70: 144-154
-Kuo MF, Paulus W, Nitsche MA. Therapeutic effects of non-invasive brain stimulation with direct currents (tDCS) in neuropsychiatric diseases. Neuroimage. 2014;85 Pt 3: 948-60
Nieber D, Schlegel S.Relationships between psychomotor retardation and EEG power spectrum in major depression. Neuropsychobiology. 1992;25:20-3.
Rogers MA, Kasai K, Koji M, et al. Executive and prefrontal dysfunction in unipolar depression: A review of neuropsychological and imaging evidence. Neurosci Res 2004;50:1-11.
Speer AM, Wassermann EM, Benson BE, et al. Antidepressant efficacy of high and low frequency rTMS at 110% of motor threshold versus sham stimulation over left prefrontal cortex. Brain Stimul. 2014;7:36-41
Yu E, Lurie P. Transcranial magnetic stimulation not proven effective. Biol Psychiatry 2010; 67: e13
Ward MP, Irazoqui PP.Evolving refractory major depressive disorder diagnostic and treatment paradigms: toward closed-loop therapeutics. Front Neuroeng. 2010;3:7.

continued **Box 14.1:** The DLPFC and Beyond

14.1.4 Comparison of Outcomes with Nonimplantable Cortical Stimulation

Both noninvasive (e.g. TMS, tDCS) and ICS treatment modalities appear to be effective and safe methods in the adjunctive treatment of major depression. Clear benefits of rTMS and tDCS include their relative ease of use and very low risk profile, as well as the absence of need for anesthesia and surgery. Although there is less data supporting its use, tDCS in particular is cost-effective and is easily attainable. ICS, on the other hand, provides the opportunity for a more potent, consistent, and accurate stimulus delivery to the target cortex. Once implanted and programmed, it obviates the need for repetitive treatment encounters or adherence to a treatment regimen. More importantly, despite stronger or accelerated dosing regimens, longer treatment courses, bilateral stimulation protocols, individually tailored stimulation frequencies, new coil geometries, application of neuronavigation and more accurate targeting, rTMS has not proved superior to ICS (30-35% remission vs 43%). Both, however, appear to fare better than medications (23-33%) and cognitive therapy (22%).

In a comparison of results from the randomized controlled trials in rTMS and tDCS with epidural cortical stimulation, it is important to note the variability in inclusion criteria in the studies and between treatment modalities. The two epidural cortical stimulation trials had rigid inclusion/exclusion criteria (Table 14.1) resulting in the most treatment refractory patient population. Furthermore, in the cortical stimulation trials, long-term efficacy and follow-up proved to have significant impact on the results; the same type of data does not exist in the rTMS and tDCS literature for an accurate comparison. Nonetheless, despite the small sample sizes, the two trials using epidural cortical stimulation had higher rates of responders and remitters, with pooled data revealing a 43% remission rate. In comparison, rTMS meta-analyses of high frequency, left DLPFC stimulation reveal lower overall response and remission rates despite a population with a comparatively less severe form of depression (Table 14.4).

A recent meta-analysis (Ren et al 2014) (n=425) found Electroconvulsive Therapy (ECT) superior in terms of remission (52.9% vs 33.6%) to both high and low frequency rTMS. ECT was superior for psychotic but equal for non-psychotic depression (high frequency rTMS). ECT had a nonsignificant advantage over HF rTMS on overall improvement in HAMD scores. However, nothing could be concluded for the longer term for all techniques and ECT is burdened by memory and verbal fluency impairment.

Table 14.4: Selected rTMS Meta-Analyses of High Frequency, Left DLPFC Stimulation

		Berlim et al 2013 (n=1371)*	**Lam et al 2008 (n=782)****
Responders	50% decrease in HDRS	29.3% (vs 10.4% sham)	19%
Remitters	HDRS<10	18.6% (vs 5% sham)	16%

* Inclusion criteria ≥10 sessions of stimulation, sham controlled

** Inclusion criteria treatment resistant depression

14.2 Future Directions

As noted previously, limitations of ICS in the treatment of depression are in individual patient variability to response. Refining the anatomical target based on functional imaging including the use of DTI, fMRI, and MEG with high-density EEG to customize electrode placement *based on individual anatomic variability* may dramatically improve results. In addition to accurate and preferably individualized anatomical targeting, patient selection is paramount in improving the overall efficacy of ICS. Higher baseline regional cerebral metabolic rate of glucose (rCMRG) in the right DLPFC has been associated with increased responsiveness to ICS for major depression (Kopell et al., 2011) and advances in neuroimaging may provide additional avenues of targeting responders.

In integrating all of these new and improving methods of cortical stimulation, non-invasive methods such as rTMS and tDCS offer the possibility of acting as invaluable screening tools in pre-assessing potential responsiveness to ICS in major depressive disorder, as well as for future psychiatric targets. TMS has already demonstrated to be useful when integrated as a screening tool for other conditions such as neuropathic pain and tinnitus (Chapters 8, 9, 15). However, if results of screening rTMS are to be accepted as a valid proxy for surgical implantation, targeting must be accurate. Recent refinements have moved the TMS field beyond the fit-for-all "5 cm rule" for localizing BA9 (i.e. stimulating the cortex 5 cm anterior to the M1 hand area in a parasagittal line): given significant anatomic variations among individuals, several patients get their stimulation over BA6 or BA8. A "6 cm rule" has been proposed (Johnson et al 2013), covering more frequently BA46. A group proposed a "9 cm rule" / F3 (10-20 EEG coordinates system) (Fitzgerald et al 2009) or F5/6 targeting (Rusjan et al 2010). Parenthetically, fMRI appears superior to neuronavigated TMS in mapping the cortical motor system, especially for the face and leg areas (Weiss et al 2012).

Also, stimulation parameters, including the frequency of stimulation, now widely variable between the methodologies, as well as the magnitude, duration, and pattern of stimulation need to be normalized. For instance, the resting motor threshold (MT) upon which intensity of rTMS stimulation is usually based is NOT the best measure for determining the minimal TMS dose required to stimulate the cortex, and doses up to 120-130% of the MT appear safe (Johnson et al 2013).

Psychiatric disorders amenable to ICS mirror to a large extent those submitted to noninvasive CS: schizophrenia (left, but not right, temporoparietal area, 1Hz rTMS: Slotema et al 2014), obsessive-compulsive disorder, autism, post-traumatic stress disorder, craving and addiction, anxiety, and several others (reviewed in Eichhammer et al 2009).

References

Berlim MT, Van den Eynde F, Daskalakis ZJ. Clinical utility of transcranial direct current stimulation (tDCS) for treating major depression: A systematic review and meta-analysis of randomized, double-blind and sham-controlled trials. J Psych Res 2013a;47:1-7.

Berlim MT, van den Eynde F, Tovar-Perdomo S, Daskalakis ZJ. Response, remission and drop-out rates following high-frequency repetitive transcranial magnetic stimulation (rtms) for treating major depression: A systematic review and meta-analysis of randomized, double-blind and sham-controlled trials. Psychol Med 2013b:1-15.

Bezard E, Boraud T, Nguyen JP, et al. Cortical stimulation and epileptic seizure: A study of the potential risk in primates. Neurosurgery 1999;45:346-350.

Bhatia KD, Henderson L, Ramsey-Stewart G, May J. Diffusion tensor imaging to aid subgenual cingulum target selection for deep brain stimulation in depression. Stereotact Funct Neurosurg 2012;90:225-232.

Eichhammer P, Langguth B, Lundgrebe M et al. Invasive and noninvasive stimulation for psychiatric conditions. In: Canavero S (ed) Textbook of therapeutic cortical stimulation. New York: Nova Science, 2009, 289-305

Fitzgerald PB, Maller JJ, Hoy KE, et al. Exploring the optimal site for the localization of dorsolateral prefrontal cortex in brain stimulation experiments. Brain Stimul. 2009;2:234-7.

Herbsman T, Avery D, Ramsey D, et al. More lateral and anterior prefrontal coil location is associated with better repetitive transcranial magnetic stimulation antidepressant response. Biol Psych 2009;66:509-515.

Johnson KA, Baig M, Ramsey D, et al. Prefrontal rTMS for treating depression: location and intensity results from the OPT-TMS multi-site clinical trial. Brain Stimul. 2013;6:108-17.

Kopell BH, Halverson J, Butson CR, et al. Epidural cortical stimulation of the left dorsolateral prefrontal cortex for refractory major depressive disorder. Neurosurgery 2011;69:1015-1029

Lam RW, Chan P, Wilkins-Ho M, Yatham LN. Repetitive transcranial magnetic stimulation for treatment-resistant depression: A systematic review and metaanalysis. Can J Psych 2008;53:621-631.

Nahas Z, Anderson BS, Borckardt J, et al. Bilateral epidural prefrontal cortical stimulation for treatment-resistant depression. Biol Psych 2010;67:101-109.

Nummenmaa A, McNab JA, Savadjiev P, et al. Targeting of white matter tracts with transcranial magnetic stimulation. Brain Stimul 2014;7:80-84.

Pathak Y, Kopell BH, Szabo A, Rainey C, Harsch H, Butson CR: The role of electrode location and stimulation polarity in patient response to cortical stimulation for major depressive disorder. Brain Stimul 2013;6:254-260.

Ren J, Li H, Palaniyappan L, et al. Repetitive transcranial magnetic stimulation versus electroconvulsive therapy for major depression: A systematic review and meta-analysis. Prog Neuropsychopharmacol Biol Psych 2014; 51C:181-189

Rusjan PM, Barr MS, Farzan F, et al. Optimal transcranial magnetic stimulation coil placement for targeting the dorsolateral prefrontal cortex using novel magnetic resonance image-guided neuronavigation.Hum Brain Mapp. 2010;31:1643-52

Slotema CW, Blom JD, van Lutterveld R, et al. Review of the efficacy of transcranial magnetic stimulation for auditory verbal hallucinations. Biol Psychiatry. 2014 (in press)

Weiss C, Nettekoven C, Rehme AK, et al. Mapping the hand, foot and face representations in the primary motor cortex Retest reliability of neuronavigated TMS versus functional MRI. Neuroimage. 2012;66C:531-542

Dirk De Ridder, Sven Vanneste, Jae-Jin Song, Berthold Langguth

15 Tinnitus

In this chapter, we will focus on cortical stimulation (CS) for the management of subjective tinnitus (see Box 15.1 for an overview).

Tinnitus (Moller et al 2011, Langguth et al 2013) is classified according to whether the perceived noise has its source within the patient's body known as objective tinnitus or *somatosounds* (for example, myoclonic contractions of the tensor tympani muscle or blood vessels) or if it is only perceivable to the patient and lacks a specific sound source, namely subjective tinnitus. Subjective tinnitus is by far the most common form. As the most common cause for tinnitus is hearing loss, subjective or non-pulsatile tinnitus is often considered as an auditory phantom phenomenon, analogous to phantom pain. There are most likely different forms of tinnitus, each with a different pathophysiological mechanism. For example tinnitus resulting from a microvascular compression of the vestibulocochlear nerve is related to ephaptic transmission between different fibers that make up the nerve, and responds to carbamazepine, in contrast to other forms of tinnitus. Some forms of cervicogenic tinnitus respond to C2 modulation by TENS or occipital nerve stimulation via implanted electrodes. Tinnitus can take the form of continuous buzzing, hissing or ringing, or a combination of these or other characteristics. It can be heard in one or both ears, but it can also be perceived holocranially. Tinnitus can occur intermittently or have a pulsatile character. The intensity of the phantom sound can vary from a subtle noise to high intensity sounds which cannot be masked by any external noise. Many patients with tinnitus also report symptoms such as frustration, annoyance, insomnia, hyperacusis, anxiety, depression, irritability and concentration difficulties and these symptoms are highly relevant for determining tinnitus severity. Thus, tinnitus represents a highly prevalent and potentially distressing condition with a wide range of symptoms that are likely to place a huge burden on patients and significantly impair their quality of life. Its socioeconomic relevance is illustrated by the dramatically increased risk for disability pension among tinnitus patients. In epidemiological surveys around the globe (Europe, USA, Japan, Africa and China), roughly one fifth of men and one sixth of women reported to perceive tinnitus, with 4.4% and 2.1%, respectively, reporting high tinnitus intensity. Tinnitus is most commonly associated with hearing loss, which explains why its prevalence increases with age, i.e. due to age-related presbycusis, but it is on the rise in young people as good. About 90% of high school students report tinnitus after leisure-induced noise exposure and about 15% have permanent tinnitus, but in most of them it is not perceived as intrusive. In addition, tinnitus is a common disability in young people resulting from warfare and was the first-most prevalent handicap for US veterans receiving compensation in 2011.

Box 15.1: TINNITUS

The concept behind the CS approach is that the areas involved in a pathologically functioning neuronal network that generates tinnitus can be visualized and that interference with this tinnitus network activity by cortical stimulation can alleviate tinnitus. The procedure follows a four-step rationale (Fig.15.1):

1. Tinnitus is thought to be related to altered activity in the auditory and frontal cortices, as well as in the amygdalo-(para)hippocampal area, anterior and posterior cingulate cortex, and insula (Fig.15.2-3).

2. The anatomical location of the tinnitus generator can be determined by functional imaging techniques (e.g. fMRI).
3. The abnormal neuronal activity can be transiently modulated by neuronavigated TMS and other non-invasive CS techniques (Vanneste et al 2011, Vanneste and DeRidder 2012, Song et al 2013)
4. If the patient responds to step 3, electrical stimulation through an electrode implanted on the same area (ICS) can provide permanent tinnitus suppression.

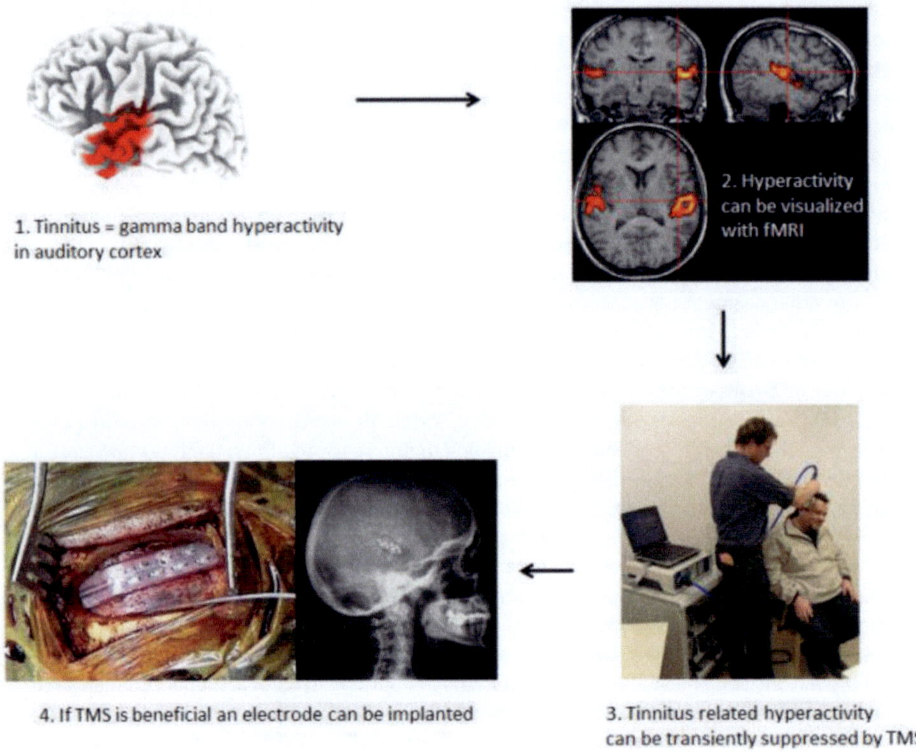

Fig. 15.1: ladder approach to auditory cortex implantation

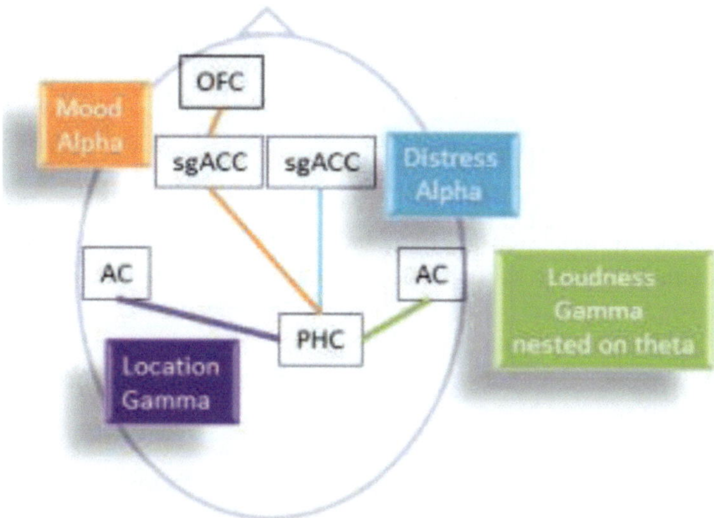

Fig. 15.2: different clinical aspects of tinnitus (e.g. loudness, distress, location, mood) are represented by different oscillatory networks which communicate at different frequencies and mutually interact in specific brain structures (hubs). AC: auditory cortex, OFC: orbitofrontal cortex, PHC: parahippocampal area, sgACC: subgenual anterior cingulate cortex

	Phase 1	Phase 2	Phase 3	Phase 4
Deafferentation	Very small bandwith	Small bandwith	Large bandwith	Very large bandwith
Audiometry	Normal to minimal hearing loss (< 20 dB)	Normal to minimal hearing loss (< 20 dB)	Normal to minimal hearing loss (< 20 dB)	Severe hearing loss (> 20 dB)
Compensation mechanism	Decrease lateral inhibition (Rajan 1998) 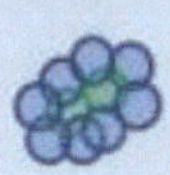	Receptive field widening (Chen 1996) 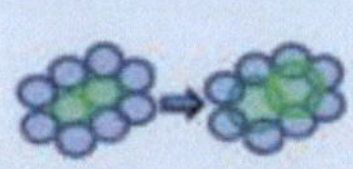	Dendritic and axonal sprouting (Hoy 1985, Hsieh 2007) 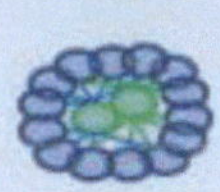	Retrieval from memory (De Ridder 2012) 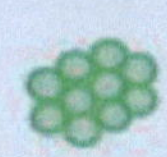
Location of compensation	Auditory cortex	Auditory cortex	Auditory cortex	(para)hippocampus

Fig. 15.3: plastic changes in tinnitus related to deafferentation. Depending on the bandwith of the deafferentation different plastic changes might occur, starting with changes in lateral inhibition, followed by widening of the receptive fields, and sprouting. These changes occur in the auditory cortex. If deafferentation occurs in a large bandwith, compensatory changes in the auditory cortex might not be sufficient to fill in the deafferentation gap, and parahippocampal mechanisms might be required. Thus in tinnitus associated with no or little hearing loss the auditory cortex might be the ideal neuromodulation target, in tinnitus with hearing loss the parahippocampus might be the ideal target for neuromodulation.

15.1 Surgical Approach and Targeting

15.1.1 Auditory Cortex

15.1.1.1 Rationale

Auditory cortex stimulation may interfere with persistent gamma band activity, which is thought to code tinnitus intensity. In a study using MEG during electrical stimulation of the auditory cortex, the stimulation increased spectral correlation across low and high gamma band activity, between alpha and beta activity, whereas delta/theta activity decreased (Ramirez et al 2009). This has been confirmed by recordings from electrodes overlying the secondary auditory cortex: maximal tinnitus suppression was obtained by current delivery exactly at the BOLD spot, elicited by tinnitus-matched sound presentation in the MRI machine (DeRidder et al 2009, 2011). The BOLD spot co-localizes with increased and coupled gamma and theta (a supposed carrier wave required for co-activation of the tinnitus network) activity, as opposed to the other electrode poles which show normal alpha peaks. These spectral changes normalize when stimulation induces tinnitus suppression, both on electrode and in source localized EEG recordings (DeRidder et al 2009, 2011). Thus, theta-gamma might be causally related to a conscious auditory phantom percept (VanDerLoo et al 2009, DeRidder et al 2009, 2011) and electrical stimulation via implanted electrodes reduces tinnitus perception by interfering with this anomalous activity embedded in a larger tinnitus network.

15.1.1.2 Target Identification

Both MSI (Magnetic Source Imaging = MEG fused with MRI) (Seidman et al 2008) and fMRI have been used for exactly localizing the auditory cortical hyperactivity. The cerebral activation induced by an external sound, that matches the tinnitus sound in frequency and presented via earphones, can be detected by fMRI. S-LORETA (Standardized low-resolution brain electromagnetic tomography) is another technique useful to capture anomalous tinnitus-related activity, but has low spatial resolution and as such cannot be employed for surgical planning. However, it may have an impact on patient selection: when comparing 5 patients who responded to auditory cortex implants with five patients who did not, sLORETA analysis demonstrated that whether or not someone is going to respond has nothing to do with differences in auditory cortex activity (De Ridder, under revision): in contrast to what was expected, differences between responders and non-responders were demonstrated in left and right parahippocampal areas for gamma, and in the left amygdala-hippocampal-parahippocampal area extending into the left insula for beta3. Variability in PET scan activation before and after rTMS failed to support the hypothesis that low-frequency rTMS improves tinnitus by reducing cortical activation at the stimulation site, questioning the utility of PET for targeting (Mannemeier et al 2011).

15.1.1.3 Modulation of Auditory Activity with rTMS

Subsequently, the exact area of the auditory cortex that is processing the tinnitus tone is stimulated by TMS. A neuronavigation system is useful for exactly localizing the target area for TMS on the patient's head. If tinnitus can be transiently suppressed by TMS of this area, an electrode is surgically placed extradurally, overlying the secondary auditory cortex exactly at the site where fMRI demonstrated hyperactivity and where TMS was successful (DeRidder et al 2009, 2011, Langguth et al 2009, Song et al 2013).

15.1.1.4 Implantation of Electrodes Over the Auditory Cortex: Technical Aspects.

Surgically implanting an extradural electrode carries a minimal risk of complications. An incision is made 5 to 6 cm above the external ear canal, based on the fMRI data: the location of the auditory cortex and the placement of the surgical incision vary among different individuals and between the left and right side in the same patient. The location of the incision in the skin is therefore guided by the fMRI. The skin incision is about 5 cm long and followed by a split of the temporal muscle. A small 1x5cm hole is made in the skull and the dura is coagulated with bipolar forceps to disconnect small sensory fibers that innervate the dura, lest the electrical stimulation cause pain by activation thereof. Thereafter, the stimulating strip –which carries 4 to 16 contacts- is placed on the exact spot with 1-2 mm accuracy based on the fMRI data and sutured onto the dura. The bone flap is placed back and secured with titanium screws and plates. After that, the lead to the stimulating electrode is tunneled to the chest where it is connected to an extension lead, and further tunneled to the abdomen where it is passed through the skin to the outside of the body. The electrode leads that exit the abdomen are connected to a stimulator, usually after 3 days, as, during the first days postoperatively, the tinnitus is often markedly decreased from intraoperative stimulation or anesthesia. During the external trial stimulation, the different electrode contacts are activated, one by one - or more than one at a time, depending on what gives the best suppression. The trial sessions are limited to one hour because it is difficult for the patient to concentrate for longer times, and a good suppressive effect can take anywhere from one day to weeks or even months. A programmable internal pulse generator (IPG) is then implanted in the abdomen or the gluteal region and the electrode is connected with a new extension lead to the IPG. The stimulation parameters (frequency, amplitude, and pulse width) can be changed postoperatively to find the best parameters for maximal tinnitus control. Stimulation is not performed continuously: switching the stimulator 5 seconds ON and 5 seconds OFF is usually sufficient. As the patient does not feel the electrical impulses, he or she does not know whether the stimulator is ON or OFF. With a given stimulation program the tinnitus reoccurs after a certain amount of time in most cases. Tinnitus recurrence can be prevented by running alternately several different stimulation programs using different electrode contacts. During the first period after the implantation, the tinnitus returns very quickly when the stimulator is turned off. However, as in another ICS protocols (see chapters 8, 10), after years of stimulation, it may take weeks before the tinnitus fully relapses when the stimulator is switched off or the battery has become drained.

Intradural (DeRidder et al 2009) and intracerebral (Seidman et al 2008) electrode placement onto and into the primary auditory cortex have been performed. However, complication risks are much higher and treatment results are not superior to the epidural approach (DeRidder et al 2009).

15.1.1.5 Outcome

Multiple small and one larger series of patients with auditory cortex electrodes have been published. 43 patients with severe treatment-resistant tinnitus (Goebel and Hiller's Scale grade 3 and 4) were implanted with a cortical electrode overlying the secondary auditory cortex. Before implantation, all patients underwent TMS test sessions on separate dates by a third party. A >20% improvement on the VAS scale on two separate occasions makes the patients eligible for implantation. Although all patients responded to TMS, 1 out of 3 patients did not respond to ICS. Among responders, perceived tinnitus loudness decreased on average by 51.3%. There was a significant, but weak, positive correlation ($r = .34$, $p < .05$) between the magnitude of relief from the TMS tests and ICS (DeRidder et al 2011).

Burst stimulation (5 stimuli of 1 ms pulse width, 1ms interpulse interval delivered at 500 Hz, 40 times a second) is more efficient than tonic stimulation: with tonic stimulation only 1 in 3 patients responded to stimulation, while with burst stimulation, half of the non-responding patients did benefit, resulting in a total response rate of 2 out of 3 patients (Fig.15.4). *Burst stimulation was specifically superior to tonic stimulation for suppressing noise-like tinnitus* (DeRidder et al 2011), analogous to what has been described for TMS. In contrast to TMS, where the suppression effect decreases with longer tinnitus duration, no correlation was found between the effect of electrical cortical stimulation and tinnitus duration for the same study population, suggesting that *ICS acts on tinnitus by a different mechanism than TMS*. Furthermore, all patients responded to TMS, as this was an inclusion criterion for implantation, and not all patients responded to the implant. Treatment effects also depended on tinnitus type. *Pure tone tinnitus* can be suppressed better than narrow band noise or the combination of pure tone and narrow band noise, and *unilateral tinnitus* better than bilateral tinnitus. This approach has been replicated by other centers with similar or different results. A French study obtained persisting 65% tinnitus reduction in a woman using an fMRI based extradural auditory cortex implant (Litre et al 2009, 2010). Another study of eight patients using a similar technique but different hardware found no permanent tinnitus suppression (Friedland et al 2007). In six out of the eight patients, temporary effects on tinnitus perception were observed. However, tinnitus distress decreased slowly over time, even without suppression of tinnitus intensity.

This may be related to the fact that an electrode with only two contacts was used which limits the way the electrodes can be programmed. The finding of decreased tinnitus distress with unchanged tinnitus intensity could possibly be explained by disruption of the phase synchronization between the 'general distress network' and the tinnitus related activity in the auditory cortex (DeRidder et al 2011b). TMS of the auditory cortex not only disrupts local ongoing activity but also long-range connections in a larger network. In some patients tinnitus suppression can be obtained, but only for short times (1 to 3 days) after which the effect wears off, even after extensive reprogramming. Perhaps, the lemniscal thalamocortical system predominantly connecting to the primary auditory cortex is less plastic than the extralemniscal system, predominantly connecting to the secondary auditory cortex (DeRidder et al 2009). In four patients an intradural electrode on the primary auditory cortex was inserted in the Sylvian fissure, stimulating gray matter of the primary auditory cortex (DeRidder et al 2009). In two patients the goal was to obtain stabilization of tinnitus suppression, because the stimulus parameters had to be reprogrammed every 2 to 3 days. In both patients the intradural positioning resulted in stabilization of tinnitus suppression. Another approach has been proposed, inserting a wire electrode in the white matter beneath layer 6 of the primary auditory cortex. This has been performed successfully, using Magnetic Source Imaging for target localization, resulting in tinnitus suppression (Seidman et al 2008).

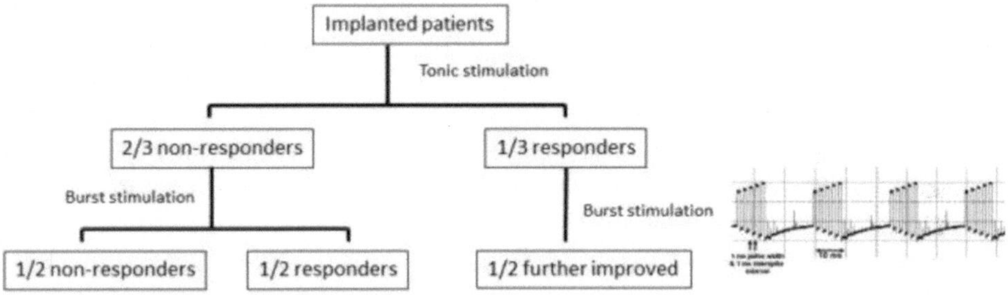

Fig. 15.4: response rate to auditory cortex stimulation: burst stimulation can rescue 50% of stimulation failures and can further improve 50% of responders to tonic stimulation.

15.1.2 Frontal Cortex

Tinnitus was among the many indications for which frontal lobotomy has been performed. In Elithorn (1953)'s study, 13 of 17 patients improved, 3 were unchanged and 1 patient's tinnitus worsened. In Beard (1965)'s series of 20 patients selected for surgery he states that "*In fact, of the 19 patients who survived the operation, 11 felt that their head noises were just the same but bothered them less and 8 felt that they had improved*". This suggests that disconnecting the frontal lobe from the rest of the brain has a particular impact on the affective component of the tinnitus. Indeed functional imaging studies using source localized EEG and MEG have shown that tinnitus distress is related to a network involving the anterior cingulate cortex (ACC), anterior insula and frontal cortex, whereas the auditory cortex is involved in the perceived tinnitus intensità (DeRidder et al 2011b, Vanneste and DeRidder 2012, Vanneste et al 2013). Other imaging studies showed that the primary hubs in tinnitus consist of the PCC, dACC, and subgenual ACC (sgACC), extending into the orbitofrontal cortex (OFC) and parahippocampal area (Schlee et al 2009, Husain and Schmidt 2014). Disconnecting frontal and auditory cortex by frontal lobotomy likely dissociated the affective component from the perceived loudness. More specifically, tinnitus distress is related to insufficient inhibition from the dorsolateral prefrontal cortex (DLPFC) and activation by the posterior cingulate cortex (PCC) (Joos et al 2012, Silchenko et al 2013). Non-invasive stimulation targeting the frontal cortex by means of tDCS can modulate tinnitus (e.g. Faber et al 2011). The tinnitus suppressing effect of stimulating the frontal cortex is mediated via the ACC and parahippocampal area, decreasing the increased gamma band activity in the auditory cortex (Vanneste and DeRidder 2011). Based on these results, a translation to invasive permanent neuromodulation was initiated, surgically targeting the DLPFC to treat tinnitus (DeRidder et al 2011).

In a patient refractory to conservative medical management and resistant to TMS of the auditory cortex, a neuronavigation-based auditory fMRI-guided frontal cortex TMS session was performed in a placebo-controlled way. A maximal tinnitus suppression of 50% was obtained reliably after stimulation of the right DLPFC. This TMS result was used as a prognostic indicator and two extradural electrodes (Lamitrode 44, SJMedical Neurodivision, Plano Tx, USA) were implanted over the spot in the DLPFC, where tinnitus frequency-matched tones induced BOLD activation in the fMRI. The tinnitus immediately improved postoperatively from VAS 7/10 to 4/10 and has progressively improved for more than one year. The initial VAS of 7/10 has decreased after 1 year to 2/10. This suggests that, in selected patients, focal extradural electrical stimulation of the DLPFC at the area of tinnitus-matched-sound elicited BOLD activation is capable of partially suppressing contralateral tinnitus. Electrophysiological data demonstrate that DLPFC stimulation by both epidural electrodes and tDCS reduces gamma band activity in the auditory cortex (Vanneste and DeRidder 2011, DeRidder et al 2011, 2013) which is abnormally increased in tinnitus (Fig.15.5).

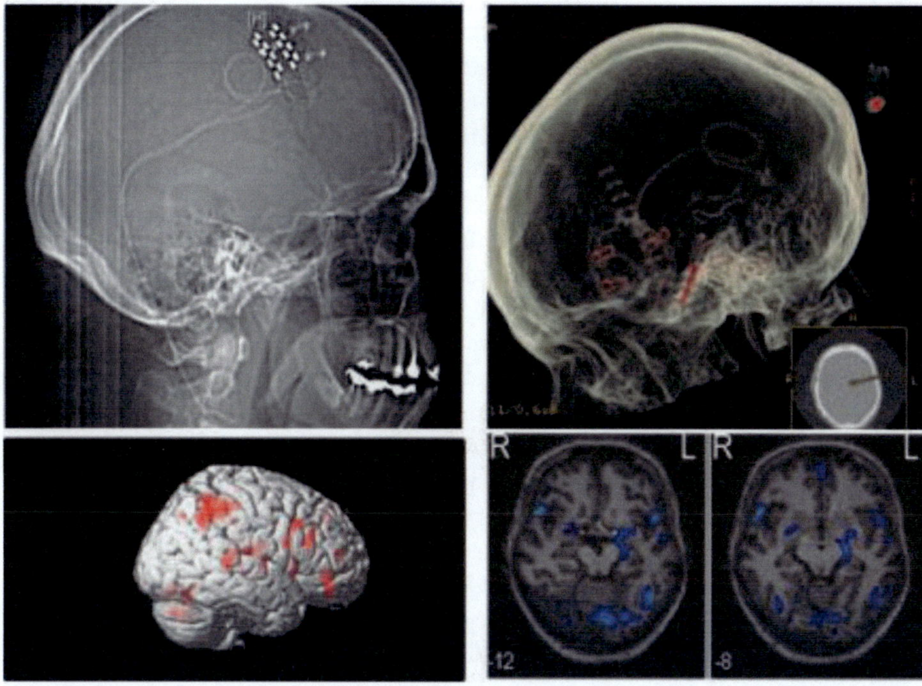

Fig. 15.5: frontal (left) and hippocampal cortical (right) stimulation for tinnitus suppression, based on tinnitus sound evoked BOLD activation.

15.1.3 Hippocampal Stimulation

The amygdala, hippocampus and parahippocampaus have been implicated in tinnitus. The auditory cortices are densely connected to the posterior parahippocampal area in a reciprocal way: this latter acts as a gatekeeper to the hippocampus and hence to the medial temporal lobe memory system, where salient information is encoded into long-term memory: a dysfunction in this mechanism is posited as an explanation for complex auditory phantom percepts such as auditory hallucinations (Diederen et al 2010) and speculatively also tinnitus: the para-hippocampus might be related to the constant updating of the tinnitus percept from memory, thereby preventing habituation. The most robust functional connectivity in resting state EEG and fMRI studies is the sgACC - parahippocampal – auditory cortex connection, which is critical in tinnitus (Maudoux et al 2012), both for distress (sgACC-parahippocampal) and loudness perception (Vanneste, under revision). Thus targeting this parahippocapal central hub should theoretically dissociate the loudness from the distress, and could thereby induce habituation to the sound, resulting in silencing the tinnitus percept.

CLINICAL CASE: a 59 year old patient has been implanted with an electrode in the amygdalohippocampal region. He presented with 5-year intractable right-sided pure tone tinnitus at 8000 Hz 10 dB SL present. He was neither responsive to medication nor to TMS. An fMRI elicited BOLD activation at the amygdalohippocampal junction only at the tinnitus matched frequency (8000 Hz), not at a control frequency (4000 Hz), suggesting a tinnitus-frequency-specific activation of this area. The technique used was the same as the one used for auditory cortex and DLPFC stimulation, i.e. an fMRI was performed with tinnitus-matched sounds and the BOLD activation in the amygdalohippocampal area was used as a target for stimulation. However, as no TMS can be performed to transiently suppress these targets, supraselective injection of amytal was performed in the anterior choroidal artery, demonstrating a transient (10 minutes) improvement in the pure tone component of the tinnitus using a technique previously described (DeRidder et al 2006). The patient experienced a transient tinnitus reduction of 30% by ipsilateral amytal injection, and by 60% on contralateral amytal injection. After contralateral injection, he also described a heavenly feeling and a disinterest in his tinnitus. A wire electrode was inserted via a posterior parietal entry under fMRI guided stereotactic conditions and inserted till the BOLD activated area in the amygdala was reached. The day after the surgery, the electrode was activated. During the first week, the tinnitus remained unchanged, but it was not perceived as annoying anymore. During the second week, its intensity decreased, but recurred in the third postoperative week, and could no longer be quelled even by intensive reprogramming. A placebo effect could not be excluded, since a blinded test had not yet been performed. On the other hand, habituation might explain the loss of effect, as also seen after auditory cortex stimulation in the Friedland et al (2007)'s study. A wire electrode limits the programming strategies, which are essential for long-lasting therapeutic success. A theoretically better option would be to insert a paddle electrode with many contacts (8 or 16) subdurally via a subtemporal approach, at the inferior part of the medial temporal lobe, covering the amygdaloparahippocampal area, thus turning deep brain stimulation into cortical stimulation (Fig.5).

15.2 Methodological Aspects

15.2.1 Non-invasive Stimulation as a Prognostic Test for Surgical Neuromodulation

TMS has been used for screening patients who might benefit from chronically implanted electrodes. However, available data question this approach. It was found that TMS is not a good predictor for deciding who is going to benefit from an implant (DeRidder et al 2011). Only patients who responded twice in a placebo controlled fashion to TMS on two separate days were implanted, but only a subgroup responded to the implant. However, TMS has some prognostic value if the patient is a responder to the implant, as a small but significant correlation was found between the amount of tinnitus suppression obtained by TMS and the amount obtained by the implant ($r = .38, p < .05$).

15.2.2 Neurostimulation Designs: burst & tonic

The stimulation design (burst versus tonic stimulation) significantly influences outcome. Tonic stimulation is not capable of suppressing noise-like tinnitus, but only pure tone tinnitus (DeRidder et al 2007, 2010). However, based on data from burst TMS (DeRidder et al 2007, 2010), changing the electrical stimulation design to burst stimulation benefited patients presenting with noise-like tinnitus (DeRidder et al 2007, 2009, 2010). Furthermore, if a patient presented with both a pure tone and a noise-like component, both components had to be relieved to yield a substantial decrease in tinnitus-related distress (DeRidder et al 2009, Langguth et al 2009): only suppressing the pure tone component, even if completely, did not benefit the patients. Indeed, burst stimulation allays almost half (13/27 or 48%) of initially unresponsive patients to tonic stimulation. Furthermore, 50% of patients who respond to tonic stimulation benefit more from burst than tonic stimulation: tinnitus suppression was 24% with tonic, versus 53% with burst stimulation. In sum, adding burst stimulation switches the outcome from poor response to an acceptable, even though far from ideal, suppression rate. A total of 2 out of 3 (29/43 or 67%) participants responded to stimulation via the implanted electrodes with an average tinnitus reduction of 53% (DeRidder et al 2011). Some participants in the study only responded to tonic stimulation. This subgroup of patients has a 52% suppression effect. So both burst and tonic stimulation have the same amount of suppression in individual patients, yet more patients benefit from burst stimulation than from tonic stimulation. Thus the question arises when to apply burst or tonic stimulation. Tinnitus duration, age, and gender were not predictive, whereas the tinnitus character was, i.e. noise-like tinnitus responds better to burst stimulation, pure tones respond equally well to burst and tonic stimulation, confirming our previously published data (DeRidder et al 2009). A previous burst TMS study demonstrated that women seem to respond better to burst TMS than men (DeRidder et al 2007), but this seems not to hold for ICS. Also, pure tone tinnitus was suppressed to a greater extent (70% tinnitus reduction) than noise-like tinnitus (40 % reduction). The worst results (only 29% reduction) were obtained in individuals who had a combination of pure tone and noise-like tinnitus.

15.3 Complications

Side effects are limited and do not occur at stimulation parameters required for tinnitus suppression. Side effects may occur when high frequency, high intensity stimulation is used. Different kinds of side effects have occurred during parameters search: a feeling of intoxication, altered spatial localization of external sounds, difficulty finding appropriate words, dizziness, vertigo and hearing perception changes (hearing perceived as being clearer - related to even their own voice), as well as out of body experiences (DeRidder et al 2009, Langguth and DeRidder 2013). Some patients with tinnitus have an associated feeling of aural pressure, the feeling as if there is water inside the ear. In all patients with successful tinnitus suppression, these associated pressure feelings decreased, however the stimulation design that best suppressed tinnitus and best suppressed pressure feelings were not always identical. Complications specific for the extradural implantation of electrodes overlying the auditory cortex are limited. Epileptic seizures occurred in 3 of the 43 patients (DeRidder et al 2011). In two patients, the fits occurred while patients were still having an external stimulator, possibly due to prolonged stimulation without enough OFF intervals: the patients are now only using programmable IPGs during the period of externalized stimulation. In a third patient, the epileptic seizure occurred during in-hospital programming. Patients with a history of epilepsy are thus best excluded from this procedure. Two major complications occurred with intradural implants. One of the 4 patients who was implanted with the electrode directly on the surface of the primary auditory cortex (DeRidder et al 2009) developed a postoperative intracranial bleeding in the superior temporal sulcus, at a distance from the Sylvian fissure, in which the electrode was inserted, with speech disturbances as a result. Moreover, the tinnitus decreased as a result of the bleeding. Another developed an intracranial abscess that required surgical evacuation, with removal of the electrode, with good outcome but worsening of the tinnitus. Thus, *this treatment should be preferentially performed extradurally, as with the extradural technique in the last 30 patients no serious complications were encountered.*

15.4 Failures

In responders vs non-responders, differences were demonstrated not in the auditory cortex, but in left and right parahippocampal areas for gamma frequency band, and in the left amygdala-hippocampal-parahippocampal area extending into the left insula for beta3 band. However, the electrodes were implanted extradurally overlying the secondary auditory cortex. Therefore we analyzed the functional connectivity between auditory cortex and hippocampal/parahippocampal area and established a difference in the functional connectivity with increased lag-phase synchronization for the delta, theta2, beta2 for responders between the auditory cortex and the hippocampus, but especially the beta3 band between the auditory cortex and parahippocampal area (De Ridder, under revision). This suggests that the mechanism of action is not via suppression of increased synchronized gamma band activity in the auditory cortex, which is hypothesized to be the final common pathway for tinnitus, but via an indirect modulation of high frequency activity (beta3 and gamma) in the parahippocampus.

Only patients who have good functional connectivity between the stimulated auditory cortex and the parahippocampal area benefit from the stimulation. Thus, combined activity (beta3 and gamma in parahippocampus) and functional connectivity (beta3 between auditory cortex and parahippocampus) measurements could be investigated in the future as response predictors to an auditory cortex implant.

15.5 Conclusion

How can results be improved?

1. Tinnitus-related plasticity changes in the inferior colliculus are mediated by BDNF (brain-derived neurotrophic factor) (Tan et al 2007). At the same time, the same Val66Met polymorphism in the BDNF gene determines whether one responds to TMS or tDCS (Cheeran et al 2008). Thus it could be of interest in the future to determine BDNF polymorphisms in patients and correlate them to the response rate to ICS.
2. Future targets to assess on the basis of neuroimaging evidence include the PCC and ACC. The ACC is involved in the salience attached to the tinnitus as well as the distress. Whereas the dorsal ACC is activated in distress in general, the subgenual ACC is related to the amount of tinnitus distress, and indirectly related to the loudness perception, via a putative noise-canceling mechanism. This noise canceling mechanism could involve the pregenual ACC, analogous to what has been described for pain: depending on the clinical picture, the sgACC, dACC or pregenual ACC could then be targeted. The PCC acts as a switch between memory encoding and memory retrieval and co-processes tinnitus-related distress. The effective connectivity from the PCC to the auditory cortex might thereby also influence the perceived loudness indirectly.
3. Burst stimulation consisting of closely spaced high frequency (500 Hz) spikes (n=5) delivered 40 times a second (40 Hz burst mode) can better suppress noise-like tinnitus than currently used tonic stimulation and can further improve the amount of tinnitus loudness suppression (DeRidder et al 2010). This bursting can lead to rerouting and multiplexing, resulting in activation of functionally connected networks, with attendant clinical benefit. Coordinated reset stimulation and pink and brown noise stimulation are other stimulation protocols worth pursuing: pink noise, for instance, mimics the frequency spectrum of normal physiological ongoing resting state activity at the level of the cortex (De Ridder, unpublished results).
4. For tinnitus too (see Chapter 17), the future rests with closed-loop stimulation. A tinnitus detector has recently been developed (Hiseni et al 2009). In tinnitus, the predominant alpha activity is replaced by theta and beta/gamma activity and the real-time detection of this electrophysiological signature in the individual brain can be exploited to stimulate only when this becomes chronic.

References

General Reviews

DeRidder D, Langguth B, Plazier M, et al. Auditory cortex stimulation for intractable tinnitus. In: Canavero S (ed) Textbook of therapeutic cortical stimulation. New York: Nova Sci.,2009, 353-361
Langguth B, DeRidder R, Eichhammer P, Hajak G. TMS for refractory tinnitus. In: Canavero S (ed) Textbook of therapeutic cortical stimulation. New York: Nova Sci., 2009, 337-352
Langguth, B., et al., Tinnitus: causes and clinical management. Lancet Neurol, 2013; 12: 920-30.
Langguth, B. and D. De Ridder, Tinnitus: therapeutic use of superficial brain stimulation. Handb Clin Neurol, 2013. 116: p. 441-67.
Moller A et al (eds) Textbook of Tinnitus. New York: Springer, 2011; 753-762.24.

Specific Studies

Beard, A.W., Results of leucotomy operations for tinnitus. J Psychosom Res, 1965. 9(1): p. 29-32
Cheeran, B., et al., A common polymorphism in the brain-derived neurotrophic factor gene (BDNF) modulates human cortical plasticity and the response to rTMS. J Physiol, 2008. 586(Pt 23): p. 5717-25.
De Ridder, D., S. Vanneste, and M. Congedo, The distressed brain: a group blind source separation analysis on tinnitus. PLoS One, 2011b. 6(10): p. e24273.
De Ridder, D., et al., Transcranial magnetic stimulation and extradural electrodes implanted on secondary auditory cortex for tinnitus suppression. J Neurosurg, 2011. 114(4): p. 903-11 (also 912-921 for part B)
De Ridder, D., et al., Dorsolateral Prefrontal Cortex Transcranial Magnetic Stimulation and Electrode Implant for Intractable Tinnitus. World Neurosurg, 2011.
De Ridder, D., et al., Remote tentorium meningioma causing sudden sensorineural deafness. Surg Neurol, 2008. 70(3): p. 312-7; discussion 318.
De Ridder, D., et al., Amygdalohippocampal involvement in tinnitus and auditory memory. Acta Otolaryngol Suppl, 2006(556): p. 50-3.
De Ridder, D., et al., Do tonic and burst TMS modulate the lemniscal and extralemniscal system differentially? Int J Med Sci, 2007. 4(5): p. 242-6.
De Ridder, D., et al., Theta, alpha and beta burst transcranial magnetic stimulation: brain modulation in tinnitus. Int J Med Sci, 2007. 4(5): p. 237-41.
De Ridder, D., et al., Burst stimulation of the auditory cortex: a new form of neurostimulation for noise-like tinnitus suppression. J Neurosurg, 2010. 112(6): p. 1289-94.
De Ridder D, Song JJ, Vanneste S. Frontal cortex TMS for tinnitus. Brain Stimul. 2013 May;6(3):355-62.
Diederen, K.M., et al., Deactivation of the Parahippocampal Gyrus Preceding Auditory Hallucinations in Schizophrenia. Am J Psychiatry, 2010. 167(4): p. 427-35.
Elithorn, A., Prefrontal leucotomy in the treatment of tinnitus. Proc R Soc Med, 1953. 46(10): p. 832-3.
Faber, M., et al., Top down prefrontal affective modulation of tinnitus with multiple sessions of tDCS of dorsolateral prefrontal cortex. Brain Stimul, 2011.
Friedland, D.R., et al., Feasibility of Auditory Cortical Stimulation for the Treatment of Tinnitus. Otol Neurotol, 2007. 28(8): p. 1005-1012.
Hiseni, S., et al., A Nano Power CMOS Tinnitus Detector for a Fully Implantable Closed-Loop Neurodevice. IEEE xplore, 2011. Conference Proceedings, BIOCAS 2009: p. 33-36.
Husain, F.T. and S.A. Schmidt, Using resting state functional connectivity to unravel networks of tinnitus. Hear Res, 2014. 307: p. 153-62.
Joos, K., S. Vanneste, and D. De Ridder, Disentangling depression and distress networks in the tinnitus brain. PLoS One, 2012. 7(7): p. e40544.

Landgrebe, M., et al., Structural brain changes in tinnitus: grey matter decrease in auditory and non-auditory brain areas. Neuroimage, 2009. 46(1): p. 213-8.

Langguth, B., et al., Neuroimaging and neuromodulation: complementary approaches for identifying the neuronal correlates of tinnitus. Front Syst Neurosci, 2012. 6: p. 15.

Langguth, B., et al., The impact of auditory cortex activity on characterizing and treating patients with chronic tinnitus--first results from a PET study. Acta Otolaryngol Suppl, 2006(556): p. 84-8.

Litre, C.F., et al., [Feasibility of auditory cortical stimulation for the treatment of tinnitus. Three case reports]. Neurochirurgie, 2010. 56(4): p. 303-8.

Litre, C.F., et al., Surgical treatment by electrical stimulation of the auditory cortex for intractable tinnitus. Brain Stimul, 2009. 2(3): p. 132-7.

Maudoux, A., et al., Auditory resting-state network connectivity in tinnitus: a functional MRI study. PLoS One, 2012. 7(5): p. e36222.

Mennemeier, M., et al., Variable changes in PET activity before and after rTMS treatment for tinnitus. Laryngoscope, 2011. 121(4): p. 815-22

Ramirez, R.R., et al., Neuromagnetic source imaging of abnormal spontaneous activity in tinnitus patient modulated by electrical cortical stimulation. Conf Proc IEEE Eng Med Biol Soc, 2009. 1: p. 1940-4.

Schlee, W., et al., Mapping cortical hubs in tinnitus. BMC Biol, 2009. 7: p. 80.

Silchenko, A.N., et al., Impact of acoustic coordinated reset neuromodulation on effective connectivity in a neural network of phantom sound. Neuroimage, 2013. 77: p. 133-47.

Seidman, M.D., et al., Direct electrical stimulation of Heschl's gyrus for tinnitus treatment. Laryngoscope, 2008. 118(3): p. 491-500

Song JJ, Vanneste S, Van de Heyning P, De Ridder D. Transcranial direct current stimulation in tinnitus patients: a systemic review and meta-analysis. Scientific World Journal. 2012;2012:427941.

Tan, J., et al., Tinnitus behavior and hearing function correlate with the reciprocal expression patterns of BDNF and Arg3.1/arc in auditory neurons following acoustic trauma. Neuroscience, 2007. 145(2): p. 715-26

Van der Loo, E., et al., Tinnitus intensity dependent gamma oscillations of the contralateral auditory cortex. PLoS ONE, 2009. 4(10): p. e7396.

Vanneste, S. and D. De Ridder, Differences between a single session and repeated sessions of 1 Hz TMS by double-cone coil prefrontal stimulation for the improvement of tinnitus. Brain Stimul 2013 Mar;6(2):155-9.

Vanneste, S., et al., Bilateral dorsolateral prefrontal cortex modulation for tinnitus by transcranial direct current stimulation: a preliminary clinical study. Exp Brain Res, 2010. 202(4): p. 779-85.

Vanneste, S. and D. De Ridder, Bifrontal transcranial direct current stimulation modulates tinnitus intensity and tinnitus-distress-related brain activity. Eur J Neurosci, 2011. 34(4): p. 605-14.

Vanneste, S., P. van de Heyning, and D. De Ridder, The neural network of phantom sound changes over time: a comparison between recent-onset and chronic tinnitus patients. Eur J Neurosci, 2011. 34(5): p. 718-31.

Vanneste, S. and D. De Ridder, The auditory and non-auditory brain areas involved in tinnitus. An emergent property of multiple parallel overlapping subnetworks. Front Syst Neurosci, 2012. 6: p. 31.

Vanneste, S., et al., Different resting state brain activity and functional connectivity in patients who respond and not respond to bifrontal tDCS for tinnitus suppression. Exp Brain Res, 2011. 210(2): p. 217-27.

Vanneste S, Congedo M, De Ridder D. Pinpointing a Highly Specific Pathological Functional Connection That Turns Phantom Sound into Distress.Cereb Cortex. 2013 Apr 30.

Vanneste S, De Ridder D. Noninvasive and invasive neuromodulation for the treatment of tinnitus: an overview. Neuromodulation. 2012 Jul;15(4):350-60.

Sergio Canavero

16 Epilepsy

Epilepsy is the third most common neurological disorder and has a prevalence of 0.5–1% worldwide. Current antiepileptic regimens are unable to provide adequate seizure control for 20–40% of patients—who are consequently labeled medically refractory. Surgical resection of a specific epileptogenic focus is capable of treating only about 60% of patients with medically refractory epilepsy. Current nonablative applications for the treatment of medically intractable epilepsy include vagus nerve stimulation (VNS), trigeminal nerve stimulation (TNS), deep brain stimulation (DBS), and more recently closed-loop stimulation systems (Rolston et al 2012, Wu and Sharan 2013). Here, I review cortical stimulation for the control of medically refractory epilepsy.

16.1 Open-Loop Cortical Stimulation

The epileptogenic zone is the minimum amount of cortex that must be resected (inactivated or completely disconnected) to achieve seizure freedom. Five "zones" have been described as those most essential to identify during pre-surgical evaluation: 1) irritative zone – the area from which spontaneous interictal spikes originate, 2) seizure onset zone – the area from which spontaneous seizures arise, 3) symptomatogenic zone – the area from which seizure symptoms and/or signs may be elicited via stimulation, 4) epileptogenic lesion – an area which is either grossly damaged (due to cortical dysplasia or tumor, for example) or is secondarily excitable due to nearby lesioned tissue, and 5) function deficit zone – an area of cortex that functions abnormally interictally. The extent of the epileptogenic zone may or may not coincide with the zone of ictal onset; in most cases, the epileptogenic zone is larger than that of the ictal onset. Furthermore, the epileptogenic zone is often dynamic, as it has been observed to migrate over the course of a patient's disease process, and in other cases remain static. Accordingly, a static epileptogenic zone will be easier to control via focal cortical stimulation. In deciding the goal for therapeutic electrical stimulation of the cortex, the main consideration is to determine what facet of the epileptic network is to be affected by stimulation. In addition, the dynamic nature of epileptogenic zones should be kept in mind as the primary area for seizure control may migrate over the course of the patient's disease progress. Finally, contacts should be less than 2 cm apart for effective epileptic control (Gwinn et al 2008). In light of these considerations, cortical stimulation (CS) becomes an option in select cases. Noninvasive CS (rTMS, tDCS) has evinced mixed results (Nitsche and Paulus 2009), while there is only one report in the literature of open-loop ICS (i.e. stimulation delivered regardless of neuronal activity) (Elisevich et al 2006). These authors implanted a strip electrode

(Resume quadripolar lead) subdurally along the axis of the dorsolateral convexity of the precentral gyrus (M1) in a man with intractable postencephalitic epilepsy with ictal onset in MI. For the five years of follow-up, cortical stimulation (2.1 mA, PW 450 µs, 50 Hz, ON 3 min/OFF10 min), with minimal alterations, successfully eliminated the jacksonian march and secondary generalization and reduced seizure frequency and intensity, with an immediate postictal return of motor function. Over time, the seizure frequency subsided by more than 90%, without adverse effects. Modeling of temporal lobe epileptogenicity suggests that a small redistribution of cerebral blood flow from non-epileptic to epileptic cortex should produce substantial reduction in temporal lobe seizure frequency in association with prolongation of inter-hemispheric prolongation time (Weinand 2000). Blood flow perturbations can be easily achieved with cortical stimulation and as such may put this theory to test.

16.2 Closed-Loop Responsive Cortical Stimulation

A closed-loop system administers stimulation only if triggered by early seizure activity. The lower doses of stimulation provided by such devices not only reduce power consumption, but also minimize the adverse reactions created by continuous stimulation, including the possibility of habituation to long-term stimulation. At the end of 2013, the first closed-loop system for the treatment of medically intractable partial epilepsy (Responsive NeuroStimulator, NeuroPace, Inc, MountainView, CA, USA) received a pre-market approval by the FDA, the target of stimulation depending on each patient's seizure focus or foci. This system is based both on progress in automated seizure detection over the past 40 years, epitomized by the International Workshop On Seizure Prediction (e.g. Jouny et al 2011) – a progress that is still ongoing in search of an ideal system- and Penfield and Jasper (1954)'s observation that in awake patients, in some cases, acute focal electrical stimulation of the exposed cortex resulted in a flattening of the local electrocortico-graphy (both normal rhythms and spontaneous epileptiform discharges) (Box 16.1). Further human trials used electrical stimulation to abort seizures by means of subdural electrodes placed for the purpose of localizing the epileptic focus for surgical excision; the clinical outcome pursued was a decrease in number of after-discharges (AD) or an increase in AD threshold (see detailed review in Mogul et al 2009).

Pulse Generator (IPG). The IPG is a hermetically-sealed neurostimulator containing electronics, battery, telemetry coil, and connector hardware that accommodates one or two 4-contact electrodes. The IPG continuously analyzes the patient's electrocorticogram (EcoG) and triggers electrical stimulation when it detects specific ECoG characteristics programmed by the clinician as indicative of interictal or ictal epileptiform activity. The IPG then stores diagnostic information that details detections and stimulations, including multichannel stored ECoGs. The IPG has the following dimensions: 41 mm wide, 60 mm long and 7 mm thick (weight 19.5 g, volume 10.5 cm3). The IPG is curved in shape to facilitate cranial implantation. It is positioned extradurally in a tailored cranial defect and held in place with a ferrule (Fig. 16.1: craniectomy with the implanted ferrule; Fig. 16.1b: IPG in place).
Electrodes. Depth electrodes are quadripolar and designed for stereotactic implantation. They are available with 3.5mm and 10mm intercontact spacings, with lengths of 30 cm and 44 cm. The individual contacts are 1.1 mm in diameter and 2.3 mm in length. Subdural strip electrodes are quadripolar with 4 mm diameter circular electrodes and intercontact spacings of 10 mm. They are available in 15 cm and 25 cm lengths. All electrodes are composed of platinum (90%) and iridium (10%).
Programmer - The programmer is a laptop computer with specialized software and a telemetry wand that communicates with the IPG. The programmer downloads diagnostic and ECoG data from the IPG. In addition, the programmer has an electrophysiology test stimulation mode, which allows real-time stimulation with simultaneous ECoG viewing.

Box 16.1: NeuroPace™ System Components

The NEUROPACE ™ system (Smith et al 2009) is capable of performing real-time seizure detection and delivering responsive electrical stimulation. The implantable components of the system include a cranially implanted neurostimulator and intracranial depth and strip leads. The neurostimulator is a battery-powered, microprocessor-controlled device that continuously monitors electrographic activity from the cortical depth and strip leads and delivers programmable electrical stimulation in response to detected events to two distinct epileptogenic zones independently. Due to techonological constraints, the sensed electrographic data are not continuously recorded; however, the neurostimulator can store segments of the electrographic data for review by the physician. The neurostimulator system has a 32-minute ECoG memory buffer. The number of ECoGs stored depends on the number of recording channels and the recording time selected. Typically, 2 bipolar recording channels are selected with a 60-second pretrigger and 30-second posttrigger duration, which allows 9 ECoGs to be stored. Any additional ECoGs overwrite the previous recordings. ECOG storage can be triggered by any of several electrographic events, including seizure onset. An important feature is the use of a personalized 'training period', in which the device is individually tuned to the patient after it has recorded seizures.

The RNS neurostimulator is designed to match typical skull thickness and curvature, and is intended for implant in a ferrule, or socket, placed in a craniectomy (Box 16.2). Up to two leads, each containing four electrodes, can be connected to the neurostimulator; each may be a depth lead or cortical (subdural) strip lead, and each has four electrode contacts, which are used for sensing and providing stimulation. To provide early seizure detection and delivery of focal electrical stimulation, leads are positioned as close as possible to the seizure focus or foci. The external components of the system include a physician programmer, a patient data transmitter and a telemetry wand. The programmer is used by the physician to program detection and stimulation settings and retrieve stored information (e.g., electrographic activity) from the neurostimulator. The data transmitter is provided to the patient to allow uploading and remote monitoring of the device between clinic visits. The telemetry wand allows wireless communication between the neurostimulator and the programmer (or data transmitter). The device data and electrographic data are uploaded via the Internet to a central patient data management system and may be reviewed by physicians using a secure Web browser.

Invasive monitoring is used in all cases to determine seizure focus localization and therefore, optimization of the location and type of closed loop electrodes used. For example, patients with a seizure focus in the left lateral temporal neocortex would receive two 1x4 subdural electrodes. If the seizure focus were left hippocampal in a patient in whom Wada memory testing revealed absence of contralateral memory support, a 1x4 hippocampal depth electrode and an ipsilateral anterior subtemporal 1x4 subdural electrode would be implanted. In general, the type and location of electrode implantation will be tailored to the individual patient. Implantation site for the IPG will be determined by the implantation site of the two electrodes. If depth electrodes alone are used, a large skin flap will be needed to expose enough skull to incorporate the IPG and its ferrule as well as the two 14 mm diameter burr holes and their burr hole rings and covers. If there was a previous craniotomy performed for invasive monitoring, this area may be re-exposed for implantation of both the subdural electrodes and the IPG and ferrule (Fig. 16.2). If a hippocampal depth electrode is implanted through an occipital entry in a case requiring repeat temporal craniotomy or repeat burr hole for implantation of a subdural electrode, then the tail of the depth electrode will need to be tunneled into the area of cranial exposure. Passing the tail of the depth electrode through the appropriate length of silastic tubing provided in the depth electrode kit will protect the electrode tail when the old or new craniotomy incision is subsequently made for subdural strip electrode and IPG placement. The patient is appropriately positioned on the operating table by attaching the base-ring to a Mayfield holder. The craniotomy incision is marked off and the surgical area is prepped and draped in a standard sterile fashion. The previously marked-off incision is infiltrated with local anesthetic and a horseshoe-shaped craniotomy flap is turned. A sterile ferrule template is provided than can be onlayed over the exposed skull to find an area where the convex contour of the template best fits that of the skull (diminishing the potential risk of bone erosion). Monopolar cutting current is used to mark off this rectangular area. A single burr hole is placed at either end of the rectangle and a Penfield 3 dissector is used to separate the dura from the skull prior to using the craniotome to cut out the rectangle of bone. A full thickness craniectomy is preferred in order to minimize protrusion of the IPG. Note that one burr hole of the craniectomy should be off center to accommodate the fixation tab that secures the IPG in the ferrule (Fig. 16.1a-b). Depth electrodes are placed using a frame-based stereotaxic system and depth electrode implant planning with a commercially available computer workstation. Frame application is carried out using IV sedation consisting of Alfentanyl and Propofol. A field block of the scalp is performed using approximately 40 cc of a 1:1 mixture of 0.25% Marcaine and 0.5% Lidocaine. Carbon fiber posts and aluminum pins are used to limit metal artifacts on the CT scan, which follows the MRI study. A contrast-enhanced, T-1 weighted, volume acquisition MRI is performed consisting of 1.3 mm axial slices with 0 mm slice gap.

Box 16.2: Technique of implantation (From Smith et al 2009)

The MRI is followed with non-contrasted axial CT with 3 mm axial slices and 0 mm slice gap. The images are transferred over the local area network to the computer workstation which is used to perform image fusion of the MRI study to the CT study. After depth electrode trajectories are generated, a probe view algorithm is used to assess (1) the proximity of any cortical vessels to the depth electrode entry and (2) the proximity of the trajectory to the ventricular system or any subependymal veins. Any appropriate adjustments to trajectories are made before actual implantation. The stereotactic arc system is attached to the base ring and a drill guide tube is then advanced through the incision down to the skull and antibiotic irrigation is flushed through the tube. The appropriate burr hole is outlined on the skull and a high-speed air-driven drill is used. The underlying dura is opened in a linear fashion in order to facilitate subsequent passage of the guide block. At this point, a 2.1 mm inner-diameter guide block is introduced and the dura and pia are cauterized with a monopolar electrode. The diameter of the burr hole must exactly match the diameter of the securing device for the implanted depth lead. Next a 14-gauge depth electrode cannula is passed through the same guide block to the target point. Intraoperative fluoroscopy verifies proper placement. The cannula and guide tube are then withdrawn. A cranial base and cap device are then implanted into the burr hole and secured by using the two self-tapping screws provided. The surgeon must align the exit groove on the base in the posterolateral direction, in the same direction that the subcutaneous portion of the lead would later be directed. An insertion tool is then passed through a large diameter guide block and inserted into the slot and the securing device. The insertion tool and guide block are then removed. The depth lead is then carefully inserted into the target point. After fluoroscopy confirmation, the stylet of the lead is removed and the distal shaft of the implanted lead is secured into the securing device. Postimplant intraoperative fluoroscopy is performed after locking the depth electrodes in place in order to assure proper positioning. If the subdural strip lead is to be placed, the dura is opened linearly and the appropriate cortical lead is inserted through the dural opening under fluoroscopy. The distal shaft of the implanted lead is safely attached to the securing device. At this point, the provided ferrule is placed on the exposed bone and the desired bony defect is outlined. The outlined bone is drilled out by high-speed air-driven drill, bony edges are smoothened, irrigated and waxed. The provided ferrule is then implanted and secured to the adjacent bone at four points with the provided self-tapping mini-screws. The IPG is connected to the distal end of the already implanted lead or leads and then is safely secured in the implanted ferrule. *To summarize*, burr holes for depth electrodes are made with a 14 mm diameter bit so that the manufacturer supplied burr hole rings, which are secured with self-tapping screws, will exactly fit. Subdural electrodes are secured with purse string 4-0 silk suture at the dural incision exit site. If the depth electrode implant is bilateral, the entire procedure is done with the patient in the stereotaxic frame using local anesthesia and i.v. Propofol and Alfentanyl. If the implant is unilateral, the tail of the depth electrode is tunneled to the planned craniotomy site, the burr hole incision is closed, and the frame removed. The area of the subsequent craniotomy incision will determine the area of skull to be clipped (avoid razors to minimize skin microtrauma and possible infection). The patient is intubated and ventilated, but the procedure may also be carried out under neuroleptoanalgesia along with field blocks of the scalp. Control of blood pressure minimizes potential intraoperative hemorrhage. The operative blood loss is generally minimal (<100 ml). At the end of the procedure, all components of the RNS neurostimulator system are connected, the skin flap is positioned for closure, and a telemetry wand (covered with a sterile camera drape) is placed over the IPG so that recording of electrode contact impedances as well as intraoperative electrocorticography (ECoG) can be performed. If impedances and ECoG recordings are satisfactory, skin closure is completed. The surgical wound is irrigated with an antibiotic solution and then closed in anatomical layers and the wound is covered with a sterile dressing. Perioperative i.v. antibiotic therapy is begun the morning of the procedure and continued 24 hours post-operatively. On the third postoperative day, the first interrogation-detection session is performed.

continued **Box 16.2**: Technique of implantation (From Smith et al 2009)

a b

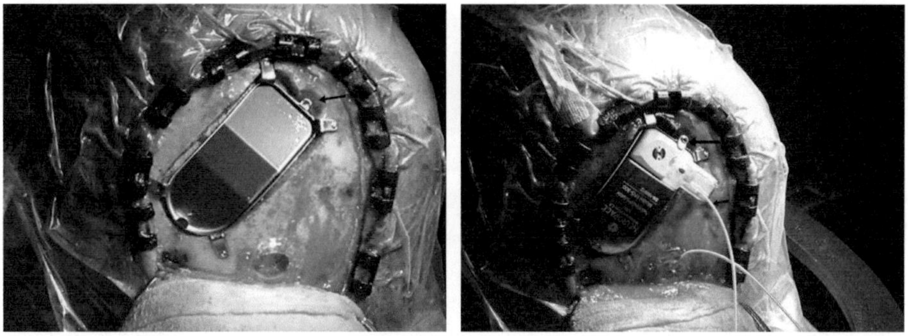

Fig. 16.1: **a** Rectangular craniectomy with implanted ferrule. Arrow points to the burr hole which will accommodate the fixation tab used to secure the IPG in the ferrule **b.** Ferrule secured in position with self tapping screws in the four tangs at the corners of the ferrule. Note the fixation tab (arrow) which is accommodated by the burr hole. Note single depth electrode (short arrow) inserted in connector port.

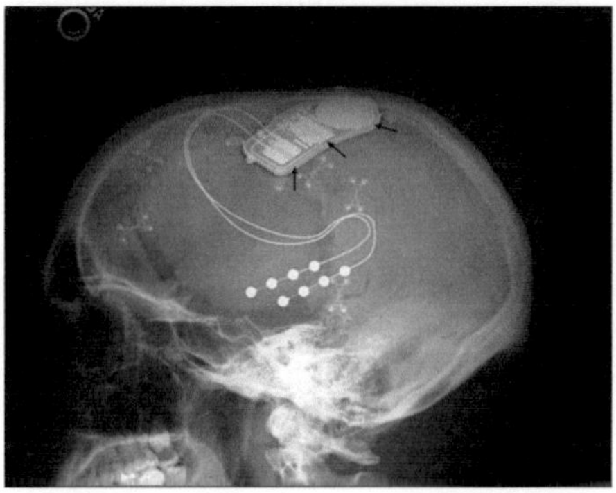

Fig. 16.2: Example of RNS with 2 4-contact subdural strip electrodes implanted over the left superior and middle temporal gyri. The three arrows (left to right) point to the connector port, microchip, and battery of the IPG.

Electrographic data storage can be triggered by detection, responsive stimulation, scheduled time of day, magnet (used by the patient to indicate a clinical event), or other events as programmed by the physician. These data allow physicians to assess detection sensitivity and effects of stimulation. The detection algorithms implemented in the RNS system are designed to be computationally efficient and are highly optimized to perform real-time seizure detection within the constraints of currently available implantable technology, such as limited power and processing capabilities. Three detection tools are provided: *area, line-length, and half-wave.* The detection tools are highly configurable and can be adjusted by the physician to optimize the sensitivity and specificity trade-off for each individual patient. Up to two independent detectors can be programmed for any two sensing channels.

The neurostimulator delivers current-controlled, charge-balanced biphasic pulses; it can be programmed by the physician to deliver stimulation frequencies ranging from 1 to 333 Hz, current amplitudes from 1 to 12 mA, and pulse-widths from 40 to 1000 μs. Any of the electrode contacts or the pulse generator housing may be programmed as anode or cathode. The stimulation montage can be configured to deliver current between any combination of electrodes and the neurostimulator case. Up to five individually configured sequential therapies of electrical stimulation may be programmed, where each therapy is composed of two independently configurable bursts. The RNS will attempt to redetect the epileptiform activity after each therapy is delivered. If the epileptiform activity is still detected, the next (sequential) therapy will be delivered. If the epileptiform activity is no longer detected, the remaining therapies will not be delivered and the episode ends. The therapy sequence will refresh with the detection of each new episode. Stimulation parameters are determined empirically, while respecting safety limits for charge density. The parameters of each therapy and each burst may be the same or varied. The RNS system has controls in place at the programmer and neurostimulator, so that current densities remain below a conservative limit of 25 μC/cm2 per phase. Furthermore, intermittent (more acute-like) stimulation may pose fewer risks to neural tissue than does continuous stimulation. The stimulation configuration is also determined empirically. Options include providing bipolar stimulation across electrode pairs or stimulating across all eight electrodes to the case of the neurostimulator. Whether stimulation is delivered to a few or many electrodes depends to some extent on the area of onset. Studies show that, unlike depth electrodes, the mean impedance of subdural strip electrodes increased over time to peak at 16-20 months and returned to baseline by 2 years (Wu et al 2013).

16.2.1 Patient Selection and Outcomes

Closed-loop stimulation is indicated for patients 18 or older with drug-resistant epilepsy who are not candidates for resective surgery. Although resection is preferred, closed-loop stimulation has also been offered to patients who decline traditional surgical options. It may be used to treat patients with bitemporal or multifocal epilepsy, but patients generally should not have more than two distinct epileptogenic foci. Because electrode implantation depends so heavily on accurate localization of seizure foci, closed-loop systems should only be implanted if the exact epileptogenic focus or foci are known, particularly if their seizures are not hippocampal in origin. This form of stimulation can also be more readily applied to eloquent brain without affecting neurologic function.

The RNS System Pivotal Clinical Investigation was a multicentered, randomized, double-blind sham stimulation controlled trial in which 191 patients were implanted across 31 institutions. This study included adult subjects 18–70 years of age with medically refractory epilepsy with an average of three or more seizures per 28 days. During the initial 12-week blinded evaluation period, an initial implantation effect was noted as the mean percentage of seizure reduction was reduced in both stimulation and sham groups: by 34.2% and 25.2%, respectively. It remains unclear if this initial effect can be attributed to the placebo effect, to anesthesia, or to some aspect of the surgical procedure itself. Over the course of the blinded period, this implantation effect was substantiated as the stimulation group continued to demonstrate seizure reduction by a mean of 41.5% at the end of the blinded period, while the sham group failed to maintain its effect, with a mean reduction of 9.4% at the end of this period. After two years, median seizure frequency was reduced by more than 50% with a responder rate of greater than 45% with stimulation. Longer term follow-up has demonstrated the sustainability of RNS, as the responder rate increases to 53% at three years after implantation. Follow-up on these 191 implanted patients presented class I evidence that closed-loop stimulation significantly reduced the frequency of disabling partial-onset seizures that were refractory not only to antieleptic drugs (AEDs), but also to VNS or resective surgeries (Morrell et al 2011). Also important are the significant improvements in overall quality of life as reported by patients receiving stimulation via the Quality of Life in Epilepsy Inventory (QOLIE-89). There was no deterioration in mood and neuropsychological function. Side effects included (among others, like implant site pain and headache) serious brain hemorrhage (2.1%) due to the implantation (no mortality, no morbidity) and infection (5.2%), but not of the brain or skull. Mortality was due in 4 cases to SUDEP (3 with implant running) and in other 2 to unrelated causes. Some patients implanted with the first generation of the system reported a transient buzzing sensation with the onset of stimulation. Fortunately, the source of this side effect was identified and there have been no such reports in patients implanted with later generations. The administration of stimulation directly to the suspected seizure focus also reduces the potential for adverse effects by sparing normal brain. In order to avoid damage to neurons from chronic stimulation, the conservative limit to the charge density is 25 $\mu C/cm^2$/phase—while it has been determined that densities of 50–60 $\mu C/cm^2$/phase can be safely delivered to human cortex for acute intermittent stimulation.

After the fifth post-implant month, all subjects received responsive stimulation in an open label period (OLP) to complete 2 years of post-implant follow-up. The percent change in seizures at the end of the blinded period was -37.9% in the active and -17.3% in the sham stimulation group ($p = 0.012$, Generalized Estimating Equations). The median percent reduction in seizures in the OLP was 44% at 1 year and 53% at 2 years, which represents a progressive and significant improvement with time ($p < 0.0001$). There were no adverse effects on neuropsychological function or mood (Heck et al 2014). Nevertheless, long-term experience beyond five years is currently very limited.

The side effects of intermittent chronic stimulation remain unclear, and it is uncertain whether or not deleterious kindling or other problematic effects will emerge.

References

Elisevich K, Jenrow K, Schuh L, Smith B. Long-term electrical stimulation-induced inhibition of partial epilepsy. Case report. J Neurosurg 2006; 105: 894-897

Gwinn RP, Spencer DD, Spencer SS, et al. Local spatial effect of 50Hz cortical stimulation in humans. Epilepsia 2008;49:1602-10.

Heck CN, King-Stephens D, Massey AD, et al. Two-year seizure reduction in adults with medically intractable partial onset epilepsy treated with responsive neurostimulation: Final results of the RNS System Pivotal trial. Epilepsia 2014; 55: 432-441

Jouny CC, Franaszczuk PJ, Bergey GK. Improving early seizure detection. Epilepsy & Behavior 2011; 22 (Suppl.1): S44-S48

Mogul DJ, Fine AS and Canavero S. Cortical stimulation for medically refractory epilepsy. In: Canavero S (ed) Textbook of therapeutic cortical stimulation. New York: Nova Sci. 2009, pp 309-318

Morrell MJ; RNS System in Epilepsy Study Group. Responsive cortical stimulation for the treatment of medically intractable partial epilepsy. Neurology. 2011;77:1295-304.

Nitsche MA, Paulus W. Noninvasive brain stimulation protocols in the treatment of epilepsy: current state and perspectives. Neurotherapeutics. 2009;6:244-50

Penfield W, Jasper H. Epilepsy and the Functional Anatomy of the Human Brain. 2nd ed. Little, Brown and Co, 1954.

Rolston JD, Englot DJ, Wang DD, et al. Comparison of seizure control outcomes and the safety of vagus nerve, thalamic deep brain, and responsive neurostimulation: evidence from randomized controlled trials.Neurosurg Focus. 2012;32:E14.

Smith J, Fountas K, Murro M, et al. Closed loop stimulation for control of focal epilepsy In: Canavero S (ed) Textbook of therapeutic cortical stimulation. New York: Nova Sci. 2009, pp 319-334

Weinand ME. Vascular steal model of human temporal lobe epileptogenicity: the relationship between electrocorticographic interhemispheric propagation time and cerebral blood flow.Med Hypotheses. 2000;54:717-20

Wu C, Evans JJ, Skidmore C, et al. Impedance variations over time for a closed-loop neurostimulation device: early experience with chronically implanted electrodes. Neuromodulation 2013: 16: 46-50

Anne Beuter

17 Closed-loop Cortical Stimulation

As illustrated in previous chapters, in open-loop cortical stimulation, parameter adjustment is a labor-intensive, trial-and-error process based on the clinical response to the last setting. Once programmed, parameters remain constant until the next follow-up visit. These limits are due in part to the absence of a feedback control system, insufficient knowledge of mechanisms of action of ICS as well as the absence of appropriate bioinspired algorithms to implement these mechanisms and guide parameter determination. This situation is slowly changing with the introduction of so-called closed-loop systems. Closed-loop brain stimulation banks on neural activities recorded in the nervous system and analyzed online to deliver appropriate electrical stimulation (Fig.17.1). Closed-loop DBS is currently being tested with cortical recording and deep stimulation (Activa® PC+S DBS http://newsroom.medtronic.com/phoenix.zhtml?c=251324&p=irol-newsArticle&id=1882373). Also, closed-loop stimulation is FDA-approved for refractory epilepsy (Chapter 16; see also Berenyi et al 2012). During the last decade, patents have been filed (e.g. Beuter and Modolo 2009) and companies have been created to design and produce the next generation of intelligent neurostimulators. Neural stimulation is the last to benefit: closed-loop control has been known and used in engineering for many decades now. In the brain, the loop can be closed at relay points located deep in the brain or superficially on the cortex (Beuter and Modolo, 2012). The rationale for closing the loop at the cortical level is that both the cortex and deep nuclei (basal ganglia, thalamus) are part and parcel of the same large-scale network of interconnected structures and this network can be entrained from any point, including indeed the easily accessible cortical mantle (Canavero, 2011).

Certainly, the cortex presents an especially challenging locale. Each cortical area contains an unknown number of networks of interconnected neurons, with a complex integration of multiple information streams originating from both hemispheres. However, due to anatomical fanning-out, the modulation of a given brain network requires a larger area of stimulation at the cortical level than at deeper sites, suggesting that less focal currents need to be delivered for cortical stimulation to obtain efficacy, without producing adverse effects (Canavero 2011). Propagating waves of electrical activity mediate specific information at specific rhythms in different cortical regions (Patten et al., 2012), e.g. propagation of beta oscillations conveys motor information from M1 in humans (Takahashi et al., 2011). The interaction of the current delivered during cortical stimulation with such propagating waves carrying physiological information between cortical regions should be avoided. This is achievable: Brittain et al (2013) showed that transcranial alternating current stimulation (tACS) delivered over M1 at pathologic tremor frequency and phase-locked to the tremor signal induces phase cancellation of the tremor rhythm. The optimal suppressive phase alignment produced 50% average reduction in resting tremor. Importantly, De Hemptinne et al (2013) observed that in patients with Parkinson's disease, the coupling between beta-phase and gamma-amplitude in M1 is exaggerated, and that this excessive coupling may be reduced by STN DBS. More specifically, peaks in gamma-amplitude in M1 are not only coupled but precede the beta-trough in the subthalamic nucleus, suggesting that M1 LFPs can be used as a control signal for automated programming of basal ganglia stimulators. Finally, the 3-D structure of the cortex with sulci and gyri results in a marked heterogeneity of neural fiber orientation, with the lowest activation threshold found at fiber endings or axonal bends, especially at the interface between the gray and white matter. This calls for neuroengineering modelization data to be integrated into the closed-loop neural analyzer (Chapters 19-20).

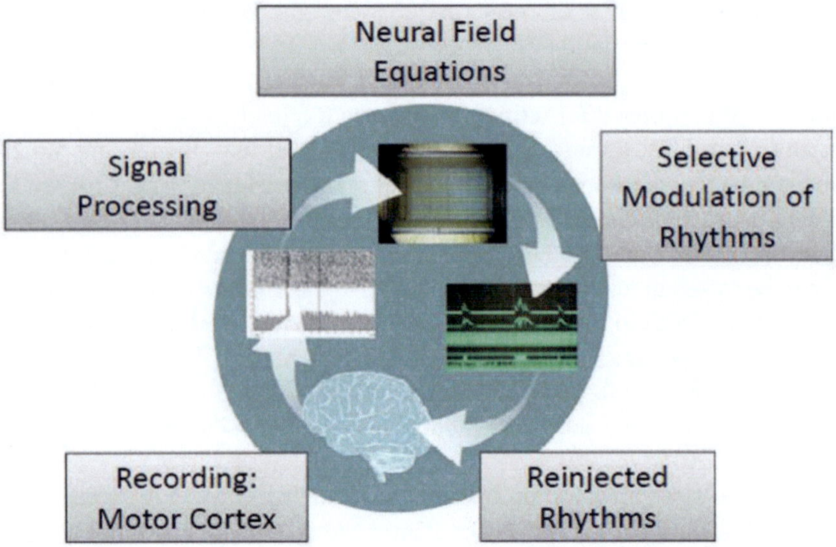

Fig. 17.1: a schematic view of the components of a closed-loop neurostimulation system.

17.1 Biomarkers

Closed-loop brain stimulation works on the assumption that a very small number of high-dimensional parameters or biomarkers can be monitored and used to parameterize the algorithm implemented in the device controller (Winslow et al 2012). There is agreement today that Local Field Potentials (LFP) recorded with macroelectrodes can be used as a suitable control variable / biomarker (Priori et al., 2013; Winestone et al., 2012 and Little et al., 2013). In Parkinson's disease, LFPs oscillate at various frequencies that are correlated with the cardinal signs of the disease such as tremor, rigidity, postural instabilities and akinesia. LFPs are robust, with reproducible time-domain, frequency-domain, linear and nonlinear features, and can be implemented on microchips (Priori et al., 2013); they can be monitored continuously during brain stimulation (Priori et al., 2005; Rossi et al., 2007, Rouse et al., 2011). The aim is to keep LFP parameters (e.g., global amplitude, spike or synchronized oscillation detection using high or low pass filtering, time-dependent spectral power in specific frequency bands) within a predetermined range, by automatically adjusting the stimulation parameters (frequency, amplitude, pulse width, cyclic or continuous stimulation, etc) to produce the desired effects, in a safe fashion and without interfering with propagating waves carrying physiological information (see above). Finally, LFP indices must correlate with the clinical (motor, cognitive, behavioral) state of the treated subjects. An appropriate battery of quantitative measures evaluating the evolution over time (weeks, months...) of the clinical symptoms must complement the classical clinical rating scales. In Parkinson's disease - for example- some LFP markers correlate with tremor, while others with bradykinesia, rigidity and even dyskinesias.

17.2 Bioinspired Modeling

Computational models of neuronal networks based on real neural circuits have become necessary tools to implement closed-loop brain stimulation (Feng et al., 2007; Schiff and Sauer, 2008; Schroll and Hamker, 2013). In the context of movement disorders, the cortical-basal ganglia-thalamo-cortical network has been addressed and modeled with a view to quell pathological activity (Rubin and Terman 2004, Pascual et al 2006, Modolo et al 2008, Modolo and Beuter, 2009ab, Modolo et al., 2009; Modolo et al., 2010abc, Modolo et al., 2012). In a multiscale biologically inspired model, Modolo et al. (2010b) proposed a method for selectively modulating cortical rhythms using a neural field approach. Continuous neural field theory provides a realistic representation of coarse-scale dynamics of cortical tissue in which non-local interactions occur with time delays and a variety of external inputs. The descriptive and, more importantly, the predictive value of neural field models have been extensively demonstrated. In this model, cortical tissue is considered as a two-dimensional continuous sheet of tissue (as opposed to a sheet of discrete elements, i.e., single neurons are densely packed), as justified by the high density of neurons in cortical tissue (Young et al., 2013); interconnected neural masses i.e., aggregates of neurons containing excitatory and inhibitory neurons, are considered as equivalent to cortical macrocolumns, and cortical tissue is described as synaptically-coupled cortical columns. Thus, a neural field is a continuous entity composed of neural masses with a connectivity function depending on the distance between two neural masses. Summation is performed over the neural field using delayed integro-differential neural field equations. Spike propagation delays and conduction speed of the fibers are taken under consideration. The general form of the function sums two exponential functions depending on the spatial range of the fibers and the strength of excitatory/inhibitory connections and gives rise to four possible connectivity patterns: local excitation, local inhibition, local excitation with lateral inhibition, and local inhibition with lateral excitation. Based on this model, the authors propose to use a two-dimensional electrode array both for cortical recording and stimulation, using a stimulation signal that is autoadaptive both in space and time. In this approach, the activity of artificial neural masses is linked with that of cortical columns, emulating cortical dynamics. The scale of the model (mesoscopic) is therefore compatible not only with the meaningful scale for information coding in M1, but also with the scale at which flat electrodes can provide stimulation to the tissue. Assumptions are made, such as considering that the connectivity function is identical in each spatial position (i.e., translationally invariant function). Also, the value of the neural field reflects the mean depolarization of cell membranes. Therefore it is assumed that all neurons in a given neural mass have a similar membrane potential. This model must be improved to include the contribution of axonal activation by electrical stimulation, and also to convert the calculated signal to a charge-balanced signal required in clinical practice to avoid brain tissue damage (see also Hess, 2013).

17.3 Underlying Physiological Control Mechanisms

As pointed out above, one direct consequence of our limited understanding of the mechanisms involved in brain stimulation is that it constrains our capacity to manipulate and control the system. One alternative comes from computational modeling (Winslow et al 2012). As a mechanism can be defined as an "*active structure that performs functions, produce regularities, underlie capacities or exhibit phenomena; doing so in virtue of the organized interaction among the mechanism's component parts, and the processes or activities these parts carry out*" (Kaplan, 2011, p 347-348), a model has explanatory power only insofar as it "maps out" aspects of the causal structure of that particular mechanism (so-called Model-Mechanism-Mapping, 3M). However, this 3M does not require a perfect correspondence or isomorphic mapping between model and mechanism, but rather it requires that some of the variables (at least one) correspond to some (at least one) identifiable component part and causal dependencies among components in the mechanism responsible for producing the target phenomenon. If this minimal degree of model-mechanism correspondence is obtained, it can be said that the model is endowed with explanatory power, and the injection of sufficient explanatory power in the model provides potentially exploitable information for manipulation and control, leading to individually tailored stimulation protocols. More to the point, the explanatory power of the Modolo et al. (2010b)'s model, although limited, comes from the fact that an artificial module mimics to some extent the behavior of the biological cortical tissue, as both are governed by similar "equations" (neural field on one side and cortical dynamics on the other side) and obey the same physical principles at a similar spatial scale. Global oscillations are modulated by a closed-loop stimulation signal triggered by, and calculated as a function of, the local mean membrane potential. Therefore, there is some correspondence between the model and the physiological system regarding the closed-loop stimulation current, i.e., the mean membrane potential, large-scale neuronal oscillations and the spatial scale at which these phenomena occur. The model predicts that to be efficient, the stimulation signal needs to be at the same frequency as the targeted pathological rhythm with a time delay dependent on neuroanatomical properties of cortical tissue. This model successfully predicts that a tremor reduction will occur with neuromodulation and recent work by Brittain et al. (2013) (see above) supports the prediction of the model (see also Nevado-Holgado et al., 2014 for new insights into the basal ganglia function).

17.4 Technological Issues

Closed-loop cortical stimulation has been advanced by recent hardware and software developments and by the emergence of novel tools to control neuronal activity with high precision in space and time. The convergence of mathematical modeling with neuro-engineering is likely to provide a new window of opportunity on disease and therapeutic mechanisms, which can be exploited for the design of next-generation "smart" neurostimulators. These devices need to be implementable in terms of size and external controllers. Various types of neuronal closed-loop controllers exist (Echauz et al 2009) including '*triggered open-loop controllers*' (such as responsive neurostimulation used to treat epilepsy) in which sensors are used to start and stop the stimulation, '*continuous feedback controllers*' using regular sensing to monitor the stimulation, '*adaptive controllers*' using feedback signals from sensors to continually adapt the stimulation parameters, and finally '*learning/intelligent controllers*'. The latter outperform all others in their ability to adjust automatically and intelligently the parameters of stimulation using fine-grained feedback (Echauz et al., 2009) and are suitable for implementation in cortical closed-loop systems.

A major issue has to do with the electrodes. Current electrodes used for cortical stimulation are not suitable for closed-loop control. Their number is too small, their size too large, and their spacing not appropriate. This is why new matrices of flexible flat electrodes are being designed (see also de Hemptinne 2013 for long-term cortical recording). Computer-based models can be used to optimize electrode placement, polarity, and geometry and to modulate efficiently the excitation properties of cortical networks (Wongsarnpigoon and Grill, 2011). Shape and rigidity of flat, flexible chronic electrode arrays suited to cortical anatomy (sulci/gyri) are becoming available, but issues remain: how to anchor them and the extent of coverage of the cortical target.

Determination of stimulation parameters is suboptimal in current open-loop systems, but novel optimization techniques have been developed that predict parameters by combining concepts of neural network modeling with nonlinear control engineering (Davidson et al., 2014). Electrodes enabling high fidelity recording with short latency are also used to deliver appropriate stimulation after reducing stimulus artifacts (Rossi et al., 2007; Al-Ani et al. 2011). The mechanisms of artifact reduction by the instrumentation must be considered (Kent and Grill, 2012). In the future a new technique, i.e., fast-scan cyclic voltammetry, could become available to wirelessly monitor and measure the production of neurotransmitters in the brain and become a concrete biological feedback to deliver precise stimulation (Van Gompell et al., 2010).

17.5 Conclusion

Cortical closed-loop neuromodulation aims at reshaping specific frequency bands without interfering with healthy physiological functioning through the development of hybrid in silico/biological coadaptive symbiotic systems. In particular, this exploits instantaneous brain activity recordings, applying an appropriate stimulation algorithm and delivering activity-dependent neuromodulation in real time contingent upon the recorded neural activity via multiple flat electrodes placed over the dura of the subject. That being said, the next generation of hardware and software integrating bioinspired algorithms will soon be available. Furthermore, it will become possible to test-simulate stimulation algorithms. Lastly, communication with the implanted device will be performed by a wireless system built to send and receive data from inside and outside the body at high speed (which would avoid current equipment implantation). Some work is still required to implement and monitor the parameters of LFPs, calibrate the stimulation parameters to the patient's individual needs and quantify the evolution of symptoms over the long run.

The possibility of adjusting parameters automatically via an adaptive system while minimizing electric stimulation delivered to brain tissues to control aberrant brain rhythms caused by the disease represents a true alternative option to current open-loop systems. Closed-loop cortical stimulation may take another few years before it enters the clinic, but when it does, it will increase the number of patients treated, improve their quality of life, and decrease the cost of the surgical intervention and the number of follow-up visits.

References

Al-Ani T, Cazettes F, Palfi S, et al. Automatic removal of high-amplitude stimulus artifact from neuronal signal recorded in the subthalamic nucleus. J Neurosci Methods 2011; 198:135–46.

Bazavan R. The brain closed-loop stimulation method with the biopotential mediation of the subthalamic nucleus for the Parkinson's disease therapy. UPB Sci Bull Series C 2013;75: 157-168.

Berényi A, Belluscio M, Mao D, et al. Closed-Loop Control of Epilepsy by Transcranial Electrical Stimulation, Science 2012; 337: 735-737

-Beuter A and Modolo J. Method and apparatus for electrical cortex stimulation EP 2 251 062 A1, WO 2010/130538 A1, CA 2 761 637, US 2012/0109252 A1, JP 2012-526572, 2009

Beuter A and Modolo J. Closed-loop control of brain rhythms. In: Mosekilde E, Sosnovtseva O, Rostami-Hodjegan A (eds). Biosimulation in Biomedical Research, Health Care and Drug Development. Wien: Springer-Verlag, 2012, p179--199

Brittain JS, Probert-Smith P, Aziz TZ, Brown P. Tremor suppression by rhythmic transcranial current stimulation. Curr Biol 2013 23:436–40.

Canavero S. Cerebral-surface. In: Arle J, Shils J (eds) Essential neuromodulation. Burlington, MA: Academic Press; 2011, p. 17–46.

Davidson CM, de Paor, AM ; Lowery, MM. Application of Describing Function Analysis to a Model of Deep Brain Stimulation Biomedical Engineering, IEEE, 2014, Volume:61 Issue:3.

de Hemptinne C, Ryapolova-Webb ES, Air EL, et al. (2013) Exaggerated phase–amplitude coupling in the primary motor cortex in Parkinson disease. PNAS USA 2013; 110: 4780-4785

Echauz J, Firpi H, Georgoulas G. Intelligent control strategies for neurostimulation. In: Valavanis KP (ed). Applications of intelligent control to engineering systems. Dordrecht Heidelberg: Springer Science + Business Media; 2009, p. 247–53.

Feng X, Greenwald B, Rabitz H, et al. Toward closed-loop optimization of deep brain stimulation for Parkinson's disease: concepts and lessons from a computational model. J Neural Eng 2007;4: L14–21.

Hess CW. Modulation of cortical–subcortical networks in Parkinson's disease by applied field effects. Front Hum Neurosci 2013 ; 7:565.

Kaplan D M. Explanation and description in computational neuroscience. Synthese 2011: 183: 339-373.

Kent AR and Grill WM. Recording evoked potentials during deep brain stimulation: development and validation of instrumentation to suppress the stimulus artifact. J Neural Eng. 2012; 9: 036004

Little S, Pogosyan A, Neal S, et al. Adaptive Deep Brain Stimulation in Advanced Parkinson Disease. Ann Neurol 2013; 74:449–457.

Modolo, J., Beuter A., Thomas A., and Legros A. Using smart stimulators to treat Parkinson's disease: re-engineering neurostimulation devices. Frontiers in Computational Neuroscience 2012 ;6, A69

Modolo J, Legros A, Thomas AL, Beuter, A. Model-driven therapeutic treatment of neurological disorders: reshaping brain rhythms with neuromodulation. Interface Focus 2011;1:61-74

Modolo J, Bhattacharya B, Edwards R, et al. Using a virtual cortical module implementing a neural field model to modulate brain rhythms in Parkinson's disease. Frontiers in Neuroscience, 2010b ; 4:45, 1-11

Modolo, J., Edwards, R., Campagnaud J., et al. Past, present and future of brain stimulation Mathematical Modeling of Natural Phenomena, 2010a; 5, 185-207.

Modolo J, Campagnaud J and Beuter A. Effect of complex delayed feedback in a neural field model. Frontiers in Computational Neuroscience. 2009; (doi: 10.3389/conf.neuro.10.2009.14.113).

Modolo, J. and Beuter A. Linking brain dynamics, neuronal mechanisms and deep brain stimulation: An integrated perspective. Med Engin Physics 2009a; 31: 615-623.

Modolo J., Beuter A. Cortical contribution to subthalamic activity during chronic electrical stimulation. Brain Stimulation 2009b; 1:300-301.

Modolo J., Henry, J., Beuter A. Dynamics of the subthalamo-pallidal complex in Parkinson's disease during deep brain stimulation. J Biol Physics 2008; 34: 351-366

Nevado-Holgado AJ, Mallet N, Magill PJ, et al. Effective connectivity of the subthalamic nucleus–globus pallidus network during Parkinsonian oscillations. J Physiol 2014; 592, 1429–1455.

Pascual A, Beuter A, Modolo J. Is a computational model useful to understand the effect of deep brain stimulation in Parkinson's disease? Journal of Integrative Neuroscience 2006; 5: 541-559.

Patten TM, Rennie CJ, Robinson PA, et al. Human cortical traveling waves: dynamical properties and correlations with responses. PLoS One 2012; 1001;7:e38392.

Priori A, Foffani G, and Rossi L. Apparatus for treating neurological disorders by means of adaptive electrostimulation retroacted by biopotentials EP 1940508 and US n. 8,078,281, 2005

Priori A, Foffani G, Rossi L, Marceglia S. Adaptive deep brain stimulation (aDBS) controlled by local field potential oscillations. Exp Neurol 2013; 245:77–86.

Rossi L, Foffani G, Marceglia S, et al. An electronic device for artefact suppression in human local field potential recordings during deep brain stimulation. J Neural Eng 2007; 4:96–106.

Rouse A, Stanslaski S, Cong P, et al. A chronic generalized bi-directional brain-machine interface. J Neural Eng 2011; 8:036018.

Rubin, J. E. & Terman, D. High frequency of the subthalamic nucleus eliminates pathological rhythmicity in a computational model. J. Comput. Neurosci. 2004; 16, 211–235.

Schroll H, and Hamker FH. Computational models of basal-ganglia pathway functions: focus on functional neuroanatomy. Front.Syst.Neurosci. 2013; 7:122

Schiff SJ and Sauer T. Kalman filter control of a model of spatiotemporal cortical dynamics. J Neural Eng 2008; 5, 1-8.

Takahashi K, Saleh M, Penn RD, Hatsopoulos NG. Propagating waves in human motor cortex. Front Hum Neurosci 2011 ; 5:40.

Van Gompel JJ, Chang SY, Goerss SJ et al. Development of intraoperative electrochemical detection: wireless instantaneous neurochemical concentration sensor for deep brain stimulation feedback. Neurosurg. Focus 2010; 29, E6.

Winestone J S, Zaidel A, Bergman H, Israel Z. The use of macroelectrodes in recording cellular spiking activity. J Neurosci Methods 2012; 206:34–9.

Winslow RL, Trayanova N, Geman D, Miller MI. Computational medicine: Translating models to clinical care. Sci. Transl. Med. 2012; 4, 158rv11.

Young N A,Collins C Eand Kaas J H. Cell and neuron densities in the primary motor cortex of primates. Front.Neural Circuits 2013 ; 7:30.

PART III: **Understading ICS**

Sergio Canavero

18 Mechanisms of Action

This chapter explores possible mechanisms of action of ICS by analyzing data from several sources.

18.1 Neuroimaging Studies

Neuroimaging studies of ICS suffer from – among many others (reviewed in Canavero and Bonicalzi 2007: pp 239-254; 2011: pp 271-272)- limited statistical power due to small number of patients, shortcomings of Region-of-Interest (ROI) measurements, inhomogeneity in patients' conditions, group analyses versus single patients, type of CS (extradural versus subdural), target and neuroimaging protocols (SPECT versus PET versus fMRI).

The data available is contradictory (see Box 18.1): whereas two groups found no cortical activation whatsoever below the electrode, i.e. in MI or SI, Saitoh's group observed M1 activation, Canavero and Bonicalzi (1995) rCBF changes in S1, Tsubokawa et al (1991) in MI, and Sol et al (2001) in S1 and M1 bilaterally. Importantly, analogous studies conducted during M1 ICS for Parkinson's disease clearly revealed cortical changes below the electrode (Canavero et al 2002). Orthodromic activity increases brain metabolism, whereas antidromic activity does not (Montgomery 2010), possibly explaining some negative studies. As concerns the thalamus, Peyron et al (2007) found no thalamic rCBF changes, whereas in their previous studies (Garcia-Larrea et al 1997, 1999, 2006) they did. Thalamic metabolic changes have been reported by Tsubokawa et al (1991), Canavero et al (1999), Saitoh et al (2004), Kishima et al (2007) and Ito et al (2011); central pain relief is accompanied by thalamic renormalization (Canavero et al 1999, Pagni and Canavero 1995, Ito et al 2011).

What is clear is that *ICS does NOT relieve neuropathic pain by primarily engaging the so-called affective axis* (e.g. the cingulate cortex) *or the opioid system*, as discussed by some authors: lesions abolishing neuropathic pain along the sensory axis (SI-thalamus) silence both the sensory complaint (pain) and the suffering that accompanies it, whereas cingulotomies and opioids, when effective (infrequently), only reduce the affective component (Canavero and Bonicalzi 2011). Studies show that M1 ICS has a preferential action on the sensory-discriminative aspect of neuropathic pain (Drouot et al 2002, Lefaucheur et al 2009). Patients submitted to ICS show better response by adding S1 as a target of M1 ICS (see Chapters 8 and 9).

Remarkably, M1 rTMS can interfere with the processing of acute laser-induced pain, even if there is an underlying chronic neuropathic pain (Lefaucheur et al 2010).

1- Tsubokawa et al (1991) studied at 4–10 days after implantation of a motor cortex stimulator 7 patients with CP with ^{131}I-amphetamine SPECT. The rCBF showed a marked increase (+150–200%) in the stimulated cortex (MI/SI) and the ipsilateral thalamic and brainstem area, along with pain abatement. The skin temperature as assessed with thermography in the painful area increased to almost the same level as that in the contralateral non-painful area.

2- Canavero and Bonicalzi (1995) found that parietal cortex stimulation renormalized a locus of SPECT hypoperfusion in the parietal cortex in one patient suffering CCP. Renormalization went along analgesia. In another CP patient, MI ECS renormalized SPECT thalamic hypoperfusion, while providing analgesia (Canavero et al 1999). In several CP patients, Canavero reported parietal and/or frontal and /or thalamic deactivation (Canavero et al 1994).

3- MI ECS has inhibiting effects on SI/MI cortex as well as contralaterally, as reported in a fMRI study of phantom pain (Sol et al 2001).

4- Saitoh et al (2004) submitted a right-sided CPSP patient to subdural M1 subdural ICS, with excellent analgesia (VAS 8 to VAS 1) after 30 minutes of stimulation. H_2(15)O PET pre- and post-stimulation revealed significant rCBF increases in left frontal areas (BA9 and 11, BA32) and the left thalamus and decreases in temporo-occipital areas (right BA22 and left BA19). The efficacy of MI CS was mainly related to increased synaptic activity in the thalamus, whereas all other changes were related to emotional processes. The same authors submitted to H_2(15)O PET (resolution: 4x4x5mm at FWHM) 6 patients during right-sided 25-40 Hz CS (3 with CP and 3 with BPA pain, all left-sided) (Kishima et al 2007). The PET study was performed 1-3 years after implantation. Stimulation was stopped more than 12 hours before PET. Six PET scans were performed before subdural MI CS. MI CS was run for 30 minutes and 6 PET scans were performed after onset of analgesia and then analyzed considering all patients together with the SPM software. Comparison of rCBF before and after MI CS showed significant rCBF increases after MI CS in the left posterior thalamus (pulvinar) and left posterior insula. No areas of significant rCBF decrease were identified. By comparing early post-MI CS scans with pre-MI CS scans, the authors found significant rCBF increases in the left posterior insula and the right orbitofrontal cortex (BA11) and significant *decreases* in the right BA9 and the *right BA4*. By comparing late post-MI CS scans with pre-MI CS scans, the left caudal ACC (BA24) showed significant increases, while comparison between early post-MI CS with late post-MI ECS scans brought out significant rCBF increases in the left SMA (BA6). Unlike the Lyon group's findings (see below), the ipsilateral (to MI ECS: right) thalamus was not affected. Results were not differentiated between central and peripheral neuropathic pain.

5- A French group (Peyron et al.1995) reported on 2 CP (both spontaneous and evoked) patients, one with a right mesencephalic infarct with left leg pain (spontaneous and evoked) and the latter with a left parietal infarct sparing the thalamus, with right hemisoma pain, bar the face. In case 1, PET at rest showed no cortical abnormality, but right thalamic hypoperfusion (-9%). During MCS, CBF was increased in brainstem, orbitofrontal cortex (OFC), right thalamus and cingulate cortex (CC): 30 minutes after discontinuation, persisting CBF changes were seen in OFC and CC. In case 2, PET at rest showed widespread CBF decrease in left parietal cortex (-35%) and hypoactivity in left thalamus (-10%), this latter being normal on MRI. During MCS, CBF was increased in brainstem, OFC, left thalamus and CC, while the parietal cortex asymmetry was unmodified. Analgesic effects in both patients lasted at least 30 minutes after stopping MCS and this went along sustained CBF changes, particularly in the thalamus. CBF increases were of the order of 7–9%. An important sustained CBF increase was seen in patient 2's brainstem, while in patient 1 it was delayed, of lesser intensity and shorter duration (patient 2, but not patient 1, also showed modulation of nociceptive flexion reflexes RIII). No change was seen in SI. Thalamic CBF changes were almost superimposable in both patients, but pain relief was satisfactory only in one patient, in whom there was also brainstem activation. CBF changes in OFC and anterior CC (ACC) were stronger and more sustained in the patient with less pain relieving effect of MCS than the other.

Box 18.1: Neuroimaging Studies of Neuropathic Pain

Garcia-Larrea et al (1997) studied 7 CPSP and 3 PNP (brachial plexus avulsion, BPA, pain) patients submitted to contralateral MI ECS (in 3 medially, i.e., subdurally). H_2(15)O PET was done before, during – 5 and 20 minutes – and 30 minutes after a 20 minute session of stimulation. Results were not differentiated between CP and BPA. There was no significant difference in regional cerebral blood flow (rCBF) between the two controls or the two stimulation conditions. The only locus of significant CBF increase during MI ECS was observed in the motor thalamus. Sizable, but insignificant CBF increases during MI ECS were seen in the left insula, BA24–32 and upper mesencephalon (plus a rCBF decrease in BA18–19 bilaterally). No significant change was seen in MI (SI could not be resolved with their machine). All changes were reversible upon stopping MI ECS, although BA24 and mesencephalic changes persisted or even increased slightly after stoppage of MI ECS. They compared 3 patients with 80–100% relief and 4 with less than 40% relief. Mean thalamic CBF was enhanced in both groups with a similar time course, albeit rCBF increase was greater in those with 80%-plus relief. In contrast, mean CBF in BA24-32 appeared to increase during MI ECS only in patients with good relief and to decrease in poor responders, even in individual analyses. The same group (Garcia-Larrea et al. 1999) evaluated 10 patients with CP and BPA (likely including the above-mentioned patients, although time from implantation to PET does not correspond). MI ECS was stopped 24 hours before PET. Four consecutive scans were first recorded (A). Then PET was recorded at 5, 15, 25 and 35 minutes after switching on MI ECS (B). MI ECS was subsequently stopped and PET recorded at 15, 30, 45, 60 and 75 minutes after MCS had been turned off (C). MI ECS (B versus A) was associated with increased rCBF in rostral ACC contralateral to the electrode. During MI ECS stoppage (C versus A) there was strong activation up to 75 minutes after MI ECS discontinuation of rostral ACC, orbitofrontal cortex, basal ganglia and brainstem. MI ECS (B+C versus A) was associated with decreased blood flow immediately below the electrode. Images of CBF changes in the brainstem did not cover the localization of the PAG. They did not find MI ECS activation of SI, a possible consequence of the spatiotemporal resolution (12 mm) limits of their PET machine. The low-threshold analysis (Z-score ^{3} 3.5) of the two-step procedure yielded some regions of significant CBF increase: the whole thalamus (ipsilateral to MI ECS), the ACC (mostly contralaterally to MI ECS, plus midline), orbitofrontal areas, a region comprising the insula and descending towards the inferomedial temporal lobe – including amygdala (exclusively contralateral to MI ECS) and the subthalamic-upper brainstem region (ipsilateral to MI ECS). The second (high-threshold) step of the analysis (Z-score ^{3}4) restricted spatially the above results and limited the anatomical region of significant CBF increase to thalamic VL ipsilateral to MCS, with extensions to VA and subthalamic region. Vc was outside the region of increased CBF in both high- and low-threshold analyses. The sequence included condition A (CBF assessed basally, 15 minutes before MI ECS with stimulator turned off for 18 hours), conditions B and C (2 consecutive scans performed respectively after 5 and 20 minutes of continuous MI ECS) and condition D (scan after 30 minutes after MI ECS discontinuation). Pain ratings during PET were 4.8 ± 2.6 during condition A, 4.3 ± 2.9 and 3.69 ± 2.8 in conditions B and C and 3.69 ± 2.8 in condition D. In spite of a trend to pain decrease from A to D, differences were not significant. As far as rCBF changes are concerned, in all cases there was an abrupt CBF increase during the first scan under MI ECS (5 minutes after onset) which remained stable during PET 20 minutes after M1 ICS onset. These effects were reversible 30 minutes after M1 ICS interruption in all sites, except in ACC where rCBF had not yet reverted to pre-stimulation values 30 minutes after MCS discontinuation: here two spots of increased rCBF appeared in right and left ACC/orbito-frontal boundaries (despite unilateral analgesia!) and stayed almost so after switching off the stimulator. No significant change related to MI ECS was observed in SI or MI. CBF decreased in BA18–19 areas and were totally reversible upon discontinuation of MI ECS. In CP and BPA patients with >80% versus <20% relief, while lateral thalamic CBF appeared to increase in all patients (albeit to a greater extent – 15% versus 5% – in those relieved), BA32 CBF increased in responders (+5% at 20 minutes), but decreased in non-responders (-10% at 20 minutes); upon close scrutiny, this does not seem a strong finding, as in their two reported CP cases this was not the case. Garcia-Larrea et al (2006) submitted to M1 ICS a patient with left facial central pain due to a left medullary infarct. Although the territory with sensory loss was much wider in the right nonpainful than in the left painful side, PET showed significant rCBF reduction in the right thalamus, contralateral to the small painful area.

continued **Box 18.1:** Neuroimaging Studies of Neuropathic Pain

40 Hz M1 ICS afforded 60% relief and PET showed renormalization of the thalamic anomaly. Peyron et al (2007) explored the post-stimulation period using an enlarged temporal window (as long as PET studies allow). 19 morphine-naïve patients suffering brain central pain (13 patients), cord central pain (4 patients) or brachial plexus avulsion (2 patients) were submitted to 35 Hz (180 µs/ 2.5V/ cyclical) MI ECS (paddle parallel to rolandic fissure) and subsequent PET scans. Analgesic drugs were not discontinued, bar fast-acting opioids for at least 12 hours before exam. PET resolution was 7 mm. Patients were blinded to M1 ICS status (ON/OFF). After acquisition of baseline scans, the next 4 scans were acquired at 5, 15, 25 and 35 min after MCS onset. MI ICS was then turned off again and 5 further scans were recorded at 15, 30, 45, 60 and 75 minutes. Data were analyzed using SPM2 software and also considered for a functional connectivity analysis (FCA), which examines the temporal correlation of neural events between distributed brain areas. Mean pain relief was 10-40% in 8 patients, 60% in 6 and >80% in 2. Results of ON versus baseline and OFF versus baseline were as follows. Only a limited activation of the pregenual ACC(anatomically connected to MI) contralateral to MI ICS was found in the ON versus baseline comparison. The large majority of activations were found in the OFF versus baseline subtraction in the ipsilateral premotor cortex, the contralateral pregenual (pg) ACC (descending pain control) and midcingulate (noxious processing) and supplementary motor (SMA) area, pallidum, putamen and PAG. Most of the rCBF changes that correlated with long-term analgesia occurred during the 75 minutes subsequent to MI ICS stoppage (after 35 minutes of effective stimulation). There was a correlation between rCBF changes and analgesia in the ON condition in midcingulate cortex (MCC) and pregenual ACC (BA32/24) contralaterally to MCS and in prefrontal cortices (BA10) bilaterally. There was a trend for the midcingulate to be activated in the ON condition with a persisting activation in the OFF condition, while the pregenual ACC still showed increased activity in the OFF condition. Regions whose rCBF increased relative to baseline during MI ECS and correlated positively with analgesia in the OFF condition (after stoppage of MCS) included a large ACC activation, extended from the posterior MCC and anterior MCC to the pregenual ACC, bilaterally, contralateral orbitofrontal cortex and SMA, ipsilateral cerebellum and posterior cingulate cortex, prefrontal cortices and basal ganglia bilaterally, hypothalamus, upper mesencephalon (PAG) and lower pons. These activations were maximal in the OFF condition and correlated with average analgesia. Unlike Saitoh's group's findings (see above), MI rCBF below the electrode was not found to change or correlate with pain scores at any time, nor was SI. In the FCA, responses that correlated with analgesia with MI ECS ON were found to correlate also with CBF changes in other subdivisions of lateral prefrontal cortices, in contralateral orbitofrontal cortex, pgACC, anterior insula, putamen and lower pons. In the OFF condition FCA, significant covariations were found between pgACC and basal ganglia, pgACC and brainstem, pgACC and posterior cingulated cortex. Basal ganglia covariated together bilaterally, but also with posterior cingulate and insular cortices. CBF changes in mesencephalon and lower pons covariated with basal ganglia and with pgACC. The authors concluded that a network comprising the ACC/OFC/medial thalamus and PAG –the same as seen during ECS induced analgesia by other procedures- appears to be the final common pathway of analgesia elicited by ECS (ACC and PAG being opioid-rich areas) and becomes activated ONLY after MI ICS is discontinued. MCC and pgACC activities did not correlate with current pain relief, but with the amount of analgesia obtained after several cycles of MI ICS. The perigenual and subgenual ACC are associated with mood alterations and the production of affective states: they are part of a "ventral affective system" involved in the identification of the emotional significance of a stimulus, production of affective states, and automatic regulation of emotional responses, and also comprise the amygdala, anterior insula and ventral striatum. The mid-posterior cingulate cortex instead is concerned with pain unpleasantness. This study failed to replicate the authors' previous finding of a significant thalamic rCBF increase, except in the FCA. They concluded that MI ICS-related thalamic activation is phasic and short-lasting, likely a trigger for other activations, and may be averaged out when 35 minutes of MI ICS are lumped together and analyzed as a whole. The same group (Maarrawi et al 2007) submitted a subgroup of the above patients (central pain 7, trigeminal peripheral neuropathic pain 1) to PET with [11C] diprenorphine PET, basally and after 2 months of chronic MI ECS. The two preoperative scans performed at 2 weeks interval did not show significant differences. Medications were kept unchanged. Data were analyzed with SPM99.

continued **Box 18.1:** Neuroimaging Studies of Neuropathic Pain

Voxel-wise comparison of preoperative and postoperative PET scans showed a significant decrease of opioid receptor binding postoperatively. Buprenorphine binding decrease (group level analysis) concerned the posterior part of the midbrain (PAG) (-25.6%), anterior middle cingulate cortex (-21.2%), lateral prefrontal cortex (-23.3%) and cerebellum (-18.3%). VAS scores decreases and binding decreases correlated significantly in PAG and anterior MCC (in PFC, there was only a trend). One CP patient got minimal relief from MI ECS (VAS 8 to 7 on MI ECS) and decreases were 16.3% in PAG, 10.3% in aMCC, 10.11% in cerebellum and 17.2% in PFC. The CP patient with the best relief (VAS 8 to 2 on MCS) showed decreases respectively of 37%, 30.3%,22.2% and 25.5%, which would seem to confirm that the magnitude of decreases significantly correlated with degree of analgesia. Yet, the largest decreases were seen at PAG and PFC levels in a patient who had a VAS 7-to-2 relief, at aMCC level in the patient with the best analgesia, at cerebellar level in one with a VAS 8-to-5 change. The authors suggest that binding decreases were not due to loss of opioid receptors (as seen in some studies of central pain), but to increased endogenous opioid secretion and resulting decreased receptor availability to exogenous diprenorphine and a possible reactive down-regulation and internalization of receptors. The authors' conclusion was that MCS triggers endogenous opioid secretion in part of the remaining medial pain system unaffected by opioid receptor loss in CPSP. The involved circuit would include MI that projects to PAG which in turn projects to ACC. In an almost duplicate paper, they (Maarrawi et al 2013) analyzed 15 patients (10 CPSP, 4 PNP, 1 mixed spinal case) submitted again to [11C] diprenorphine (D) PET pre (twice)- and post-MCS and matched the findings against a group of 11 healthy (!!!) subjects. Correlation of opioid binding with pain relief after 7 months of MCS was significant, especially contralaterally to pain, within the cingulate (anterior and perigenual) cortex, orbitofrontal cortex, mesencephalon, contralateral insula, PAG and cerebellum. Correlations between mean binding potential values in these areas and the percentage of pain relief for paroxysmal and continuous pain ratings were significant in contralateral and ipsilateral insula, ACC/MCC, OFC, thalamus and PAG. These correlations held for both CP and PNP. Patients with binding potential lower than the range of controls (healthy patients!!!) in the thalamus, PAG and contralateral insula did not obtain benefit from MCS (pain relief <30%). These conclusion are nixed by poor opioid responsiveness of CP (Canavero and Bonicalzi 2011). They (Garcia-Larrea et al. 1999) also recorded CO_2 laser-evoked potentials (LEPs) and flexion nociceptive reflex (RIII) in a subgroup of these same patients. LEPs (amplitude and latency of each component) and RIII (surface) were studied with M1 ICS turned off, on and at least 30 minutes after M1 ICS interruption. LEPs were obtained after stimulation of both the painful and the intact side, while RIII was obtained after stimulation of the painful side only. In one patient, after stimulation of the non-affected side, LEP amplitudes of the vertex component decreased significantly during active stimulation. In the group as a whole, after stimulation of the non-affected side, LEP amplitudes tended to decrease under M1 ICS, although not statistically significantly. RIII was not modified in the three conditions. Electrophysiological responses did not correlate with VAS. There was a lack of any significant acute change in SEPs during MI ECS in any of the recorded patients with central lesions. None of the 4 patients whose nociceptive reflexes remained unmodified by M1 ICS was satisfied with the attained analgesia. Although the 7 patients with CP had sizable epidural SEPs during intraoperative monitoring, only 4 retained scalp-recorded SEPs of enough amplitude to permit assessment of M1 ICS effects. Parietal somatosensory responses up to 50 ms post-stimulus did not exhibit any significant change in amplitude, latency or topography in relation to M1 ICS. Thus, significant modulation of spinal nociceptive reflexes was seen during MI ECS in 3/7 patients, while it was unchanged in 4. Modification thereof corresponded in every case to attenuation of the responses during M1 ICS. Two of 3 patients with M1 ICS-related reflex attenuation experienced good to very good relief, while the third reported >60% abatement of allodynia during M1 ICS, but only 30% of spontaneous pain.

5-Ito et al (2011) assessed 4 CPSP patients who responded to MCS to pre- (within 1 week before MCS) and post- (2 weeks after MCS, stimulation OFF) stimulation 18F-FDG PET. A semiquantitative analysis was conducted (NEUROFLEXER software/NEUROSTAT template) on 17 regions of interest both in the cerebrum, brainstem and cerebellum. The only significant asymmetry was found in the thalamus (basal ratio: 0.81, ratio during analgesia: 0.89). In particular, the improvement in CMR-Glu asymmetry was noteworthy in 3 cases without thalamic injury. The therapeutic effect was proportional to the improvement of the PET asymmetry.

continued **Box 18.1:** Neuroimaging Studies of Neuropathic Pain

18.2 Neurophysiology Studies

Katayama et al (1988) recorded descending volleys from the spinal extradural space after direct stimulation of the exposed cortex in anesthetized patients during neurosurgery. They described recruitment of probable D (irect) and I(ndirect) waves, with D waves having the lowest threshold for monopolar anodal (rather than cathodal) stimulation.

An opposite result was reported by Hanajima et al (2002), who found that, in awake pain or movement disorders patients, chronic stimulation through a quadripolar strip electrode placed directly on the arachnoid in the subdural space over M1 appears to activate low threshold (short chronaxie and refractory period) neural elements – probably myelinated axons- likely at cortical level. These, in turn, may activate corticospinal neurons (producing detectable effects on motoneurons) and inhibitory neurons in the cortex. The facilitation was larger (lower threshold) with cathodal (-) than with anodal (+) monopolar stimulation (which excluded corticospinal neuron axons) in most, but not all, patients (3.9:1 ratio, range 0.9-11.1). Anodal stimulation was less effective, maybe because in the awake state interneurons are better activated.

Di Lazzaro et al (2004) compared the pattern of activation produced by TMS and extradural electrical stimulation of MI in a single awake patient who had both a cortical extradural electrode implanted over the motor area parallel to the central sulcus for treatment of face central pain, and an extradural electrode inserted into the spinal extradural space. The recordings showed that suprathreshold extradural M1 stimulation can evoke multiple descending waves: an I1 and an I2 wave, with the same latency as magnetic postero-anterior stimulation, together with a delayed I3 wave. ICS also evoked an earlier probable D wave that had a slightly later onset than that after lateromedial TMS stimulation. It might be that the D wave evoked by ICS originates closer to the cell body of the pyramidal neurons than the conventional D wave, perhaps at the initial segment rather than at some distance down the axon. Thus, extradural stimulation of M1 can produce repetitive excitation of corticospinal neurons. The order of recruitment of the volleys, and the latency of the D and I3 waves may be slightly different from that seen after TMS. This suggests that there may be subtle differences in populations of cortical excitatory and inhibitory neurons activated by the two forms of stimulation, presumably related to differences in the focality and distribution of the electric field produced by the two methods of stimulation. It was suggested that, in order to improve clinical effects of rTMS, changing the orientation of the coil by 90° (from postero-anterior to latero-medial) may make it more "ICS-like" and thus more effective. However, these authors did not study the descending volleys generated by bipolar EMCS at lower stimulus intensities, as used for chronic therapeutic stimulation.

Yamamoto et al (2007) investigated the corticospinal motor evoked potential (MEP) as an intraoperative index for the placement of stimulation electrodes in the epidural space over M1. A grid of plate electrodes was placed in the epidural space to cover M1, S1, and premotor cortex employing a magnetic resonance imaging-guided neuronavigation system in two patients with CPSP. The D-wave of the corticospinal MEP was recorded with a flexible wire electrode placed in the epidural space of the spinal cord during anodal monopolar stimulation of each plate electrode under general anesthesia. The grid electrode was fixed in position with dural sutures and the craniotomy closed. The effect of pain reduction induced by anodal monopolar stimulation of the same plate electrodes was examined using the visual analogue scale (VAS) on a separate day in the awake state without anesthesia. Comparison of the percentage VAS reduction and the recorded amplitude of the D-wave employing the same stimulation electrode revealed significant correlations in both cases. The grid electrode was then replaced with two paddle electrodes over the hand and foot areas, and the optimum positions were identified by D-wave recording before electrode fixation. Both patients reported satisfactory pain alleviation with lower stimulation voltages than usually required for patients with similar symptoms, i.e. the site of stimulation producing the best pain relief corresponded to the location of the cortical contacts evoking the largest D-waves. However, these D-waves were produced during a screening phase by using 0.2-ms duration monophasic rectangular stimuli delivered at very low frequency (2 Hz) and high (suprathreshold) intensity (30 mA). These parameters of cortical stimulation are fully unusual for chronic therapeutic M1 ICS. Therefore, these authors did not demonstrate that therapeutic M1 ICS elicited D-waves, but only that recording D-waves to suprathreshold anodal stimulation could help to determine the optimal site for chronic stimulation.

Lefaucheur et al (2010) studied the descending volleys in two anesthetized patients with peripheral hand neuropathic pain successfully treated by M1 ICS (2 quadripolar leads perpendicular to the central sulcus, 40Hz, 60 μs, 2V), who also had an implanted epidural cervical electrodes for spinal cord stimulation. Recordings were carried out under general anesthesia. Drugs had not been weaned prior to recordings. Low-intensity cathodal M1 ICS produced I2-waves, reflecting transsynaptic activation of corticospinal tract fibers. Conversely, low-intensity anodal M1 ICS produced D-waves, reflecting direct activation of corticospinal tract fibers. These D-waves were delayed by 0.6–0.8 ms compared to those produced by lateromedial-oriented TMS. A similar delay (0.4 ms) was observed by Di Lazzaro et al. (above) using high-intensity bipolar M1 ICS. Compared to TMS, M1 ICS could recruit slower conducting fibers or excite corticospinal fibers at a more proximal site. Low-intensity bipolar EMCS mostly produced I3-waves and not a combination of D- and I2-waves. These results suggest that bipolar stimulation is not simply a "bifocal" stimulation that would have corresponded to the addition of the responses to monopolar anodal and cathodal stimulations. Anodal and cathodal electrical fields likely overlap and the neuronal activity produced near the anode and near the cathode, respectively, can interact with each other (Manola and Holsheimer 2009) The magnitude of these interactions depends on the center-to-center distance between the electrodes. The bipolar M1 ICS configuration providing optimal chronic pain relief produced mostly late I-waves at low intensity (below motor threshold) and also D- and early I-waves at high intensity (above motor threshold). As stimulus intensity increased, the induced electrical field likely spread and went deeper into the brain, recruiting more fibers. These results confirmed modelization studies in which M1 ICS could produce analgesia by recruiting horizontal fibers in the upper cortical layers of precentral gyrus rather than by directly exciting the pyramidal tract (Manola and Holsheimer 2009). The descending volleys produced by the optimal M1 ICS configuration for pain treatment are closer to those produced by PA-oriented TMS than LM-oriented TMS: indeed, LM-oriented TMS preferentially recruits D-waves at low intensity, whereas PA-oriented TMS recruits I-waves. Thus, M1 ICS and PA-oriented TMS likely activates similar neural circuits and this latter may truly act as a tool to predict the outcome of subsequent M1 ICS. AP-oriented TMS should be even more effective, since it evokes later I-waves than PA-oriented TMS, at least in some patients (Di Lazzaro et al 2009). The conclusions of this study are weakened by observing that the descending volleys generated by M1 ICS were not compared to those in patients in whom M1 ICS failed, and the effects recorded could have thus been purely unspecific. Moreover, nothing could be said about possible influences of M1 ICS on the brainstem or cord, since recordings were effected in response to single pulses, whereas M1 ICS for pain relief is performed at 40 Hz.

18.3 Modelization Studies

Several attempts at modelizing the effects of ICS have been made (see Chapters 19-20 for detailed discussion). However, their limits are immediately apparent if one considers the daunting task of simultaneously factoring in the multitude of parameters that are at work in the living human brain, many of which are unknown.

The belief that only a cathode can activate cortical neural tissue and that the anode placed over the cortex is indifferent seems to be wrong (Manola and Holsheimer 2009). Although the stimulation of nervous tissue generally occurs in the vicinity of the cathode, this is not true in ICS due to the different orientations of cortical nerve fibers (parallel and perpendicular to the laminae) and to the large size of the epidural lead electrodes: thus various populations of axons can be activated under either the cathode or the anode (horizontal fibers vs perpendicular fibers), making bipolar stimulation bifocal (thus, in M1 ICS with a perpendicular position of the paddle, S1 is engaged). A large motor response is evoked when either anodal stimulation is applied on M1 or cathodal stimulation is applied on the central sulcus, according to the orientation of cortical nerve fibers in the stimulus-induced electric field. When the MEP amplitude is high in anodal stimulation, it will be lower in cathodal stimulation and viceversa. When the electrode covers the lip of CS, anodally and cathodally evoked MEPs may have similar amplitudes. Also, despite the large center-to-center distance of the cathode and the anode in a quadripolar strip (=/> 10 mm), some overlap of the corresponding stimulus-evoked field is still present: due to this overlap, the electrical fields in the cortex below the cathode and the anode are different from real monopolar fields, and elicited neural activities will most likely differ from monopolar ones. In other words, when MI ICS is applied bipolarly, the neural activity evoked near the cathode may affect the activity near the anode -and vice versa- via their intracortical connections (likely an inhibitory interaction).

According to Arle et al. (2008)'s model of ICS for pain control, 'subthreshold' M1 ICS only excites the horizontal inhibitory fibers coursing horizontally within the exposed parts of the M1 gyrus, and these in turn lead to local inhibition, and subsequent lack of layer 5 excitation, of S1 (thus inhibiting SI by providing less excitation as well)(see also Drouot et al 2002): in particular, during stimulation, the mean firing rate in S1 is decreased by 40.5% (Shils et al 2008). Many of the horizontal fibers are from the predominantly inhibitory layer 1-3 stellate interneurons. The significant change in activity is centered only within the topographically oriented region which is coding for the 'painful' stimulus coming from sensory thalamus. In other words, the computational representation of a 'painful' stimulus arising through sensory thalamic cells and carried on to S1 is inhibited by M1 ICS acting on just the inhibitory interneurons of M1. This is in line with Manola and Holsheimer (2009)'s studies, in which the neural elements most likely stimulated by M1 ICS were superficial horizontal fibers of the largest diameter. Higher amplitudes would also stimulate excitatory layer V pyramidal cells (for instance) in M1, in addition to the inhibitory interneurons: this increased activity would override the inhibition and lead to motor unit driving, which indeed does occur clinically, through vertically oriented fibers. M1 ICS stimulates both horizontal and vertically oriented fibers, rather than directly hyperpolarizing them, as has been reported (Hanajima et al 2002).

According to Wongsarnpigoon and Grill (2009, 2012)'s modelization studies of (now defunct) NorthStar Neuroscience's stimulating array, bipolar stimulation increases thresholds compared to monopolar stimulation for neurons beyond the stimulating electrode, with thresholds lowest beneath the electrodes (i.e. focuses injection of charge). Although current passes through the region of the cortex between the electrodes as it travels from the anode to the cathode, thresholds for excitation of neurons directly between the two electrodes are greater than beneath the electrodes. This is the case also when the electrodes straddle M1, with thresholds lowest beneath the electrodes, and not in the crown of M1 between the electrodes. The two electrodes stimulate two distinct populations of neurons, but it is unclear if and how activation of one population affects the other. The conclusion is that monopolar stimulation would be more prudent. Importantly, if the electrode is placed perpendicularly to the central sulcus to straddle two gyri, as done by some groups, this configuration leads to substantially lower thresholds in the adjacent gyrus compared to stimulation with the lead oriented over and parallel to M1 and this could have clinically relevant effects beyond what is intended. Thus, these authors advise against perpendicular positioning across the rolandic fissure (or any other) unless one is sure ICS of the adjacent gyrus is innocuous (which is arduous to guarantee anywhere in the cortex). In other words, the counter-electrode during bipolar ICS does more than simply return the current to the stimulator and bipolar ICS can produce different outcomes from monopolar stimulation singly for the anode or the cathode. Selective stimulation (straddling electrodes) of neurons located deep within a sulcus appears exceedingly difficult with ICS: this means that, while the hand area is generally targeted in many ICS procedures, sulcal neurons cannot be directly activated without co-activation of neurons on the crowns and lips of M1 and S1. However, in TMS, despite the gyral crown of the cortex being subjected to a larger magnetic field magnitude, the sulcal bank of M1 has larger cerebral CBF responses (Krieg et al 2013). However, the importance of localization is not well understood. In certain disorders, stimulating a wide area of the cortex may be more beneficial than targeting a small area, a fact confirmed by ICS cases in which focal stimulation benefited widespread body pain or in PD where benefit is pansomatic. Another important observation is that thresholds beneath the electrode are directly related to electrode diameter, i.e. larger electrodes reduce the spatial selectivity of stimulation beneath the electrode. Spatial selectivity is also influenced by inter-electrode spacing: reducing the spacing (7 mm vs 10 mm) increases thresholds (larger amplitudes are needed to produce an effect) throughout most of the cortex for bipolar stimulation. This affects the ability to perform current steering, a technique where stimulation is delivered through multiple independent sources to direct the flow of current and focus stimulation on a specific region between the electrodes.

18.4 Conclusion

In sum, ICS directly engages the underlying stimulated cortex and only thereafter other brain regions (including the thalamus) connected anatomically. The effects of ICS appear to be produced by activation of horizontal fibers located in the superficial layers of the cortex and in the vicinity of the origin of the pyramidal tract corresponding to the targeted region, but not by direct activation of the pyramidal tract in case of M1 ICS. Both the cathode and the anode have effects.

References

Arle JE, Mei LZ, Shils JL. Modeling parkinsonian circuitry and the DBS electrode: I. Biophysical background and software. Stereotact Funct Neurosurg 2008;134:1-15.
Canavero S, Pagni CA, Castellano G, Bonicalzi V. SPECT and central pain. Pain. 1994;57:129-31.
Canavero S, Bonicalzi V. Cortical stimulation for central pain. J Neurosurg 1995; 83: 1117
Canavero S, Bonicalzi V, Castellano G, et al. Painful supernumerary phantom arm following motor cortex stimulation for central post-stroke pain. Case report. J Neurosurg 1999; 91: 121-123

Canavero S, Paolotti R, Bonicalzi V, et al. Extradural motor cortex stimulation for advanced Parkinson disease. Report of two cases. J Neurosurg. 2002;97:1208-11

Canavero S, Bonicalzi V. Central pain syndrome. Pathophysiology, diagnosis and management. Cambridge: Cambridge University Press, 2007 (1st ed), 2011 (2nd ed)

Di Lazzaro V, Oliviero A, Pilato F, et al. Comparison of descending volleys evoked by transcranial and epidural motor cortex stimulation in a conscious patient with bulbar pain. Clin Neurophysiol. 2004;115:834-8

Di Lazzaro V, Proficue P, Pilato F, et al. Mechanisms of action. In: In: Canavero S (ed) Textbook of therapeutic cortical stimulation. New York: Nova Science, 2009, pp 57-68

Drouot X, Nguyen JP, Peschanski M, et al. The antalgic efficacy of chronic motor cortex stimulation is related to sensory changes in the painful zone. Brain 2002; 125: 1660-1664

Garcia-Larrea L, Peyron R, Mertens P, et al Positron emission tomography durino motor cortex stimulation for pain control. Stereotact Funct Neurosurg 1997; 68: 141-148

Garcia-Larrea L., Peyron R., Mertens P., et al. Electrical stimulation of motor cortex for pain control: a combined PET-scan and electrophysiological study. Pain 1999; 83: 259—273

Garcia-Larrea L, Maarrawi J, Peyron et al. On the relation between sensory deafferentation, pain and thalamic activity in wallenberg's syndrome: a PET-scan study before and after motor cortex stimulation. Eur J Pain 2006; 10: 677-688

Hanajima R, Ashby P, Lang AE, Lozano AM. Effects of acute stimulation through contacts placed on the motor cortex for chronic stimulation. Clin Neurophysiol 2002; 113: 635-641

Ito M, Kuroda S, Shiga T, et al. Motor cortex stimulation improves local cerebral glucose metabolism in the ipsilateral thalamus in patients with poststroke pain: case report. Neurosurgery. 2011;69:E462-9.

Katayama Y, Tsubokawa T, Maejima S, et al. Corticospinal direct response in humans: identification of the motor cortex during intracranial surgery under general anaesthesia. J Neurol Neurosurg Psychiatry 1988;51:50–59

Kishima H, Saitoh Y, Osaki Y, et al. Motor cortex stimulation in patients with deafferentation pain : activation of the posterior insula and thalamus. J Neurosurg 2007; 107: 43-48

Krieg TD, Salinas FS, Narayana S, et al. PET-based confirmation of orientation sensitivity of TMS-induced cortical activation in humans. Brain Stimul 2013;6:898-904

Lefaucheur JP, Drouot X, Cunin P, et al. Motor cortex stimulation for treatment of refractory peripheral neuropathic pain. Brain 2009; 132:1463-71

Lefaucheur JP, Jarry G, Drouot X, et al. Motor cortex rTMS reduces acute pain provoked by laser stimulation in patients with chronic neuropathic pain. Clin Neurophysiol 2010; 121: 895-901

Lefaucheur JP, Holsheimer J, Goujon C et al. Descending volleys generated by efficacious epidural motor cortex stimulation in patients with chronic neuropathic pain. Exp Neurol 2010; 223: 609-614

Maarrawi J, Peyron R, Mertens P, et al. Motor cortex stimulation for pain control induces changes in the endogenous opioid system. Neurology 2007; 69: 827-834

Maarrawi J, Peyron R, Mertens P, et al. Brain opioid receptor density predicts motor cortex stimulation efficacy for chronic pain. Pain. 2013;154:2563-8.

Manola L, Holsheimer J. A neuroengineering model of extradural cortical stimulation. In: Canavero S (ed) Textbook of therapeutic cortical stimulation. New York: Nova Science, 2009, pp 91-112

Montgomery Jr EB. Deep Brain Stimulation Programming. New York: Oxford University Press, 2010

Pagni CA, Canavero S. Functional thalamic depression in a case of reversibile central pain due to a spinal intramedullary cyst. J Neurosurg 1995; 83: 163-165

Peyron R, Garcia-Larrea L, Deiber MP, et al. Electrical stimulation of precentral cortical area in the treatment of central pain: electrophysiological and PET study. Pain. 1995;62:275-86

Peyron R, Faillenot I, Mertens P, et al. Motor cortex stimulation in neuropathic pain. Correlations between analgesic effect and hemodynamic changes in the brain. A PET study. Neuroimage 2007; 34: 310-321

Saitoh Y, Osaki Y, Nishimura H, et al. Increased regional cerebral blood flow in the contralateral thalamus after successful motor cortex stimulation in a patient with poststroke pain. J Neurosurg. 2004;100:935-9.

Shils JL, Mei L, Arle JE. A computational approach to the investigation of motorcortical stimulation of the treatment of pain. Mov Disorders 2008; 23 (S1): S380-1

Sol JC, Casaux J, Roux FE, et al. Chronic motor cortex stimulation for phantom limb pain: correlations between pain relief and functional imaging studies. Stereotact Funct Neurosurg 2001; 77: 172-176.

Stepniewska I, Preuss TM, and Kass JH. Thalamic connections of the primary motor cortex (MI) of owl monkeys. The journal of comparative neurology 1994;349:558-582.

Tsubokawa T., Katayama Y., Yamamoto T., et al. Treatment of thalamic pain by chronic motor cortex stimulation PACE, Pacing Clin. Electrophysiol 1991; 14: 131—134

Yamamoto T, Katayama Y, Obuchi T, et al. Recording of corticospinal evoked potential for optimum placement of motor cortex stimulation electrodes in the treatment of post-stroke pain. Neurol Med Chir (Tokyo) 2007;47:409-14

Wongsarnpigoon A, Grill W.M. Optimization of parameter selection and electrical targeting. In: Canavero S (ed) Textbook of therapeutic cortical stimulation. New York: Nova Sci. 2009, 69-90

Wongsarnpigoon A, Grill W.M. 2012. Computer-based model of epidural motor cortex stimulation: effects of electrode position and geometry on activation of cortical neurons. Clin Neurophysiol 123, 160-172.

Hyoung-Ihl Kim, Donghyeon Kim, Hyeon Seo, Sung Chan Jun

19 Modelization: Overview

Following the implantation of an ICS system, clinicians must decide which electrode on a multi-electrode lead will deliver stimulation, which electrode will serve as the return electrode during bipolar stimulation, or whether to deliver monopolar stimulation (when available) and also program the stimulation parameters, including amplitude, frequency, polarity and pulse width. The large number of potential combinations of stimulation parameters results in excessively long programming sessions and suboptimal treatment. Only infrequently symptoms are alleviated immediately upon application of ICS with the appropriate parameters, e.g. pain and tremor; for parkinsonian akinesia, dystonia, stroke, depression, effects take days, weeks and even months to build up. Although amplitudes are typically set at a fixed percentage of the motor threshold, this is quite pointless for stimulations outside M1. That's why efforts have been directed towards modelizing the effects of ICS in order to make the procedure speedier and more effective.

Electricity used to stimulate the cortex may affect cortical functions, but it has not been easy to demonstrate the invisible electrical current flow distributed underneath and around the electrodes. To understand the underlying electrical field/current density (EF/CD) distribution generated by electrical stimulation of the brain, a few early, cadaveric studies measured electrical fields; however, researchers were not convinced that the results accurately reflected EF/CD in the brain (Rush and Driscoll, 1968). Currently, the effect of cortical stimulation is exclusively inferred from behavioral and/or physiological outcomes measured by electroencephalography (EEG), magnetoencephalography (MEG), electromyography (EMG), and functional magnetic resonance imaging (fMRI). The inferred values are more reliable than the cadaver studies; however, they require further clarification to validate the measurement values. Further, electrical cortical stimulation is a dynamic event that involves multiple structures of the brain in continuously changing states. Therefore, a single tool or combination of current research tools does not easily reflect variable consequences following cortical stimulation. Consequently, computer-based, neuroengineering modelling has been introduced to provide the EF/CD such mapping. To date, neuroengineering models have been successfully used not only to probe the action mechanism of cortical stimulation, but also to predict the effect of cortical stimulation.

Virtual results obtained from these neuroengineering models are widely accepted more and more for measuring and evaluating the efficacy of cortical stimulation in clinical contexts, but future modification or improvement in cortical neuromodulation technology is contingent on the appropriate utilization of the neuroengineering models.

Currently, cortical responses to electrical stimulation can be predicted by measuring two factors: formation of EF/CD (see Box 19.1) and intrinsic neuronal response to stimulation. The EF/CD distribution by cortical stimulation can perturb the cortical functions and alter physiological or behavioral responses.

Electrical field and current density are frequently used as synonyms in cortical stimulation research. However, the two terms differ in several ways. Exposure to an electrical source induces the electrical field (expressed in V/m or mV/m); the result of inducing the electrical field is current density (expressed in A/m^2 or mA/m^2) inside the body. If the conductivity (expressed in S/m) is the same for all of the body's tissues, the electrical and current density values are the same. However, if every type of tissue has its own conductivity, the values are different, with the relationship between electrical field and current density expressed as

Current density = Tissue conductivity × Electrical field

Therefore, current density may be changed depending on how each tissue conducts the same electrical field. Nonetheless, the magnitudes of the electrical field and the current density are proportional to each other, and they are often used together to represent the magnitude of the electrical field in the tissues that has been induced by cortical stimulation.

Box 19.1: Electrical field and current density

Intrinsic neuronal response refers to the different neuronal response specific to each parameter of electrical stimulation of the brain. Table 19.1 summarizes four types of computational neuroengineering models that have been exclusively used to evaluate these two factors during cortical stimulation procedures: simple concentric spherical models, high-resolution three-dimensional (3D) realistic head models, motor cortex compartment models, and neuronal circuit models. Concentric spherical and 3D realistic head models are often used to demonstrate the EF/CD, whereas motor cortex compartment and neuronal circuit models are used to represent the intrinsic neuronal or circuit responses.

It is difficult to make a one-to-one comparison of these models. Table 19.2 compares a few parameters of the four neuroengineering models. The 3D realistic head model is becoming the standard neuroengineering model to estimate the induced EF/CD, because this model accommodates more stimulation-related variables such as tissue heterogeneity and anisotropic conductivity. By demonstrating the EF/CD, the concentric spherical and 3D realistic head models both help researchers determine the best target for cortical stimulation.

Table 19.1: Overview of neuroengineering models for cortical stimulation and their applications

Model	Construction of Model	Type of stimulation	Aims of Investigation	Relevant References
Concentric spherical model	Three to five layered concentric shells	TMS	Electrical field /current density distribution induced by TMS Secondary electrical field magnitude	(Datta et al., 2008; Deng et al., 2011)
		tDCS/ TES/ electroconvulsive therapy	Spatial distribution of magnitude and direction of current density Inter-electrode position, size and shape of electrode Optimal electrode positioning for high focality of stimulation	(Faria et al., 2011; Im et al., 2008; Miranda et al., 2013)
3D Realistic head model	Isotropic	TMS	Current in the brain induced by TMS and anatomical change following stroke or cortical atrophy Geometry of magnetic coil Gyral geometry on electrical field	(Tachas and Samaras, 2013; Thielscher et al., 2011; Wagner et al., 2008)
		tDCS	Current density with electrode configuration Electrode configuration in relation with focality of transcranial stimulation Effect of skull defect and lesion on CD Brain current flow in stroke	(Datta et al., 2011; Dmochowski et al., 2013; Edwards et al., 2013)
		ECS	Current density distribution in relation with amplitude, shape of electrode, reference electrode, and polarity	(Kim et al., 2011)
	Anisotropic	TMS	Anisotropic conductivity distribution and distortion of electrical field during TMS	(Opitz et al., 2011)
		tDCS/ electroconvulsive therapy	Effect of anisotropic tissue conductivity on spatial distribution of induced electrical field Antidepressant effect with montage and size of electrode	(Bai et al., 2014; Lee et al., 2012; Shahid et al., 2013)
Motor Cortex Compartment Model	Extruded slab	TMS	Elucidation of physical mechanism and actual stimulation site by TMS	(Salvador et al., 2011)
		ECS	Stimulation response in relation with neuronal orientation, polarity, and CSF thickness, electrode position, etc.	(Manola et al., 2007; Wongsarnpigoon and Grill, 2008, 2011, 2012; Zwartjes et al., 2012)
Neuronal Circuit Model	Cortico-basal ganglia	ECS		(Kang and Lowery, 2013; Rubin and Terman, 2004)

Table 19.2: Comparison of neuroengineering models for cortical stimulation

Parameter	Concentric spherical model	3D realistic head model	Motor cortex compartment model	Neuronal circuit model
Coverage of anatomical structure	Tissue layers overlying brain and gross cortical and subcortical brain	Wider and detailed cortical and subcortical structure	Mostly motor cortex	Structures in cortico-basal ganglia circuit
Reflection of tissue heterogeneity	Moderate	Good	Poor	N/A
Neuronal orientation	Poor	Moderate	Good	N/A
Anisotropic Conductivity	Poor	Good	Poor	N/A
Current density measurement	Moderate	Good	Limited	N/A
Electrode configuration	Moderate	Good	Limited	N/A
Estimation of stimulation parameters	Moderate	Moderate/good	Good	Good
Translational application	Extent of current flow across tissue layers; determine CS target	Determine CS target with EF/CD	Optimization of stimulation parameters	Interaction b/w cortex and basal ganglia

On the other hand, anatomical-physiological factors are known to produce different neuronal responses, depending on the stimulation parameters. For instance, neuronal orientation to the electrical field, size of the nerve fiber, structure of the neuronal circuit, and response to different frequencies may influence the neuronal response to cortical stimulation. Also, there is a discontinuity in stimulation thresholds at the white matter-gray matter boundary. The motor cortex compartment and neuronal circuit models have been proposed to address these issues. In the motor cortex compartment model, single or multiple neurons are modelled to represent the neuronal response to polarity, electrode size and position, and neuronal orientation. The neuronal circuit model explores the response of subcortical structures (basal ganglia and subthalamus) to cortical stimulation. Specifically, this model helps predict the effect of cortical stimulation in Parkinson's disease patients.

19.1 Neuroengineering Models : Pros and Cons

19.1.1 Concentric Spherical Model

The concentric spherical model is the simplest neuroengineering model. It consists of conducting spheres with three to five shells representing the scalp, skull, cerebrospinal fluid, gray matter, and white matter (Fig.19.1). The thickness and conductivity of each shell, or layer, are incorporated in the modeling (Table 19.3).

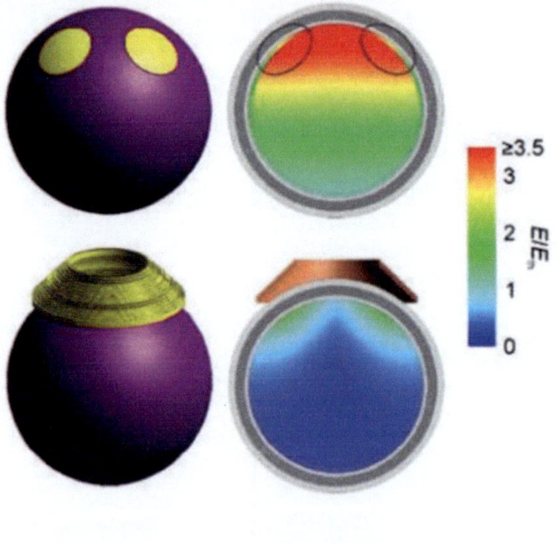

Fig. 19.1: Examples of concentric spherical model. Upper row fig.s demonstrate the electrode position in tDCS and the expected electrical field generated. Lower row fig.s show the position of the magnet in TMS and the expected electrical field. (Modified from Deng et al., 2011, with permission)

Table 19.3: Head parameters used in generating concentric spherical models and 3D realistic head models

Parameter	Thickness (mm)	Conductivity (S/m)
Scalp	5.60	0.33
Skull	7.08	0.0083
Dura	N/A	0.065
Cerebrospinal fluid	3.00	1.79
Gray matter	3.00	0.33
White matter	67.8	0.14
Sponge pad	N/A	0.14

An electrode or magnet placed over the head can be modelled to reproduce the layers' shapes and geometry of the electrode or magnet. This model is useful to estimate the electrical field in the brain induced by non-invasive means (TMS, TES, ECT). The concentric spherical model also allows the researcher to directly compare the configuration and geometry of different electrodes without a concomitant complexity of the head. However, the model does not represent the complex geometry, non-uniform thickness, and heterogeneous conductivity of each tissue layer or the complex morphology of the skull and eye cavity and orifices (which are all potential paths for electrical current). Moreover, this model does not consider the cortical geometry and subcortical structures in the brain or the tissue anisotropy addressed in most spherical models. Therefore, *this model may be underestimating the strength of cortical stimulation for both electrical and magnetic stimulation.*

19.1.1.1 3D Realistic Head Model

Recent advances in computer and finite element modelling (FEM) technology and software have accelerated the use of the 3D realistic head model to elucidate the effect of cortical stimulation (see Box 19.2). 3D realistic modelling has become a popular tool because this model has several advantages. The model more accurately predicts stimulation-induced EF/CD, and it better simulates stimulation-related parameters in the brain. Recently, use of this intricate model has expedited the development of a new strategy for cortical stimulation. The 3D realistic head model holds promise for studying cortical stimulation more easily than before.

To construct a volume conductor model of the head, multiple steps of data processing are required, including segmentation, mesh generation, electrode configuration, tissue property assignment, and finally establishment of the 3D realistic head model (fig.2).
Perform image segmentation to locate the boundaries and objects with same characteristics.
Use T1 and T2-weighted MRI data to reconstruct the skull and scalp boundary.
Use T1 image for cortical (brain) segmentation.
If a neural stimulator is implanted in the chest, the chest area may be also be involved.
Generate volume meshes for each segmented tissue such as scalp, skull, gray matter, white matter, CSF space and sulcus, ventricles, and chest wall.
Combine a variety of electrode factors (size, shape, montage, inter-electrode distances, etc.) and types of stimulation (TMS, tDCS, and ECS, subdural cortical stimulation, etc.) with the volume mesh.
Incorporate electrical conductivity of each tissue layer into the model (Table 3).
The result is a 3D realistic head model that reflects the EF/CD distribution. The model has been generated based on the assumption that each layer has uniform conductivity; however, anisotropic conductivity can be added to reflect the direction of flow by using diffusion tensor imaging (DTI).

Box 19.2: Procedure for making a 3D realistic head model (Kim et al 2011; Seo et al 2012)

This model accommodates the complex environment of the brain, which can influence current flow. Especially useful is that the gyri/sulci structures, scalp and cerebrospinal fluid (CSF) shunting, and electrode configuration and sizes can be incorporated along with skull thickness during cortical stimulation, resulting in more accurate simulation of current flows than provided by the concentric spherical model. Individualized, high-resolution imaging has been applied to the realistic head model; this approach shows the potential to overcome the challenges presented by anatomical differences among diverse subjects. However, *most realistic head models continue to have limitations in implementing the structural details, such as individual neuronal orientation to cortical surface, anatomical connections, and continuously changing brain activities.*

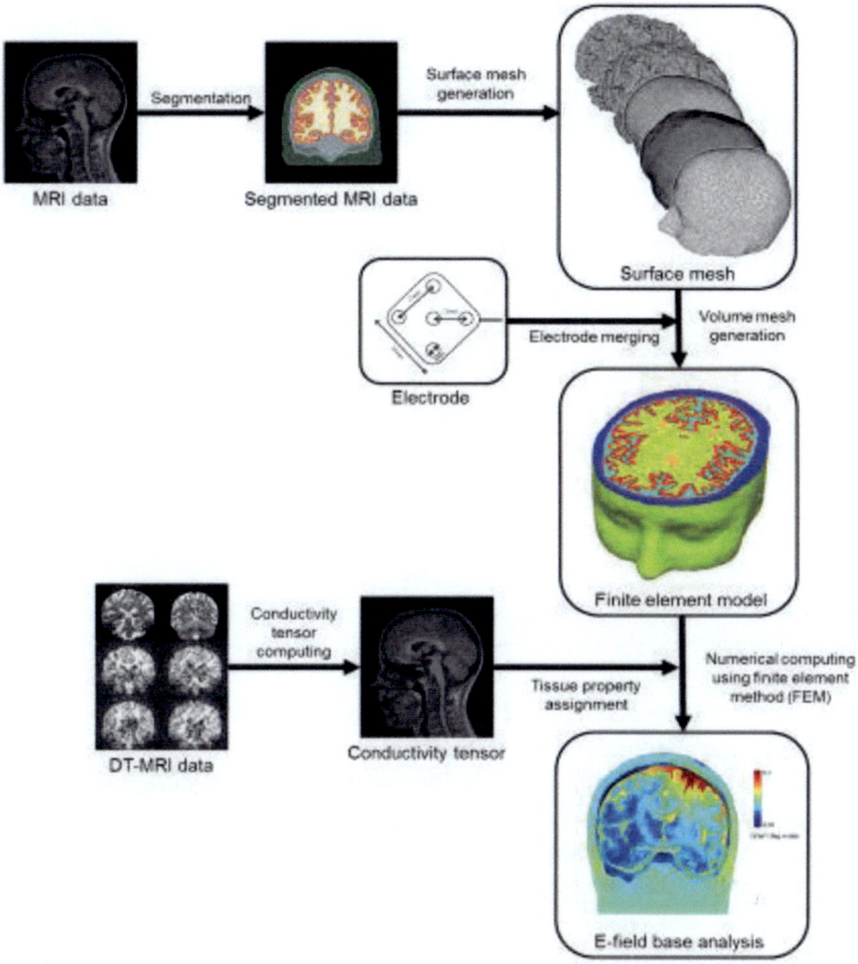

Fig. 19.2: Construction of a 3D realistic head model, including segmentation, mesh generation, establishment of head model, and tissue property assignment.

19.1.2 Motor Cortex Compartment Model

The motor cortex compartment model has been used to delineate the mechanism of motor cortex stimulation by TMS or extradural CS. Researchers have long debated the question of which cells are excited during M1 stimulation and were thus motivated to create this model to exclusively explain the stimulation effect in M1 and adjacent cortices. Recently, this model has been strengthened with the neural component and optimized to determine the neuron-specific response to cortical stimulation in Parkinson's disease (Zwartjes et al., 2012) (Fig.19.3).

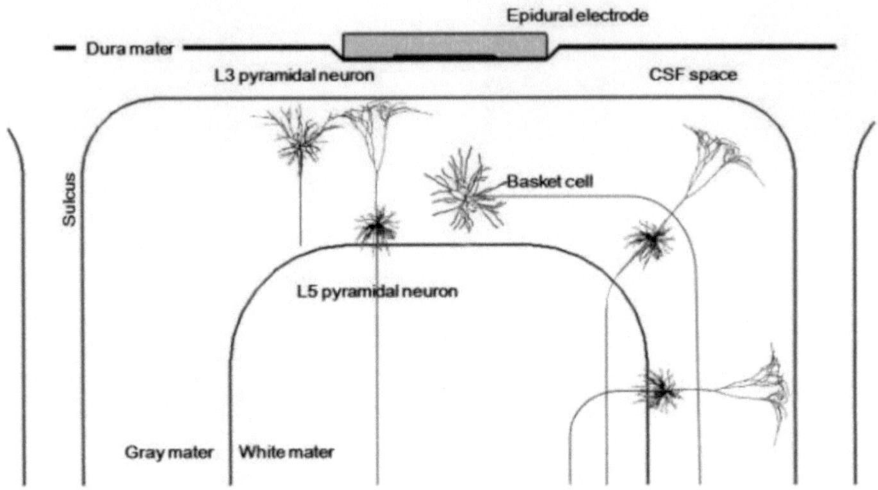

Fig. 19.3: Motor cortex compartment model. Note that the pyramidal neurons and basket cells are oriented vertically and horizontally to cortical surface, respectively.

The motor cortex compartment model incorporates the characteristics of the different neurons. Since the pyramidal and basket cells in the cortex respond to different polarity of the stimulation, the model helps researchers differentiate the neuronal response as a function of the polarity of cortical stimulation. In addition, the cortical folding produces a different orientation of neurons when an electrical field is applied at the crown, lip, and bank of gyrus and around the bottom of the sulcus, up the opposite bank on the postcentral gyrus. For example, electrical properties and geometries of layer 3 and 5 pyramidal neurons are implemented at different angles to represent the different neuronal orientations (Fig.19.3). The strong tangential electric field is known to stimulate the neurons, mostly in the crown of a gyrus or the pyramidal neurons in the walls of the sulcus (Manola et al., 2005; Wongsarnpigoon and Grill, 2009, 2012). Therefore, placing the electrode on the crown and lips of the gyrus activates the neurons at lower amplitude. However, stimulation over the sulcus requires an increased amplitude to excite the neurons in the precentral gyrus. Based on this concept, the influence of electrode position, polarity, and amplitude of ICS is calculated to show the threshold and the site of initiation of action potentials.

This model is useful to figure out the effect of M1 ICS used to control central pain and Parkinsonian symptoms. As several types of neurons are modelled together, the model can show the neuronal responses for different stimulation parameters. The limitation of this model is that the *accurate anatomies of the gyrus and sulcus are not reflected in this box-type cortex*. Thus, variable morphology (shape, depth, and width) of the gyrus and sulcus may not be modelled. Further, because the modelling is confined to the motor cortex and the adjacent precentral and postcentral gyri, it is difficult to interpret the spread of stimulation and changes in the threshold of stimulation due to background cortical activity change.

19.1.3 Neuronal Circuit Model

Cortical stimulation affects not only the cortical areas of the brain but also subcortical structures such as the basal ganglia. This model is based on the basal ganglia circuit, which consists of the cortex, striatum, external and internal segments of the globus pallidus, subthalamic nucleus (STN), and thalamus (Fig.19.4). Specifically, the model includes axons projecting from the cortex to STN (hyperdirect pathway) and axons projecting to direct and indirect pathways in the cortex–basal ganglia circuit. To implement the electrical properties, membrane potentials of the neurons in each component are incorporated to match the firing properties of the basal ganglia and thalamic neurons. Additionally, the model applies the plateau potential responsible for long-lasting bursts in the STN neuron. This model is useful for predicting the effect of cortical stimulation on the STN and basal ganglia in the movement disorders setting; however, it is *not able to explain current flow and distribution in the context of realistic anatomical space.*

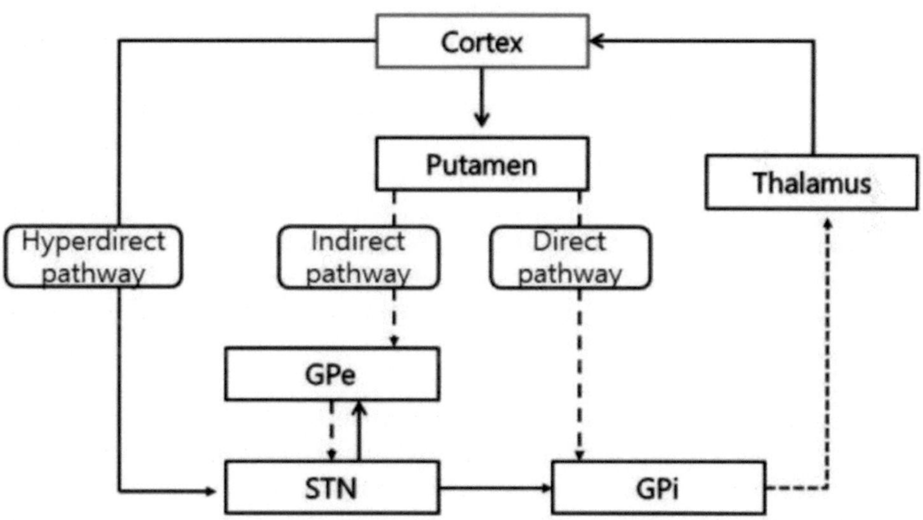

Fig. 19.4: Cortico–basal circuit model showing the connection between cortex and basal ganglia. Excitatory connections are indicated with a solid line and inhibitory connections with a dashed line. GPe: gobus pallidus externa, Gpi: globus pallidus interna, STN: Subthalamic nucleus,

19.2 Validation of the Models

Emerging technologies are typically validated through multiple series of rigorous testing, analyses, and demonstrations. In line with this, neuroengineering models have undergone many trials to prove their feasibility and accuracy. For example, Rush and Driscoll (1968) measured the voltage distribution in an electrolytic tank containing a human half skull and found that the estimated current density agrees well with concentric spherical models. In a trial of direct intracranial measurement of TMS-induced electrical field in the human cortex, Wagner et al (2004) measured TMS-induced current densities in a patient with implanted depth electrodes for epilepsy monitoring. They recorded a maximum current density of 12 A/cm^2 at a depth of 1 cm from scalp surface with an intensity of 7% of the maximal stimulator output. This human experiment showed that the measurement of current densities were in accordance with current theoretical models. This method is useful for validating the accuracy of a subject-specific 3D realistic head model in predicting the CD distribution.

19.3 Application of Models

There is a general agreement that electrical stimulation of the brain, regardless of stimulation methods, produces the EF/CD leading to neuronal activation. Therefore, EF/CD distribution is the primary concern in planning cortical stimulation and the purpose of neuroengineering models is to generate a virtual EF/CD map, in order to guide targeting and parameters selection.

Since the site of neuronal activation is predicted by peak electrical field magnitude (cortical current density) in the cortical neurons,it is critical to generate the electrical field at the targeted area of the brain in which neuronal population is excited or inhibited. Figure 19.5 shows factors that may influence the formation of EF/CD in cortical stimulation. Neuroengineering models provide a virtual map of EF/CD influenced by a convergence of factors, including brain morphology–related, tissue conductivity–related, electrode-related, and stimulation-related factors. Most of the brain morphology–related and tissue conductivity–related factors are implemented while establishing the neuroengineering models. Therefore, more accurate prediction of EF/CD is possible if a more precise model is established by incorporating potential and individual variables. These include electrode and stimulation factors, among others.

Electrode factors include the electrode configuration and geometry, shape, size, inter-electrode distance, and the location of the reference electrode (e.g. Wongsarnpigoon and Grill, 2009, 2012). Stimulation factors include the amplitude, polarity, frequency, and direction of current (AC, DC, and pulsed) (Manola et al., 2007; Wongsarnpigoon and Grill, 2008; Zwartjes et al., 2012). Both sets of factors (described below) can determine the focality and magnitude of EF/CD in the model. Thus, simulation of these factors prior to application of therapeutic stimulation provides an essential guide to determine the target of cortical stimulation. Further calculation of the EF/CD strength required to excite the cortex (mostly motor cortex) in neuroengineering models provides important data towards optimization of parameters of stimulation.

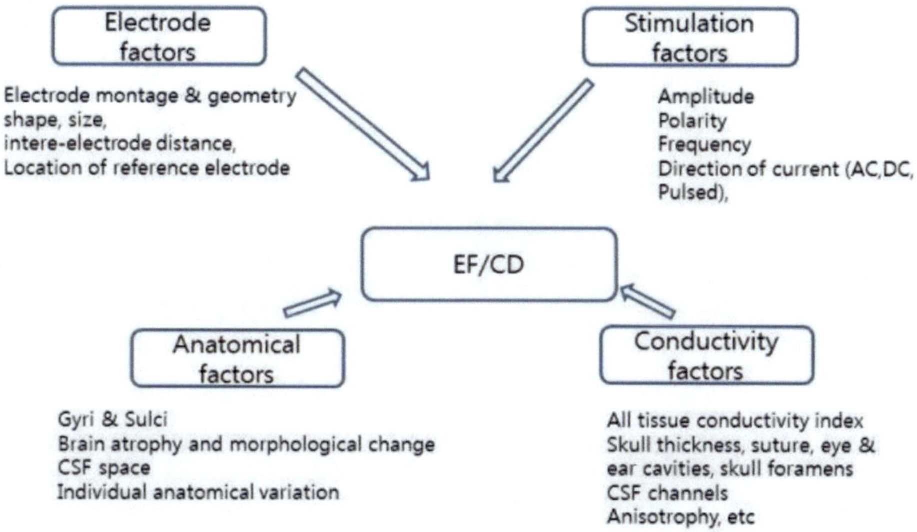

Fig. 19.5: Factors affecting the extent and direction of the EF/CD generated by cortical stimulation

19.4 Electrode Factors

19.4.3.1 Electrode Size and Numbers

The electrode channels the current flow between the source of electricity and target neurons. Therefore, the size and numbers of electrodes are relevant to determine the width of the brain target involved in the intended ICS procedure (Fig.19.6). In ICS, a paddle electrode containing multiple disc electrodes is preferred (Kim et al., 2011). Neuroengineering models such as the 3D realistic head model clearly show the extent of EF/CD under and around the electrode: in the gyri under the center of the electrode, the electrical field increases with decreasing electrode size. If two electrodes are used, the maximum value of the electrical field always occurs in the gyri between electrodes, and the electrical field value increases faster with decreasing electrode size (Miranda et al., 2013).

19.4.3.2 Electrode Configuration

The EF/CD related to the electrode configuration can be well simulated using a 3D realistic head model. Electrode configuration is important to increase the focality and direction of the electrical field. Different electrode montages result in distinct distribution patterns of electrical field, with variations of electrical field strength (Kim et al., 2011). (Fig.19.6,19.7). Therefore, an appropriate combination of electrode position and inter-electrode distance is likely to increase the electrical field in the target area. In ICS, the electrode is usually placed over the target areas and the electrical field is generated around the electrodes. However, the electrode configuration determines an anatomically different EF/CD distribution in the cortical and subcortical areas (Fig.19.7). It is important to carefully plan the electrode configuration to cover the intended areas: *the simple placement of the electrode on the cortex may be not enough to stimulate the desired area of the brain.*

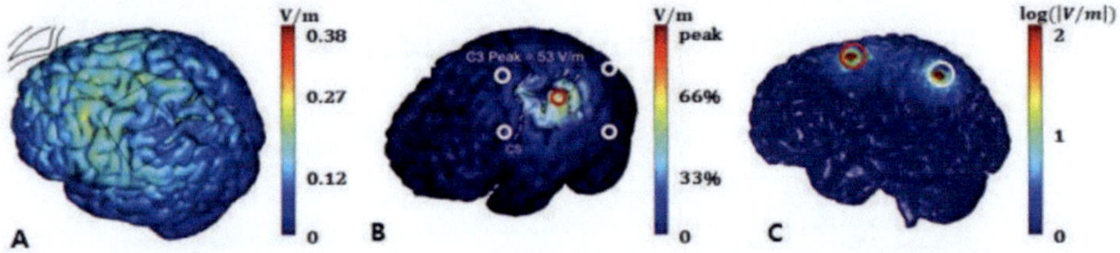

Fig. 19.6: Examples of EF/CD generated by conventional tDCS, high-definition tDCS, and ECS. Note difference in the size and numbers of electrode used in the cortical stimulation. Also note that focalities and strengths of EF/CD are different depending on the methods of cortical stimulation tools. (Modified from Miranda et al., 2013, and Edwards et al., 2013, with permission)

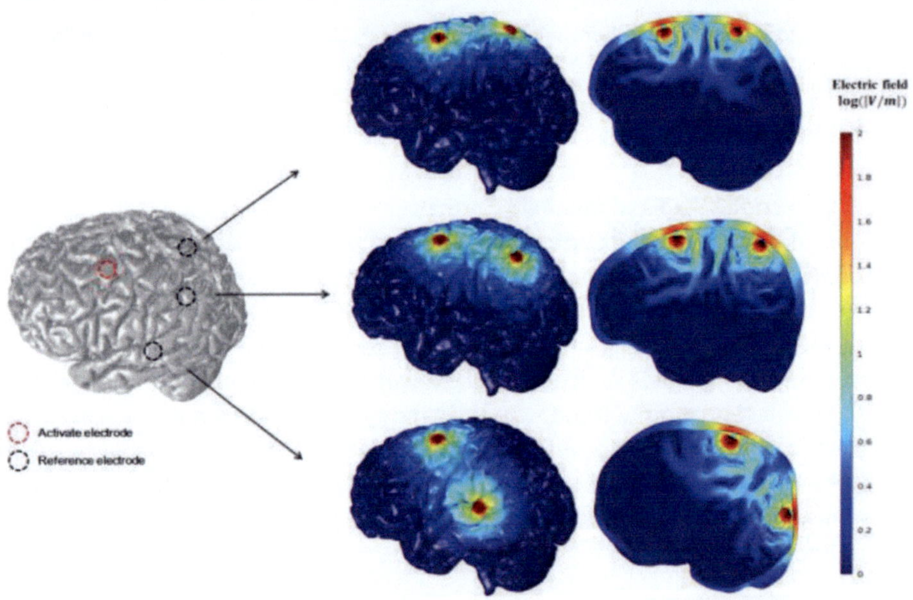

Fig. 19.7: Extent and strengths of EF/CD induced in the cortical surface by different electrode configurations and shapes in transcranial stimulation. Total electrode current was adjusted to produce a 0.328 mV/mm peak electrical field, 1 mm below the cortical surface. (Modified from Datta et al., 2008, with permission)

Measurement of the EF can be extended to include the chest, since the neural stimulator (which often acts as a reference electrode) is usually implanted in the upper chest (Kim et al., 2011). Figure 19.8 demonstrates the extended EF to the upper chest, showing that the EF size depends on the side of the chest where the neural stimulator is located. In this comparison, the side of the implanted neural stimulator did not affect the EF/CD distribution in the brain.

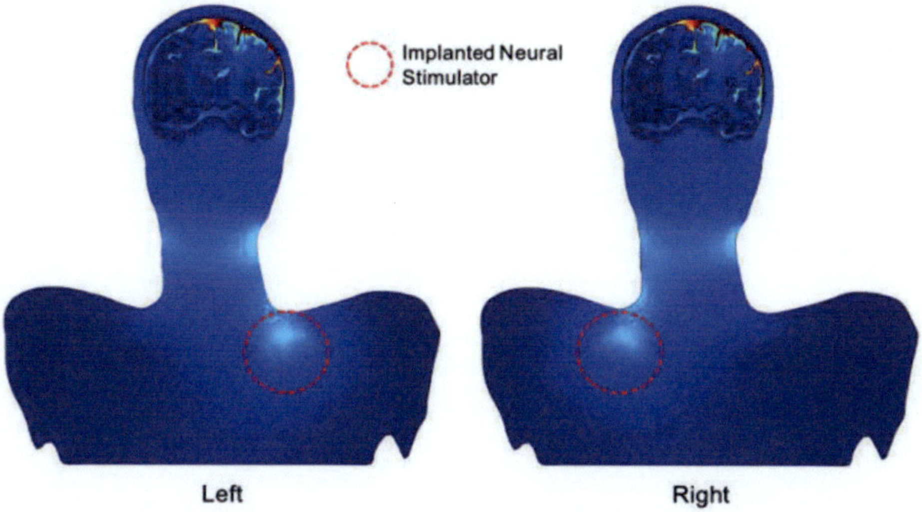

Fig. 19.8: Influence of the location of a neural stimulator chest implant on intracerebral EF/CD. Note that the location did not affect the EF/CD measurements within the brain.

19.4.3.3 Electrode Shape

The influence of the electrode shape can be predicted in a 3D realistic head model. Figure 19.9 compares the EF/CD distribution among bipolar, tripolar, belt, and ring electrodes in tDCS using concentric spherical head models (Datta et al., 2008). Increasing the proximity of two electrodes increases the focality of EF/CD with reduced surface EF/CD. A tripolar electrode at similar distances produces a comparable peak focality with lowered radial bi-directionality. The belt electrode configuration results in radial EF/CD with reduced magnitude of surface EF/CD. The concentric-ring configuration produces the highest spatial focality and unidirectional radial modulation (Datta et al., 2008). This kind of simulation is very helpful in designing new types of electrodes (see also Wei and Grill 2009). We found a very small difference between the disc and ring type of electrodes, although the former seems more effective than the latter.

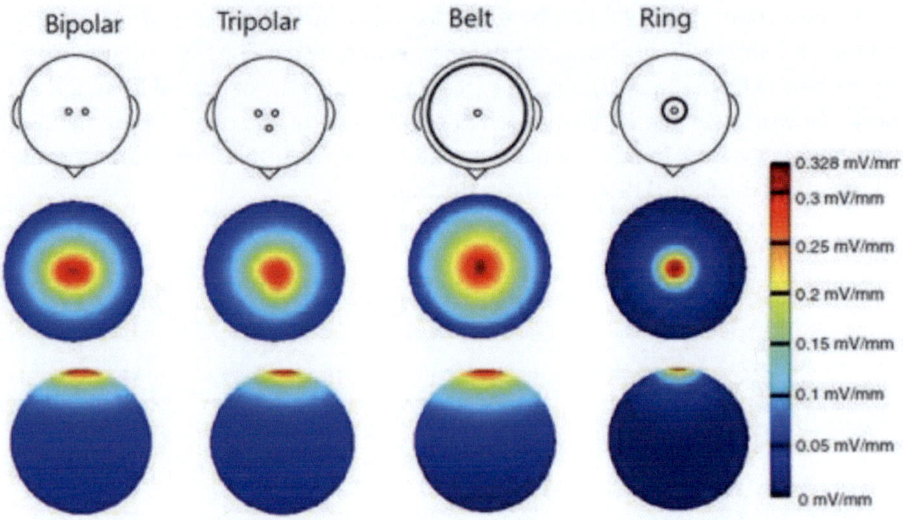

Fig. 19.9: Influence of stimulation amplitude on the EF/CD. The simulation was performed in ECS using a paddle electrode containing five disc electrodes. Note that EF/CD is increasing with increased amplitude.

19.4.1 Stimulation-Related Factors

19.4.1.1 Amplitude of Stimulation

The EF/CD related to stimulation amplitude is well simulated by a 3D realistic head model. CD may be variably distributed in depth and extent by the amplitude of the stimulation (Kim et al., 2011). If a fixed current is used, as in conventional tDCS, this is less of an issue. However, in ICS, a change in amplitude is critical to determine the extent of EF/CD in the target areas. In the specific case of stroke or brain injury, where brain anatomy is disrupted, the extent and volume of EF/CD must be optimized to provide better electrical targeting or to recruit the potential areas for offsetting the damaged area. Figure 19.10 evinces what occurs by changing EF/CD as the amplitude of stimulation is increased in a 3D realistic head model. As expected, the volume and depth are proportionally increased by increasing the amplitude. If simulation is performed in subjects who have experienced anatomical changes before treatment, it becomes possible to adjust the optimal amplitude of stimulation.

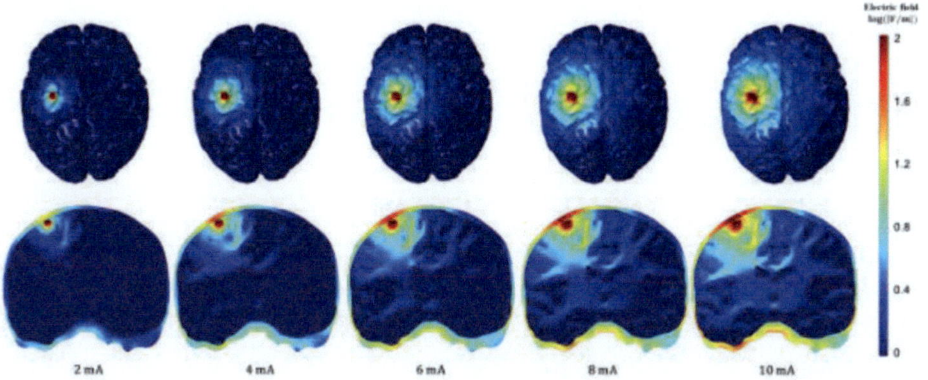

Fig. 19.10: Different EF/CD maps obtained by varying electrode configurations in ECS. An active electrode was placed in the premotor cortex and reference electrodes in the superior parietal, inferior parietal, and superior temporal areas.

19.4.2 Polarity of Stimulation

The neuronal response related to polarity of the stimulation is well simulated using a motor cortex compartment model, because this model incorporates different kinds of neurons and their axons. Neurons in the brain are arranged in a unique pattern and are oriented in particular directions relative to the cortical surface. To demonstrate the relationship between neuronal orientation and neuronal response to different polarity of stimulations, a motor cortex compartment model is often used because the model is convenient to implement the different neurons and their axons. In the cortex, the pyramidal and basket cells are known to be the major neurons to respond clinically to cortical stimulation. The pyramidal neurons lie perpendicular to the surface of the brain and have long axons that run vertically into the subcortical white matter below the cortex. The basket cells are oriented parallel to the pial surfaces and have relatively short axons that run within the grey matter. Zwartjes et al. reported that *cathodal (inhibitory) stimulation selectively activates basket cell axons*, while *pyramidal neurons are selectively targeted using anodal (excitatory) stimulations* from the modelling study of ICS (Fig.19.11) (Zwartjes et al., 2012). Also, *the polarity and amplitude that are most effective at one location on the cortex may be less effective (or ineffective) at another location just a few millimeters away.* Kim et al (2011) and Seo et al (2012) found that *unipolar stimulation can be more effective than bipolar stimulation for functional recovery* and subdural stimulation injects more current in the cortex than epidural stimulation.

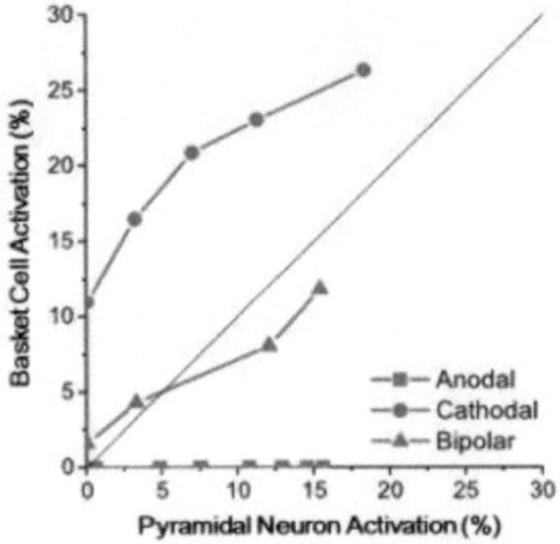

Fig. 19.11: Activation patterns of pyramidal neurons and basket cells using different polarities of stimulation. Note that basket cells are most selectively activated during cathodal stimulation, while pyramidal neurons are most influenced by anodal stimulation. Bipolar stimulation affects both types of cells, but selective activation for each cell type is lower. (Modified from Zwartjes et al., 2012, with permission)

19.4.2.1 Frequency of Stimulation

In ICS, rapid accumulation of excitatory postsynaptic potentials (EPSP) or inhibitory postsynaptic potentials (IPSP) due to higher frequency is likely to drive the tonic subthreshold depolarization or hyperpolarization of the target neurons (Wongsarnpigoon and Grill, 2008). Therefore, an appropriate frequency should be selected based on the calculation of potential benefit using cortical stimulation. In this sense, the neuronal (cortical–basal ganglia) circuit model may be useful to determine the optimal frequency of cortical stimulation to suppress the unwanted oscillatory activity. Kang and Lowery (2013) reported that increased gain through the hyperdirect pathway resulted in the interaction of neural oscillations at different frequencies in the cortex and STN under simulated dopamine depletion conditions, leading to the emergence of synchronized oscillations at a new intermediate frequency. Therefore, research on cortical stimulation with varying frequencies will help determine the optimal parameters of cortical stimulation, e.g. in Parkinson's disease patients.

19.5 Conclusion

Cortical neuromodulation holds great promise for treating neurological and psychiatric disorders that may not be well controlled with medication. Nevertheless, *researchers have yet to elucidate the mechanisms of action and the full gamut of clinical applications: the disparity between theoretical expectations and real effects in cortical stimulation remains to be resolved.*

Neuroengineering models generate a virtual EF/CD map, which may be directly linked to ICS targeting. Considering that the EF/CD map can be changed by different parameters of stimulation, stimulation parameters can be modified in the neuroengineering models to induce the appropriate neuronal response. Neuroengineering models thus provide the foundation to overcome the barriers to better understanding the role of ICS. However, despite their usefulness, *current neuroengineering models are limited, as they do not reflect the anatomical details of cortical and subcortical structures, tissue heterogeneity, and functional connections among the brain structures. In the single patient,* only more intricate models will allow researchers not only to more accurately plan cortical stimulation but also to more consistently predict stimulation effects. At the same time, neuroengineering plays a key role in developing more efficient electrode geometries (Golestanirad et al 2013).

Acknowledgements: This work was supported by a grant from the Institute of Medical System Engineering (iMSE) and GIST-Caltech Collaborative Fund (K03912) from GIST; additional support was provided by the Basic Science Research Program through the National Research Foundation of Korea, funded by the Ministry of Science, ICT [Information and Communications Technology] and Future Planning (201301067890) and by the National Research Foundation funded by the Korean Government (NRF-2010-0026438)

References

Antal, A., Boros, K., Poreisz, C., et al. Comparatively weak after-effects of transcranial alternating current stimulation (tACS) on cortical excitability in humans. Brain Stimul 2008; 1, 97-105.

Antal, A., Polania, R., Schmidt-Samoa, C., et al. Transcranial direct current stimulation over the primary motor cortex during fMRI. Neuroimage 2011; 55, 590-596.

Bai, S., Dokos, S., Ho, K.A., et al. A computational modelling study of transcranial direct current stimulation montages used in depression. Neuroimage. 2014; 87:332-44

Brown, J.A., Lutsep, H.L., Weinand, M., et al. Motor cortex stimulation for the enhancement of recovery from stroke: a prospective, multicenter safety study. Neurosurgery 2006; 58, 464-473.

Datta, A., Baker, J.M., Bikson, M., et al. Individualized model predicts brain current flow during transcranial direct-current stimulation treatment in responsive stroke patient. Brain Stimul 2011; 4, 169-174.

Datta, A., Bansal, V., Diaz, J., et al. Gyri-precise head model of transcranial direct current stimulation: improved spatial focality using a ring electrode versus conventional rectangular pad. Brain Stimul 2009; 2, 201-207, 207 e201.

Datta, A., Elwassif, M., Battaglia, F., et al. Transcranial current stimulation focality using disc and ring electrode configurations: FEM analysis. J Neural Eng 2008; 5, 163-174.

Datta, A., Zhou, X., Su, Y., et al. Validation of finite element model of transcranial electrical stimulation using scalp potentials: implications for clinical dose. J Neural Eng 2013; 10, 036018.

Deng, Z.D., Lisanby, S.H., Peterchev, A.V. Electric field strength and focality in electroconvulsive therapy and magnetic seizure therapy: a finite element simulation study. J Neural Eng 2011; 8, 016007.-

Dmochowski JP, Datta A, Huang Y, et al. Targeted transcranial direct current stimulation for rehabilitation after stroke. Neuroimage. 2013;75:12-9

Edwards, D., Cortes, M., Datta, A., et al. Physiological and modeling evidence for focal transcranial electrical brain stimulation in humans: a basis for high-definition tDCS. Neuroimage 2013; 74, 266-275.

Faria, P., Hallett, M., Miranda, P.C. A finite element analysis of the effect of electrode area and inter-electrode distance on the spatial distribution of the current density in tDCS. J Neural Eng 2011; 8, 066017.

Ferdjallah, M., Bostick, F.X., Jr., Barr, R.E. Potential and current density distributions of cranial electrotherapy stimulation (CES) in a four-concentric-spheres model. IEEE Trans Biomed Eng 1996; 43, 939-943.

Golestanirad L, Pollo C, Graham SJ. Analysis of fractal electrodes for efficient neural stimulation. EMBC 2013 35th Annual Int.Conference of the IEEE, 3-7 July 2013, 791-794

Im, C.H., Jung, H.H., Choi, J.D., et al. Determination of optimal electrode positions for transcranial direct current stimulation (tDCS). Phys Med Biol 2008; 53, N219-225.

Im, C.H., Park, J.H., Shim, M., et al. Evaluation of local electric fields generated by transcranial direct current stimulation with an extracephalic reference electrode based on realistic 3D body modeling. Phys Med Biol 2012; 57, 2137-2150.

Kim, D., Jun, S.C., Kim, H.I. Computational study of subdural and epidural cortical stimulation of the motor cortex. Conf Proc IEEE Eng Med Biol Soc 2011, 7226-7229.

Kirsch, D.L., Smith, R.B. The use of cranial electrotherapy stimulation in the management of chronic pain: A review. NeuroRehabilitation 2000; 14, 85-94.

Lee, W.H., Deng, Z.D., Kim, T.S., et al. Regional electric field induced by electroconvulsive therapy in a realistic finite element head model: influence of white matter anisotropic conductivity. Neuroimage 2012; 59, 2110-2123.

Lee, W.H., Kim, T.S. Methods for high-resolution anisotropic finite element modeling of the human head: automatic MR white matter anisotropy-adaptive mesh generation. Med Eng Phys 2012; 34, 85-98.

Manola, L., Holsheimer, J., Veltink, P. et al. Anodal vs cathodal stimulation of motor cortex: a modeling study. Clin Neurophysiol 2007; 118, 464-474.

Manola, L., Roelofsen, B.H., Holsheimer, J., et al. Modelling motor cortex stimulation for chronic pain control: electrical potential field, activating functions and responses of simple nerve fibre models. Med Biol Eng Comput 2005; 43, 335-343.

Miranda, P.C., Lomarev, M., Hallett, M. Modeling the current distribution during transcranial direct current stimulation. Clin Neurophysiol 2006; 117, 1623-1629.

-Miranda, P.C., Mekonnen, A., Salvador, R., et al. The electric field in the cortex during transcranial current stimulation. Neuroimage 2013; 70, 48-58.

Nagarajan, S.S., Durand, D.M. Analysis of magnetic stimulation of a concentric axon in a nerve bundle. IEEE Trans Biomed Eng 1995; 42, 926-933.

Nagarajan, S.S., Durand, D.M., Warman, E.N. Effects of induced electric fields on finite neuronal structures: a simulation study. IEEE Trans Biomed Eng 1993; 40, 1175-1188.

Nathan, S.S., Sinha, S.R., Gordon, B., et al. Determination of current density distributions generated by electrical stimulation of the human cerebral cortex. Electroencephalogr Clin Neurophysiol 1993; 86, 183-192.

Nitsche, M.A., Liebetanz, D., Tergau, F., et al. [Modulation of cortical excitability by transcranial direct current stimulation]. Nervenarzt 2002; 73, 332-335.

-Nitsche, M.A., Paulus, W. Transcranial direct current stimulation--update 2011. Restor Neurol Neurosci 2011; 29, 463-492.

Opitz, A., Windhoff, M., Heidemann, R.M., et al. How the brain tissue shapes the electric field induced by transcranial magnetic stimulation. Neuroimage 2011; 58, 849-859.

Rubin, J.E., Terman, D. High frequency stimulation of the subthalamic nucleus eliminates pathological thalamic rhythmicity in a computational model. J Comput Neurosci 2004; 16, 211-235.

Rush, S., Driscoll, D.A. Current distribution in the brain from surface electrodes. Anesth Analg 1968; 47, 717-723.

Salvador, R., Silva, S., Basser, P.J. et al. Determining which mechanisms lead to activation in the motor cortex: a modeling study of transcranial magnetic stimulation using realistic stimulus waveforms and sulcal geometry. Clin Neurophysiol 2011; 122, 748-758.

Seo, H., Kim, D., Jun, S.C. A comparative study of the 3D precentral gyrus model for unipolar and bipolar current stimulations. Conf Proc IEEE Eng Med Biol Soc 2012, 1892-1895.

Shahid, S., Wen, P., Ahfock, T. Assessment of electric field distribution in anisotropic cortical and subcortical regions under the influence of tDCS. Bioelectromagnetics. 2013

Suihko, V. Modelling the response of scalp sensory receptors to transcranial electrical stimulation. Med Biol Eng Comput 2002; 40, 395-401.

-Tachas, N.J., Samaras, T. The effect of head and coil modeling for the calculation of induced electric field during transcranial magnetic stimulation. Int J Psychophysiol. 2013

Terney, D., Chaieb, L., Moliadze, V., et al. Increasing human brain excitability by transcranial high-frequency random noise stimulation. J Neurosci 2008; 28, 14147-14155.

Thielscher, A., Opitz, A., Windhoff, M. Impact of the gyral geometry on the electric field induced by transcranial magnetic stimulation. Neuroimage 2011; 54, 234-243.

Wagner, T., Eden, U., Fregni, F., et al. Transcranial magnetic stimulation and brain atrophy: a computer-based human brain model study. Exp Brain Res 2008; 186, 539-550.

Wagner, T., Fregni, F., Fecteau, S., et al. Transcranial direct current stimulation: a computer-based human model study. Neuroimage 2007; 35, 1113-1124.

Wagner, T., Gangitano, M., Romero, R., et al. Intracranial measurement of current densities induced by transcranial magnetic stimulation in the human brain. Neurosci Lett 2004; 354, 91-94.

Wei XF, Grill WM. Analysis of high-perimeter planar electrodes for efficient neural stimulation. Front Neuroeng. 2009 Nov 10;2:15.

Wongsarnpigoon, A., Grill, W.M. Computational modeling of epidural cortical stimulation. J Neural Eng 2008; 5, 443-454.

Wongsarnpigoon, A., Grill, W.M. Effects of stimulation parameters and electrode location on thresholds for epidural stimulation of cat motor cortex. J Neural Eng. 2011;8:066016.

Wongsarnpigoon A, Grill W.M. Optimization of parameter selection and electrical targeting. In: Canavero S (ed) Textbook of therapeutic cortical stimulation. New York: Nova Sci. 2009, 69-90

Wongsarnpigoon, A., Grill, W.M. Computer-based model of epidural motor cortex stimulation: effects of electrode position and geometry on activation of cortical neurons. Clin Neurophysiol 2012; 123, 160-172.

Zwartjes, D.G., Heida, T., Feirabend, H.K. et al. Motor cortex stimulation for Parkinson's disease: a modelling study. J Neural Eng 2012; 9, 056005.

Elena Rossi, Alberto Priori, Sara Marceglia

20 Modelization: Theoretical Aspects

Non-invasive cortical stimulation methods (TMS, tDCS) are known to have limitations, including the shunt of the current due to high impedance barriers (scalp and skull) and the difficulty in providing continuous therapies without interfering with normal daily activities, since the stimulating devices are not implanted in the patient (Priori and Lefaucheur 2007). Conversely, extradural cortex stimulation (ECS) and subdural cortex stimulation (SCS) use surgically implantable stimulation systems consisting of electrodes placed epidurally or subdurally and connected to a subcutaneous pulse generator. They have the potential to provide a continuous treatment without limiting patient's activities. In general, cortical stimulation consists of injecting electrical current or voltage through electrode(s) into the head or directly to the brain. The applied field can variously induce a modulated neuronal activation (neuronal firing), a synchronization of neuronal populations, or a change in neuronal excitability. The aim of modeling is to represent the spatial distribution and amplitude of the electrical field injected and to interpret its impact on target brain areas. These studies can improve ECS/SCS clinical outcomes by optimizing electrode design, device implantation and stimulation parameters selection, thus reducing side effects and improving outcomes.

20.1 Computational Modeling Priciples

In physics, Maxwell's equation can represent the behavior of the electrical field within the head or brain and we can get, in a quasi-stationary condition, the following Laplace equation defined in the computational head model:

$$\nabla\bullet(\sigma\nabla\varphi)=0 \text{ in } \Omega \tag{2.I}$$

where: scalar electric potential; ∇: gradient vector; and σ: tissues' conductivity.

The quasi-static approximation is a valid assumption for typical neural stimulation parameters (Bossetti et al 2008).

This approximation cannot be accurately applied to cases involving Transcranial Magnetic Stimulation (TMS) because the magnetic field generated does not remain constant over time. With cases of TMS, it is necessary to consider the Maxwell-Faraday equation:

$$\nabla x\, E = -\frac{\partial B}{\partial t} \tag{2.II}$$

where B is the magnetic field generated by the coil and E the electric field induced into the tissue.

The ideal solution for the Maxwell's equations is analytic, without approximations and continuous in time and space. Unfortunately, from a computational viewpoint, the solution to the purely analytical electromagnetic problem is too expensive and also the modelling of the sources and the transmission medium cannot be completely realistic. For these reasons, the numerical solution of the electromagnetic problem is usually implemented by a computational model. This solution is discrete in the time and in the frequency domains, and it is always affected by approximations. In fact, the numerical solution of differential equations requires the discretization of time and space in appropriate mesh grids consisting of a finite number of elements in which the partial derivatives are replaced by finite differences (that are their numerical approximation). Finite Element Method (FEM), Boundary Element Method (BEM), Finite Integration Technique (FIT) are examples of methods that can be used for the numerical solution of Maxwell's equations.

20.2 Head Model and Tissue Connectivity

The characterization of electrical properties of brain tissue is a fundamental issue for computational modelling methods. Within biological tissues, electric fields drive currents with ohmic (resistive) and displacement (capacitive) components. Ohmic currents are generated by the movement of free charges, such as unbound extracellular sodium and potassium ions, and are measured in terms of electrical conductivity of the medium. Displacement currents are generated by the polarization of paired charges, such as ionic double-layers that surround cellular membranes and/or macromolecules embedded in cellular membranes. *Electrical permittivity* is the measure of this polarization. Impedance measurements in ex-vivo tissues revealed that displacement currents are orders of magnitude smaller than ohmic (Wagner 2004, 2007). In-vivo recordings of the electromagnetic fields generated in brain tissues by TMS (Tay, 1992; Tay et al., 1989) and DBS (Miocinovic et al., 2009) suggest that the stimulatory fields are influenced by both tissue capacitance and resistance. This suggests that past theories of brain stimulation may not fully describe fundamental biophysical processes occurring in neural tissues, which could conversely influence the predicted response and the safety consideration that guide the clinical use of brain stimulation (Wagner et al., 2007). Furthermore, coupled displacement and ohmic mechanisms in the neural tissue could lead to frequency dependent filtering of the applied stimulatory fields, or endogenously generated fields, thus changing the expected distributions. Wagner et al (2014) recorded the in-vivo impedances of brain tissues during neurosurgical procedures and used these results to construct magnetic resonance image (MRI) guided computational models of TMS and DBS. Their results are relevant also to other CS techniques since they are all based on tissue conductivity parameters. They measured the conductivity, σ, and permittivity, ε, values of tissues, in the frequency range from 10 to 50000 Hz, in anesthetized animals that can be used for comparison to the current ex-vivo estimated values. Then they evaluated how these tissue properties affected TMS and DBS stimulatory fields: they constructed MRI guided FEMs of the human head based on the individual tissue impedance properties recorded in-vivo and compared their results with FEMs based on classical ex-vivo impedance values. The recorded impedance properties of the skin, skull, gray matter, and white matter differed substantially compared to past tissue impedance values used for characterizing the fields of neurostimulation. Conductivities were generally within the range of past reported magnitudes used for brain stimulation studies, with a slightly greater frequency response, but permittivities differed greatly in magnitude and frequency response to values typically implemented in neurostimulation modeling ((IFAP), 2007; Foster and Schwan, 1996; Gabriel et al., 1996; Wagner et al., 2004, 2007). Such sizeable differences in the overall permittivity values can be due to the alteration of tissue impedance properties in ex-vivo models where cell are degenerated and/or death. Overall, Wagner et al. (2014) demonstrated that the living tissue carries currents through both dipole and ionic mechanisms, in a frequency-dependent manner. They found also significant alterations of the TMS and DBS field distributions in the brain when comparing the solutions from the in-vivo tissue impedance recordings with those from past ex-vivo values commonly used for modeling brain stimulation. Predicted stimulation thresholds were consistently higher for the in-vivo models compared to those resulting from the ex-vivo tissue systems. The in-vivo systems higher thresholds were due to the increased tissue impedance attenuation of the stimulatory electric fields. The application of these parameters estimated in-vivo may change the results obtained in modeling the effects in other CS techniques and should be considered in future modeling studies.

20.3 Models of Implantable Cortical Stimulation (ICS)

ICS systems consist of epidurally or subdurally placed electrodes connected to an implantable pulse generator. The main difference between epidural cortical stimulation (ECS) and subdural cortical stimulation (SCS) is the electrode placement, right above the dura mater (ECS) and right beneath the dura mater (SCS) respectively. Compared to SCS, ECS is less invasive and safer in inducing seizures (Bezard et al. 1999). However, SCS has more focality and less loss of current, yielding higher efficiency. Conversely, ECS is strongly influenced by the thickness or conductivity of the dura mater (Wongsarnpigoon and Grill 2008). Subdural stimulation is more focused with lower current intensities compared to ECS; SCS however has a higher complication rate due to epileptic seizures, intracerebral hemorrhages and wound infections. In general, stimulation devices can deliver the output current in two different ways: current controlled or voltage controlled stimulation. In current-controlled devices, the user specifies the device output in units of Amperes and the current output will be kept constant while the voltage will be adjusted to keep the current intensity at the desired level. Conversely, in voltage-controlled devices, the user specifies the device output in units of Volts, and the output voltage will be kept constant while the output current will change according to the tissue impedance. Whereas non-invasive cortical stimulation methods (tDCS and TMS) have been extensively investigated using computational models, there is a lack of reports studying SCS likely due to difficulties in model generation. As explained in Kim et al (2011), the current density distribution (CDD) in invasive CS can be estimated by solving the Laplace equation (2.I) with the following assumptions:

- the Neumann boundary condition is applied to the upper boundary on skull because the electric flux through skull is negligibly small:

$$n \cdot J = 0 \text{ on } \partial\,\Omega_{\text{upper}} \tag{4.I}$$

where n is the normal vector to the boundary

- The Dirichlet boundary condition is applied to the remaining outer boundaries in the model and the upper boundary on electrode (s) surface:

$$V = 0 \text{ on } \partial\,\Omega_{\text{other}} \tag{4.II}$$

$$V = V_0 \text{ on } \partial\,\Psi_{\text{upper}} \tag{4.III}$$

where V_0 is considered as an input value.

In the case of voltage controlled stimulation, when voltage is injected through the electrode and kept constant, the corresponding total current induced over the model can be estimated with the following equation:

$$0 = \int_{\Omega} \nabla \cdot (\sigma \nabla V) dr = \int_{\partial\Omega} (\sigma \nabla V) \cdot n \, dS$$
$$= \int_{\partial\Omega upper} (\sigma \nabla V) \cdot n \, dS + \int_{\partial\Omega other} (\sigma \nabla V) \cdot n \, dS - \int_{\partial\Psi upper} (\sigma \nabla V) \cdot n \, dS$$

where n is outward normal vector on the boundary. Since in invasive CS the vector n is directed inward, the third term changes in sign. Hence, considering the boundary conditions, the current induced by voltage input to the electrodes (output current) is estimated by:

$$I_{\text{output}} = \int_{\partial\Psi upper} \sigma \frac{dV}{dn} \, dS = \int_{\partial\Omega other} \sigma \frac{dV}{dn} \, dS \tag{4.IV}$$

The total output current is the sum of all currents flowing out of the model's boundaries below the electrode.

20.3.1 Extradural ICS Models

Different studies using human motor cortex finite element models (including detailed anatomical structures such as gyrus and sulci) estimated the spatial distribution of the stimulation potential in the cortical tissue, that, combined with compartmental neuron models for the simulation, could also be used to estimate the subsequent response of neural elements. These studies demonstrated that many factors can influence the neurons excitability during ECS. The combination of conductor volume models with compartmental neuronal models allowed researchers to evaluate the effects of ECS on neuronal excitation.

20.3.1.1 Electrode Design

Electrode design is a crucial factor that influences the power supplied by the implanted pulse generator (IPG). In order to avoid frequent surgical replacement of battery-depleted IPGs, the electrode design has to reduce power usage. Surgical leads used for ECS have heterogeneous geometry: FEMs can be useful to better understand the impact of electrode's material, geometry, shape and lead's location on device efficiency.

According to Ohm's Law the power consumed by electrode and tissue is equal to

$$i^2 \text{x}\, Z_{\text{load}}$$

where i is the stimulation current and Z_{load} is the load impedance (series combination of tissue resistance, interface impedance of the working and the return electrodes). Different materials can be used to reduce the electrode impedance. Moreover, by suppressing tissue encapsulation of the implanted electrode during the inflammation process, also the stimulation thresholds can be reduced. The electrode geometry can influence the efficiency of the stimulation by decreasing the power necessary to achieve the same level of cortical excitability. In fact the activation function f of neurons can be considered (Rattay, 1989) proportional to the second spatial derivate of the extracellular potential V_e:

$$f_x \propto \frac{\Delta^2 V_e}{\Delta x^2} = \frac{\Delta J_x}{-\sigma \Delta x}$$

this means that the activating function in the x direction is proportional to the derivative of the current density (J). Wei and Grill (2009) investigated the effects on stimulation efficiency of different electrode geometries. In order to increase the spatial non-uniformity of J, they increased the electrode perimeter (using a serpentine shape) without changing the electrode area. They created FEM models of different electrodes and, to quantify stimulation efficiency, each resulting potential was coupled with cable models of a population of axons. They demonstrated that increasing the perimeter of the electrode results in an increase of the activation function of neurons underneath. Thus, the stimulation efficiency of planar disk electrodes can be improved by high-perimeter designs. However, before this new electrode geometry can be introduced for clinical use, safety aspects have to be considered, as higher current densities on the electrode surface may induce tissue damage (Kronberg and Bikson, 2012). In the specific case of ECS, changing electrode geometry could also mean varying the distance between contacts of the same epidural lead, the diameter of each electrode or the width of the substrate. The inter-electrode spacing (ISI) can influence not only the spread of stimulation but also the stimulation thresholds: a reduction of the distance between electrodes increases the threshold in motor cortex during bipolar stimulation and decreases it during equipolar stimulation. Also, the diameter of each electrode can influence the threshold amplitude in the underlying gyri. Substrate width has little influence on the threshold of the neurons around the edge of the substrate (Wongsarnpigoon et Grill, 2012).

20.3.1.2 Electrode Position

MEP recording experiments (Wongsarnpigoon et Grill, 2011) showed that the excitability threshold of neurons are lower in primary sites as compared to secondary sites, so that the electrode location over the primary area can reduce the stimulation intensity necessary for cortical excitation (with a consequent reduction of battery consumption). Efficiency of ECS depends not only on the distance of the neuronal populations from the electrode (Wei and Grill 2009), but also on the relative position between the electrode and the underlying sulci or gyri, because deep neurons within sulci have larger stimulation thresholds than those on the crown and lips of the gyri. In general, stimulation thresholds are lowest on the crown or lip of the precentral gyrus beneath the active electrode (Wongsarnpigoon et Grill, 2012). Also the rotation of the lead placed over the central sulcus can alter the stimulation threshold in adjacent gyri (Wongsarnpigoon et Grill, 2012). Wongsarnpigoon and Grill (2008) additonally carried out different simulations varying the thickness of tissues in an extruded slab model of the precentral gyrus, characterized by an anisotropic conductivity in the white matter. Their results showed that, by placing the ECS electrode directly above the gyrus, about half of the stimulus current flowed through the crown of the gyrus while the current density was lower along the banks deep in the sulci.

20.3.1.3 Electrode Polarity

In order to investigate the effect of polarity on the stimulation threshold during ECS, a 3D model of the motor cortex was developed (Wongsarnpigoon et Grill, 2012) and the electric potentials within the cortex were calculated. Since the polarity was expected to affect the responses depending on the neuron orientations, the model was characterized by an anisotropic conductivity: inside the white matter the electrical conductivity was higher in the axial direction because the orientation of the fibers in this tissue is mostly perpendicular to the skull. In order to determine the excitation thresholds, the estimated potentials were applied to a compartmental model of cortical neurons: pyramidal cells (PCs) of layer 3 (L3) and 5 (L5) and thalamocortical axons (TCAs). Anodal and cathodal stimulations had opposite effects. For cathodal stimulation of L3 PCs, thresholds were lower on the bank of the precentral gyrus than on the crown. Anodal thresholds were lower than cathodal ones on the crown of the precentral gyrus for L3 and L5 PCs, and higher for TCAs. Neurons could be activated by opposite stimulation polarity, according to the orientation of their axons relative to the electrode, as the site of action potential generation is the terminal of the axon. The results of this study demonstrated that thresholds were affected more by neuron orientation than by the reciprocal position between neurons and electrodes. Wongsarnpigoon and Grill (2008, 2012)'s data confirm previous computer modeling studies (Manola et al. 2005) that described a polarity-conditioned excitation of nerve fibers arranged parallel or perpendicular to the electrode surface. These fibers were excitable only by cathodal (parallel) or anodal (perpendicular) stimulation respectively. The same results were obtained using a more detailed compartmental neuron model including the axon, soma and dendritic trunk (Manola et al. in 2007). In general, the introduction of a soma-dendritic model reduced the estimated excitation threshold compared to the simulation results using the simpler axonal model. They however confirmed that anodal stimulation excited neural elements perpendicular to the electrode surface and cathodal stimulation neural element parallel to the electrode surface. Despite different models, the two approaches were consistent in describing the effects of anodal and cathodal stimulation. These models however were made only with separate and independent neurons: a more detailed model with interneurons would be useful to better understand the communication between neurons during anodal and cathodal ECS. Other useful information about the effects of stimulation polarity comes from MEP recording experiments in animals, as done by Wongsarnpigoon and Grill (2011): excitation thresholds for anodal and cathodal ECS were equal when the stimulation electrode was placed over the primary site, whereas over the secondary site cathodal thresholds were significantly lower than anodal thresholds for evoking a response in primary muscle. These result suggest that, *during therapeutic ECS, the polarity and amplitude that are most effective at one location of the cortex may be less effective a few millimeters away.*

20.3.1.4 Monopolar and Bipolar Stimulation

Even though available ECS devices do not yet allow clinicians to fully control the montage (monopolar, bipolar or equipolar), FEM studies reveal that the choice of montage can influence ECS outcomes. During monopolar stimulation, all the electrodes have the same polarity, whereas during bipolar stimulation some electrodes act as anodes (positive polarity) and others as cathodes (negative polarity). Bipolar ECS, employed in most clinical applications, is believed to induce a more focal stimulation over a specific cortical area due to the proximity of the anode and the cathode. Indeed, results from FEM simulations (Wongsarnpigoon et Grill, 2011, 2012) evince that bipolar stimulation increases neuronal threshold compared to monopolar stimulation for neurons beyond the electrodes. The lowest thresholds were identified in the region beneath the electrodes. The non-passive return electrode may be responsible for the different outcomes observed using bipolar and monopolar stimulations. This result was observed in studies where monopolar ECS of human motor cortex induced larger EMG responses than during bipolar stimulation (Holsheimer et al. 2007). Moreover bipolar or equipolar stimulation produces a confounding effect because the two electrodes stimulate different populations of neurons. During bipolar and equipolar stimulation, one of the two electrodes is sometimes placed on an adjacent gyrus in order to minimize interaction between neurons. However, this configuration is characterized by a lower threshold in the adjacent gyrus compared to the stimulation with the leads parallel to the pre-central gyrus, thus leading to possible ECS side effects. For these reasons, modeling suggests that *the simplest method of stimulation is monopolar or equipolar over the target.*

20.3.1.5 Stimulation Waveform

The stimulation waveform delivered to the tissue depends on the stimulation type (voltage- or current- controlled), the stimulation frequency, and the number of pulses delivered per time unit. The effects of stimulation type were investigated by Wongsarpigoon and Grill (2008). The neuronal activating function was found to be inversely proportional to the thickness of CSF and dura during voltage controlled stimulation. In case of current controlled stimulation, instead, they found influences only from the thickness of cerebrospinal fluid (CSF) and not from the dura. This means that in *current controlled ECS, treatment outcomes are less affected by individual anatomical features*. However, the thickness of the CSF layer between the dura mater and the cortex beneath the electrode always influences the distribution of the electrical field and the excitation threshold due to its highest electrical conductivity (Manola et al. 2005). A possible explanation of the different level of activation obtained with current controlled or voltage controlled stimulation could be the difference in shape of voltage and current waveforms, due to the capacitive behavior of tissues and the electrode-tissue interface (Merrill et al. 2005). ECS was delivered in anesthetized animal (Wongsarnpigoon et Grill, 2011) in order to investigate the effect of two stimulation parameters (stimulation frequency and number of pulses per train) on the threshold for evoking motor responses. Thresholds were measured for monopolar anodal and cathodal ECS over the primary site and were defined as the amplitude necessary to evoke EMG responses. The result was that the threshold for evoking EMG responses is inversely related to both the parameters analyzed.

20.3.2 Subdural SCS Models

Whereas selective stimulation of neurons located deep within sulci is very difficult with ECS, subdural stimulation (SCS) may allow more localized stimulation of deep neurons in sulci: the location of the electrodes on the cerebral surface and beneath the dura mater reduces the loss of current in the cerebral spinal fluid (CSF). SCS is generally less frequently used than ECS even though it is more focal. Again, FEM studies can be useful to investigate the effect of different factors on SCS efficiency.

20.3.2.1 The Electrode Factor: Design, Position and Polarity

Kim et al (2012) investigated the effects of three SCS electrode types (disc, ring, and covered-disc) and the stimulation condition (voltage controlled vs current controlled stimulation) in bipolar subdural cortical stimulation (SCS). In the covered-disc, all the sides of the electrode were covered by a substrate; only a metal internal disc on the bottom face of the cylinder was in contact with the cortex. This electrode model is more realistic because the SCS devices used in clinic include an array of electrodes characterized by metal contacts insulated with silicone membranes in order to avoid current leakage into the CSF. Using a MRI-derived 3D realistic head FEM model, the authors proposed three efficiency measures to compare the effectiveness of the stimulation between different stimulation conditions:

- effective depth of penetration: diameter of the region having current density above the effective threshold (for the motor cortex is $2.5 A/m^2$ at frequency 50Hz, Kowalski et al. 2002).
- effective volume: the volume of the region with current density exceeding the effective threshold
- amount of CSF leakage current: amount of current that flows out to cerebrospinal fluid. CSF leakage current can be computed by the following equation:

$$\iiint_{\Omega} Jnorm\, dV$$

where Ω is the cerebrospinal fluid domain and J_{norm} is the magnitude of the current density. If CSF leakage current is high, much of the current flows to cerebrospinal fluid but not the cortex. Therefore, cerebrospinal fluid leakage current should be reduced in order to have an effective stimulation.

With voltage-controlled stimulation, there was no difference in effectiveness between the disc and ring electrodes. However the minimum leakage current in CSF was obtained with covered-disk electrodes. At the same time this electrode type reduced the volume and the depth of penetration compared to uncovered electrodes, because the substrate layer increased the electrode impedance and consequently reduced the output current. On the contrary, during current-controlled stimulation, the current from the covered-disc did not diffuse in the CSF and penetrated deeper into the cortex, reaching larger stimulation areas. So this study demonstrated that *the optimal SCS condition is a current-controlled stimulation using covered electrodes in order to reduce the current shunt effect into the cerebral spinal fluid and to maximize the efficiency of the stimulation.* For subdural cortical stimulation optimization, substrate design seems to be a crucial factor, because it can avoid leakage current into the cerebrospinal fluid, but it can also manipulate the amount of output current and the effects of stimulation, especially during voltage controlled stimulation. Both electrode grid location and the activated electrode pair influence the current distribution inside the cortex. Modeled bipolar stimulation with various electrode pairs active inside the subdural electrode grids demonstrated that each current density distribution generated was unique and highly dependent on the distance of the active pair from a gyrus or sulcus (Agarwal et al. 1994).

20.3.2.2 Stimulation Type and Waveform

Seo et al (2013) investigated the effects of monopolar and bipolar SCS on neurons' activation thresholds using a pyramidal neuronal model coupled with a realistic 3D head model (FEM model based on MRI data). Two electrodes were disposed over the gray matter beneath the dura mater and covered with a substrate (conductivity equal to 0.1×10^{-9} S/m); their polarity during monopolar simulation was positive (anodic). This study demonstrated that during monopolar stimulation the neuron excitation threshold was the same underneath both the electrodes, the threshold being lower in the crown. During bipolar simulation, neurons underlying the anode revealed comparable thresholds to the monopolar case, whereas, in the other location, neurons' excitation threshold was higher due to the cathodic influence. In accordance with previous studies (Manola et al. 2005, Manola et al. 2007, Wongsarnpigoon et Grill, 2012) cathodal stimulation preferably excited neurons parallel to the electrode surface. Compared to the extruded slab model (where the thickness of gray matter and depth of sulci were uniform), the estimated thresholds were higher in the realistic head model. According to MRI data, the distance between each electrode and the bottom of the sulcus was not equal and this could be the reason of the difference in estimating the excitability thresholds. Experiments in animals with subdural stimulation of the motor cortex demonstrated that thresholds for visually observed evoked movements were inversely related to the number of pulse per train (NP) and stimulation frequency with thresholds plateaued at 200 Hz (Lilly et al 1952). These results are consistent with ECS experiments.

20.3.3 Comparing ECS and SCS

The first comparison between ECS and SCS was conducted by Kim et al (2011). They developed 3D computational models for respectively epidural and subdural stimulation of the precentral gyrus. For each model, two types of electrode, a disc and a ring electrode, were used and the current density distributions (CDD) were analyzed to compare ECS and SCS. They simulated voltage controlled stimulations so the corresponding current induced could be estimated as I_{output}. The total output current

(I_{output}) in ECS was the sum of currents flowing through the boundaries of the dura mater, CSF, gray matter, and white matter. I_{output} in SCS was the sum of currents flowing out of the boundaries of CSF, gray matter, and white matter, since SCS electrodes were located below the dura mater. Exploring the extent of current density distribution for each CS over various input voltages (1 V, 1.5 V, 2 V, 2.5 V, 3 V), Kim et al showed that SCS produced total output currents about four times larger than those of ECS when the input was 1 V. SCS had effective volumes that were about 6 times larger on average than those of ECS. The difference between effective volumes in the gray and white matter increased with the increase of injected current. *SCS therefore penetrated deeper into the brain than ECS on voltage controlled stimulation.* In terms of current penetration, SCS yielded an average penetration about 3.4 times higher than ECS. The overall difference between the disc and ring electrodes was negligible. This suggested that the ring type can be an advantageous alternative to the disc electrode without significantly reducing effectiveness, since the area available in the middle of the ring can be used for a pH sensor or a sensor for monitoring neural responses to stimuli. *SCS seems hence more effective than ECS for the amount of current both entering the brain cortex and penetrating in depth.* However, SCS requires implanting an electrode beneath the dura mater, while ECS is less invasive. Seo et al (2012) compared ECS and SCS during both monopolar and bipolar stimulation. In this case too, a simple geometrical model restricted to the precentral gyrus was used, but the authors did not find significant differences in the current density distribution between ECS and SCS. The authors described a deeper and wider penetration of the stimulation current during unipolar CS with respect to bipolar CS, in both the epidural and subdural cases. Therefore unipolar stimulation could to be more effective for functional recovery than bipolar. Results from these two studies are opposite, because Seo et al (2012) simulated a constant current condition, whereas Kim et al (2011) compared ECS and SCS under constant voltage condition: this corresponds to different output currents due to different tissue conductivities under the electrode. Hence, *the advantages in terms of penetration and effective volumes of SCS compared to ECS are consistently reduced when using current-controlled stimulation. Current-controlled stimulation can be used in ECS to maximize its effects while keeping the benefits of lower complications and easier electrode positioning.*

20.4 Comparison with Models of Non-Invasive Cortical Stimulation

During both invasive and non-invasive cortical stimulations (CS) there are two critical factors influencing the activation of the target brain tissue: the induced electric field strength and its spatiotemporal distribution. Accurate methods for estimating the brain volumes activated by CS and modeling the interaction between the electric field and the neurons are essential for the optimization of stimulation parameters and for the repeatability of electrode positions. In the last decade several FEM studies of non-invasive CS were conducted in order to analyze which mechanisms lead to activation of neurons using different stimulation parameters and montages for transcranial Direct Current Stimulation (tDCS) or Transcranial Magnetic Stimulation (TMS). This is the same unsolved issue as for epidural and subdural cortical stimulation. Yet, comparing FEM results in the case of invasive and non-invasive CS, it is possible to extract some common behaviors. One is the impact of gyral geometry on the induced electrical field inside the cortex (Datta et al. 2012). Thielscher et al (2011) used FEM characterized by a high-resolution volume mesh, constructed from T1-weighted structural MR images, in order to obtain an anatomically accurate modeling of the gyrification pattern. Their results demonstrated that the field strength induced by TMS in the gray matter increased up to 51% when the induced currents were perpendicular to local gyrus orientation. This effect was mainly restricted to the gyral crowns and lips, and did not extend into the sulcal walls. This enhancement effect might in part underlie the dependency of stimulation thresholds on coil orientation, as commonly observed in TMS motor cortex studies. In contrast to the clear-cut effects of the gyrification pattern on the induced field strength, current directions were predominantly influenced by the CSF–skull boundary. This latter result has to be considered with caution because charge accumulation and conductivity differences in tissues borders (for instance skin/skull, skull/cerebrospinal fluid, cerebrospinal fluid/gray matter, and gray matter/white matter interfaces) were shown to introduce significant distortions to electric fields generated by TMS in the brain (Chen and Mogul 2010). Another commonality with ECS modeling studies (Wongsarnpigoon and Grill 2012) was the identification of the action potentials initialization area: neurons were especially excitable at the white matter - gray matter boundary. This low threshold zone can be caused by the discontinuity of electrical conductivities, so future studies are necessary to avoid incorrect interpretation of FEM results due to distortions, as in the case of TMS studies. The demonstration that the origin of the low threshold zone is not caused by electrical field distortions injected into the model suggests the development of models characterized by pathological alteration of tissue conductivity (such as ischemic tissue damage) for further improving surgical CS outcomes. FEM results can be validated by performing neurophysiological recordings during motor mapping experiments or analyzing subject behaviors during task performance. In case of non-invasive CS, FEM results were compared with both MEPs and working memory tasks. Opitz et al (2013) measured motor evoked potentials (MEPs) elicited by single-pulse TMS over the motor cortex with different coil orientations and in different locations. Results of neurophysiological recordings and those of personalized modeling (MRI-based FEM simulations) were correlated, thus validating this new approach. Kim et al. (2013) investigated the relationship between the behavioral outcomes of a simple working memory (WM) task and the current density value at the dorsolateral prefrontal cortex (DLPFC) induced by tDCS and simulated using FEM models from individual MRI data. Their results showed that participants with enhanced WM task performance after tDCS had a significantly larger current density on DLPFC. This outcome suggests that the inconsistent behavioral outcomes of tDCS might be *partially due to the anatomical differences among subjects*. This might also apply to ICS, but further studies must yet be conducted. More realistic human head models should be developed that include tissue anisotropy and individual anatomical differences. In case of non-invasive CS, simulations demonstrated that personalized FEM can improve the spatial targeting accuracy of stimulation. Indeed, both heterogeneity and anisotropy of the conductive medium influence the spatial distribution of the electric field, thus affecting the stimulation site (Miranda et al. 2003). Individual FEM model can be based on subject's structural MRI and DTI image data, describing both anatomical and anisotropic conductivity properties (Opitz et al. 2013). Inter-individual neuroanatomical characteristics can alter CS outcomes, even if the same stimulation protocol (electrode montage and stimulator setting) is used over different subjects. The stimulation montage and parameters defined by the operator and by the subject-specific anatomy can both influence the amount of electrical current that reaches the target area in the brain and the responsiveness of the subject to the treatment. Currently, there is still limited knowledge for the optimization of the "dose" which can be controlled by the operator (Bikson et al., 2008; Peterchev et al., 2012). However, the distribution of current flow in the brain depends not only on the stimulation dose, but also on the underlying anatomy/tissue properties. The same dose applied to different subjects may result in different brain current flow patterns (Chaieb et al., 2008). Furthermore, if one of the subjects has compromised anatomy (i.e., lesions or skull defects), this may lead to activation of other various brain regions and thus to inconsistent clinical outcomes (Wagner et al. 2007, Datta et al. 2010). In the case of non-invasive CS, the use of personalized FEM was crucial for the estimation of the amount of stimulation current that penetrates over the scalp and skull barriers: inter-individual variation of the amount of hairs on the scalp, of the thickness of the skull and of the shape of the head has to be considered during the optimization of non-invasive CS. For ICS, personalized FEM could be useful to improve the modeling of neurons' population localization and orientation or connectivity based on individual MRI data. This new approach may be essential for the investigation of the effects of cortical pathological lesions on surgical CS outcomes. Finally, in case of tDCS, FEM studies provided a quantitative comparison between different electrode montages described in the literature. Since the exact mechanisms through which tDCS acts are still unclear (Creutzfeldt et al 1962, Purpura et al 1965), the electrode montage can vary consistently also for the treatment of the same pathology. In particular, the position of the return electrode influences the treatment outcomes because it is not passive. For this reason, there are two categories of tDCS montages using respectively intra or extra-cephalic references (Parazzini et al. 2013a, 2013b). Similarly, the effect of the return electrode has to be considered for bipolar ICS: future simulations with highly detailed FEM of the cortex, including synaptic connections, beneath the electrode pair could be useful to better describe the behavioral connection of the two populations of neurons activated respectively by the anode and by the cathode.

20.5 Conclusions

FEM models are an essential tool for the optimization of both invasive and non-invasive CS and suggest future FEM studies for ICS, in order to better describe the shunt effect of the stimulation current inside the cerebrospinal fluid (CSF) and to reduce CSF leakage currents. In case of tDCS, this effect was demonstrated using FEM: a large amount of stimulation current spreads inside the scalp making the stimulation less focal. In order to assist the surgeon in his choice of monopolar or bipolar ICS, further FEM studies investigating the effect of the return electrode location are necessary for the optimization of the montage. FEM simulations demonstrated that outcomes of non-invasive CS are inconsistent among subjects, even if identical protocols are applied, due to inter-individual anatomic variation at the scalp and skull level. In the case of invasive CS the anatomical variation is less, but the electrode position and orientation are more crucial factors for the efficiency of the treatment.

FEM studies for ECS and SCS have revealed important information about the effect of various factors on the treatment outcomes. First of all, the orientation of the neurons can have a greater influence on neurons activation threshold than the location of neurons with respect to the electrode. This result suggests that during therapeutic ECS, the polarity and amplitude that are most effective at one location of the cortex may be less effective a few millimeters away. Moreover the level of activation obtained with current controlled or voltage controlled stimulator settings differ. Since FEM studies demonstrated that all the considered factors (electrode design, location, polarity and stimulator setting) can influence neuronal excitability during ICS, this investigational technique can be used for the research of optimal parameters combinations, in order to reduce the side effect and increase the efficiency of implantable device. However FEM results have to be validated by performing neurophysiological recordings during motor mapping experiments or analyzing the behavior of the subjects during task performance.

Most computational studies for the optimization of CS parameters have used very simple geometrical models, such as extrusion slab partial head models, in order to estimate the distribution of current density and potential induced in the cortex at the level of the precentral gyrus. Their combination with compartmental neuronal models allowed the estimation of stimulation thresholds of neurons during CS. Future simulations with more realistic human head models, characterized by anisotropic tissue conductivities and based on individual MRI data, coupled with neuronal models are needed to confirm the estimated thresholds. Finally, FEM models could also include simulations of synaptic connections between the several neurons represented, which would allow not only the investigation of the mechanisms that determine the stimulation of an individual neuron, but also the prediction of the response due to synaptic interactions between neurons in the network (Salvador et al. 2011).

References

Agarwal VS, Thakor NV, Lesser RP, et al. Modeling electrical stimulation of the human cerebral cortex. Proceedings of 16th Annual International Conference of the IEEE Engineering in Medicine and Biology Society 1994, Vol.1, pp.185-186

Bezard E, Boraud T, Nguyen JP. Cortical stimulation and epileptic seizure: A study of the potential risk in primates. Neurosurgery. 1999;45:346-50.

Bikson M, Bulow P, Stiller JW, et al. Transcranial direct current stimulation for major depression: a general system for quantifying transcranial electrotherapy dosage. Curr Treat Options Neurol. 2008;10:377-85.

Bossetti CA, Birdno MJ, Grill WM. Analysis of the quasi-static approximation for calculating potentials generated by neural stimulation. J Neural Eng. 2008;5:44-53.

Chaieb L, Antal A, Paulus W. Gender-specific modulation of short-term neuroplasticity in the visual cortex induced by transcranial direct current stimulation. Vis Neurosci. 2008;25:77-81.

Chen M, Mogul DJ. Using increased structural detail of the cortex to improve the accuracy of modeling the effects of transcranial magnetic stimulation on neocortical activation. IEEE Trans Biomed Eng. 2010;57:1216-26.

Creutzfeldt OD, Fromm GH, Kapp H. Influence of transcortical D-C currents on cortical neuronal activity. Exp. Neurol. 1962; 5: 436– 452.

Purpura DP, McMurtry JG. Intracellular activities and evoked potential changes during polarization of motor cortex. J. Neurophysiol. 1965; 28:166–185.

Datta A, Bikson M, Fregni F. Transcranial direct current stimulation in patients with skull defects and skull plates: high-resolution computational FEM study of factors altering cortical current flow. Neuroimage. 2010;52:1268-78.

Datta A, Truong D, Minhas P, et al. Inter-Individual Variation during Transcranial Direct Current Stimulation and Normalization of Dose Using MRI-Derived Computational Models. Front Psychiatry. 2012;3:91.

Foster KR, Schwan HP. Dielectric properties of tissues. In: Polk C and Postow E (Eds) Biological Effects of Electromagnetic Fields. CRC Press, New York 1996, pp. 25–102.

Gabriel C, Gabriel S, Corthout E. The dielectric properties of biological tissues: I. Literature survey. Phys Med Biol. 1996;41:2231-49.

Holsheimer J, Lefaucheur J P, Buitenweg J R, et al. The role of intra-operative motor evoked potentials in the optimization of chronic cortical stimulation for the treatment of neuropathic pain Clin. Neurophysiol. 2007; 118: 2287–96.

Kim D, Jun SC, Kim HI. Computational study of subdural and epidural cortical stimulation of the motor cortex. Conf Proc IEEE Eng Med Biol Soc. 2011;2011:7226-9.

Kim D, Seo H, Kim HI, et al. The computational study of subdural cortical stimulation: a quantitative analysis of voltage and current stimulation. Conf Proc IEEE Eng Med Biol Soc. 2012;2012:867-70.

Kim JH, Kim DW, Chang WH, et al. Inconsistent outcomes of transcranial direct current stimulation (tDCS) may be originated from the anatomical differences among individuals: a simulation study using individual MRI data. Conf Proc IEEE Eng Med Biol Soc. 2013;2013:823-5.

Kowalski T, Silny J, Buchner H. Current density threshold for the stimulation of neurons in the motor cortex area. Bioelectromagnetics. 2002;23:421-8.

Kronberg G, Bikson M. Electrode assembly design for transcranial Direct Current Stimulation: a FEM modeling study. Conf Proc IEEE Eng Med Biol Soc. 2012;2012:891-5.

Lilly J C, Austin G M and Chambers W. Threshold movements produced by excitation of cerebral cortex and efferent fibers with some parametric regions of rectangular current pulses (cats and monkeys) J. Neurophysiol. 1952;15: 319–41.

Manola L, Roelofsen BH, Holsheimer J, et al. Modelling motor cortex stimulation for chronic pain control: electrical potential field, activating functions and responses of simple nerve fiber models. Med Biol Eng Comput. 2005;43:335-43.

Manola L, Holsheimer J, Veltink P, et al. Anodal vs cathodal stimulation of motor cortex: a modeling study. Clin Neurophysiol. 2007;118:464-74.

Merrill DR, Bikson M, Jefferys JG. Electrical stimulation of excitable tissue: design of efficacious and safe protocols. J Neurosci Methods 2005;141:171-98.

Miranda PC, Hallett M, Basser PJ. The electric field induced in the brain by magnetic stimulation: a 3-D finite-element analysis of the effect of tissue heterogeneity and anisotropy. IEEE Trans Biomed Eng 2003;50:1074–85.

Opitz A, Legon W, Rowlands A, et al. Physiological observations validate finite element models for estimating subject-specific electric field distributions induced by transcranial magnetic stimulation of the human motor cortex. Neuroimage. 2013;81:253-64.

Parazzini M, Rossi E, Rossi L, et al. Numerical estimation of the current density in the heart during transcranial direct current stimulation. Brain Stimul. 2013;6:457-9.

Parazzini M, Rossi E, Rossi L, et al. Evaluation of the current density in the brainstem during transcranial direct current stimulation with extra-cephalic reference electrode. Clin Neurophysiol. 2013;124:1039-40.

Peterchev AV, Wagner TA, Miranda PC, et al. Fundamentals of transcranial electric and magnetic stimulation dose: definition, selection, and reporting practices. Brain Stimul. 2012;5:435-53.

Priori A, Lefaucheur JP. Chronic epidural motor cortical stimulation for movement disorders. Lancet Neurol. 2007; 6:279-86.

Rattay F. Analysis of models for extracellular fiber stimulation. IEEE Trans Biomed Eng. 1989;36:676-82.

Salvador R, Silva S, Basser PJ, et al. Determining which mechanisms lead to activation in the motor cortex: a modeling study of transcranial magnetic stimulation using realistic stimulus waveforms and sulcal geometry. Clin Neurophysiol. 2011;122:748-58.

Seo H, Kim D, Jun SC. A comparative study of the 3D precentral gyrus model for unipolar and bipolar current stimulations. Conf Proc IEEE Eng Med Biol Soc. 2012; 2012:1892-5.

Seo H, Kim D, Jun SC. Comparison of neuronal excitation between extruded slab partial head model and full head model in subdural cortical stimulation. Conf Proc IEEE Eng Med Biol Soc. 2013;2013:241-4.

Thielscher A, Opitz A, Windhoff M. Impact of the gyral geometry on the electric field induced by transcranial magnetic stimulation. Neuroimage. 2011;54:234-43.

Wagner TA, Zahn M, Grodzinsky AJ, et al. Three-dimensional head model simulation of transcranial magnetic stimulation. IEEE Trans Biomed Eng. 2004;51:1586-98.

Wagner T, Valero-Cabre A, Pascual-Leone A. Noninvasive human brain stimulation. Annu Rev Biomed Eng. 2007;9:527-65.

Wei XF, Grill WM. Analysis of high-perimeter planar electrodes for efficient neural stimulation. Front Neuroeng. 2009;2:15.

Wongsarnpigoon A, Grill WM. Computational modeling of epidural cortical stimulation. J Neural Eng. 2008;5:443-54.

Wongsarnpigoon A, Grill WM. Effects of stimulation parameters and electrode location on thresholds for epidural stimulation of cat motor cortex. J Neural Eng. 2011;8:066016.
Wongsarnpigoon A, Grill WM. Computer-based model of epidural motor cortex stimulation: effects of electrode position and geometry on activation of cortical neurons. Clin Neurophysiol. 2012;123:160-72.

List of Figures

List of Boxes

List of Tables

Bei Fragen zur Produktsicherheit wenden Sie sich bitte an:
If you have any questions regarding product safety,
please contact:

Walter de Gruyter GmbH
Genthiner Straße 13
10785 Berlin
productsafety@degruyterbrill.com